INFLAMMATION IN TUMORIGENESIS AND CANCER TREATMENT

Translational Immunology

INFLAMMATION IN TUMORIGENESIS AND CANCER TREATMENT

Volume 9

From Molecular Mechanisms to Personalized Therapeutic Strategies

Edited by

CHUNXIANG ZHANG

Department of Cardiology, The Affiliated Hospital of Southwest Medical University, Luzhou, Sichuan, P.R. China

MOWEI KONG

Department of Cardiology, The Affiliated Hospital of Southwest Medical University, Luzhou, Sichuan, P.R. China

Series Editor

NIMA REZAEI

ELSEVIER

ACADEMIC PRESS

An imprint of Elsevier

Academic Press is an imprint of Elsevier
125 London Wall, London EC2Y 5AS, United Kingdom
50 Hampshire Street, 5th Floor, Cambridge, MA 02139, United States

ISBN: 978-0-443-36649-9

For Information on all Academic Press publications
visit our website at https://www.elsevier.com/books-and-journals

Publisher: Andre Wolff
Acquisitions Editor: Wendi Baker
Editorial Project Manager: Nayanika Saikia
Production Project Manager: Gomathi Sugumar
Cover Designer: Arumugam Kothandan

Typeset by MPS Limited, Chennai, India

Contents

Section III

Translational research and therapeutic targets

5. Micro/nanoplatforms for modulating programmed cell death and tumor inflammation

Xilong Wu, Huanran Qu and Yundi Wu

6. Micro/nano-enabled immunometabolic regulation in inflammatory tumors

Xilong Wu, Ruocan Liu and Yundi Wu

Section IV

Biomarkers and personalized medicine

7. Biomarker discovery and validation in inflammatory cancer research

Xiangfeng Guan

8. Personalized medicine utilizing biomarkers

Jingsong Shen and Zheng Xie

Section V

Clinical implications and therapeutic strategies

9. Inflammation and tumor microenvironment

Meng Xia

10. Antineoplastic potential of nonsteroidal antiinflammatory drugs

Arkadiusz Surażyński, Magda Chalecka and Jerzy Palka

11. Immunotherapy and inflammation management

Yuyu Xie, Mowei Kong and Junfeng Yu

List of contributors

Xilong Wu School of Biomedical Engineering, School of Pharmaceutical Sciences, Key Laboratory of Tropical Biological Resources of Ministry of Education, Hainan University, Haikou, P.R. China; State Key Laboratory of Digital Medical Engineering, Hainan Engineering Research Center for Drug Screening and Evaluation, Collaborative Innovation Center of One Health, Hainan University, Haikou, P.R. China

Magda Chalecka Department of Medicinal Chemistry, Medical University of Białystok, Bialystok, Poland

Xiangfeng Guan Department of Cardiology, The Affiliated Hospital of Southwest Medical University, Luzhou, Sichuan, P.R. China

Mowei Kong Department of Cardiology, The Affiliated Hospital of Southwest Medical University, Luzhou, Sichuan, P.R. China

Ruocan Liu School of Biomedical Engineering, School of Pharmaceutical Sciences, Key Laboratory of Tropical Biological Resources of Ministry of Education, Hainan University, Haikou, P.R. China; State Key Laboratory of Digital Medical Engineering, Hainan Engineering Research Center for Drug Screening and Evaluation, Collaborative Innovation Center of One Health, Hainan University, Haikou, P.R. China

Jerzy Palka Department of Medicinal Chemistry, Medical University of Białystok, Bialystok, Poland

Huanran Qu School of Biomedical Engineering, School of Pharmaceutical Sciences, Key Laboratory of Tropical Biological Resources of Ministry of Education, Hainan University, Haikou, P.R. China; State Key Laboratory of Digital Medical Engineering, Hainan Engineering Research Center for Drug Screening and Evaluation, Collaborative Innovation Center of One Health, Hainan University, Haikou, P.R. China

Shuai Shao Department of Cardiology, The Affiliated Hospital of Southwest Medical University, Luzhou, Sichuan, P.R. China

Jingsong Shen Department of Cardiology, The Affiliated Hospital of Southwest Medical University, Luzhou, Sichuan, P.R. China

Arkadiusz Surażyński Department of Medicinal Chemistry, Medical University of Białystok, Bialystok, Poland

Cong Wang School of Biomedical Engineering, School of Pharmaceutical Sciences, Key Laboratory of Tropical Biological Resources of Ministry of Education, Hainan University, Haikou, P.R. China

Yundi Wu School of Biomedical Engineering, School of Pharmaceutical Sciences, Key Laboratory of Tropical Biological Resources of Ministry of Education, Hainan University, Haikou, P.R. China; State Key Laboratory of Digital Medical Engineering, Hainan Engineering Research Center for Drug Screening and Evaluation, Collaborative Innovation Center of One Health, Hainan University, Haikou, P.R. China

Meng Xia Department of Cardiology, The Affiliated Hospital of Southwest Medical University, Luzhou, Sichuan, P.R. China

Yuyu Xie Department of Dermatology, Chengdu Fifth People's Hospital, Chengdu, Sichuan, P.R. China

Zheng Xie Orthopaedics of Zigong Fourth People's Hospital, Zigong, Sichuan, P.R. China

Junfeng Yu Department of Dermatology, Chengdu Fifth People's Hospital, Chengdu, Sichuan, P.R. China

Yang Yu Department of Cardiology, The Affiliated Hospital of Southwest Medical University, Luzhou, Sichuan Province, P.R. China

Chunxiang Zhang Department of Cardiology, The Affiliated Hospital of Southwest Medical University, Luzhou, Sichuan, P.R. China; Key Laboratory of Medical Electrophysiology, Ministry of Education, Institute of Cardiovascular Research, Luzhou, Sichuan, P.R. China; Basic Medicine Research Innovation Center for Cardiometabolic Diseases, Ministry of Education, Southwest Medical University, Luzhou, Sichuan, P.R. China; Nucleic Acid Medicine of Luzhou Key Laboratory, Luzhou, Sichuan, P.R. China

Xingwei Zhao Department of Cardiology, The Affiliated Hospital of Southwest Medical University, Luzhou, Sichuan Province, P.R. China

Acknowledgments

In the course of completing this book, Mowei Kong was fortunate to receive invaluable support and assistance from many individuals and organizations. First and foremost, Mowei Kong would like to express his sincere gratitude to Prof. Xilong Wu. With his exceptionally profound expertise in the field of materials science, Prof. Wu provided essential academic guidance and intellectual leadership for this work. He broadened the perspectives presented in this book, enriching its depth and scope, and made the most significant and outstanding contributions to both its overall conception and detailed content.

Mowei Kong would also like to extend his heartfelt thanks to Elsevier for choosing to collaborate with him on this project. Throughout our coordination and communication, Bhavya Rattan and Wendi Baker demonstrated remarkable professionalism, patience, and dedication. Their support in manuscript preparation, publication processes, and overall coordination was invaluable, ensuring the smooth completion of this book.

Mowei Kong is sincerely grateful to all of them for their contributions.

SECTION I

Foundational concepts

CHAPTER

1

Introduction

Mowei Kong[1] *and Chunxiang Zhang*[1,2,3,4]

[1]Department of Cardiology, The Affiliated Hospital of Southwest Medical University, Luzhou, Sichuan, P.R. China [2]Key Laboratory of Medical Electrophysiology, Ministry of Education, Institute of Cardiovascular Research, Luzhou, Sichuan, P.R. China [3]Basic Medicine Research Innovation Center for Cardiometabolic Diseases, Ministry of Education, Southwest Medical University, Luzhou, Sichuan, P.R. China [4]Nucleic Acid Medicine of Luzhou Key Laboratory, Luzhou, Sichuan, P.R. China

1.1 Basic concepts of inflammation and cancer

Inflammation is commonly regarded as an adaptive response of the body to resist the harmful consequences of infections, tissue damage, or other noxious stimuli. It is generally triggered by exogenous stimuli, such as infections, injuries, or allergens. In most cases, these stimuli are eventually eliminated, and the inflammation subsides, allowing tissue repair to occur. This type of inflammation is known as acute inflammation (Furman et al., 2019). However, if the stimuli are not promptly removed, inflammation may evolve into a low-grade, persistent chronic inflammation.

Inflammation is a highly coordinated defense response of the body to external stimuli, such as infections, trauma, or harmful factors, with functions of eliminating pathogens and repairing damaged tissues. Inflammation includes two phases: acute and chronic. Acute inflammation has a rapid onset and short duration, mediated by neutrophils, and is typically characterized by redness, swelling, heat, pain, and functional impairment, which are the five cardinal signs of inflammation proposed by Celsus. Chronic inflammation progresses slowly, lasts longer, and involves mainly monocytes, macrophages, and lymphocytes, often accompanied by tissue structural changes and fibrosis. Although inflammation is protective to the body, uncontrolled or persistent inflammation may damage tissues, leading to various chronic diseases and even inducing tumor development. Therefore inflammation is not a single physiological process but a double-edged sword with both protective and destructive properties.

The core of the inflammatory response is defined by an elaborate set of events. These commence at a point at which pathogen-associated molecular pattern (PAMPs) or damage-associated molecular pattern (DAMPS) bind to the pattern recognition receptors (PRRs) found on immune cells that underlie the innate immune system. This leads to downstream

Inflammation in Tumorigenesis and Cancer Treatment
DOI: https://doi.org/10.1016/B978-0-443-36649-9.00013-X

signaling cascades, which include toll-like receptor (TLR)/MyD88–mediated NF-κB activation that, in turn, induces the expression of proinflammatory cytokines like interleukin-1(IL-1), interleukin-6(IL-6), and tumor necrosis factor-alpha (TNFα), heightening the inflammatory response, while the JAK/STAT pathway is involved in controlling cytokine responses. At the same time, inflammasomes (e.g., NLRP3) activate caspase-1, cleaving and activating IL-1β and IL-18, amplifying local inflammation (Chen et al., 2018). Chronic persistent inflammation leads to the overproduction of reactive oxygen species (ROS), enhanced DNA damage, and inhibited apoptosis, which can eventually cause carcinogenesis under certain circumstances.

Existing studies have shown that the development of cancer is often accompanied by a certain degree of inflammatory response. Persistent tissue inflammation caused by various stimuli can promote the occurrence of tumors and accelerate their progression (Mantovani et al., 2008). For example, chronic infection with *Helicobacter pylori* is associated with gastric cancer and lymphoma (Stolte, 1992); schistosomiasis infection is also considered one of the factors contributing to the high incidence of bladder cancer (Gelfand et al., 1967); approximately 90% of liver cancer cases are closely related to chronic infection with hepatitis B or C virus (Rook & Dalgleish, 2011); and persistent infection with human papillomavirus (HPV) is one of the important causes of the high incidence of cervical cancer in women (Abbasifarid et al., 2021). In addition, chronic inflammatory responses caused by environmental factors, such as asbestos exposure, smoking, and ultraviolet radiation, are also closely related to the occurrence of various cancers, including lung cancer and skin cancer (Mossman et al., 2006). Besides exogenous stimuli, chronic inflammation caused by other factors, whether infectious or noninfectious, is also associated with the occurrence and development of tumors. For example, enteritis, pancreatitis, esophagitis, or chronic inflammation caused by aging may all increase the risk of tumor development (Gudkov et al., 2011; Goldstein et al., 2011).

Clinical research has further confirmed that chronic inflammation is highly correlated with the occurrence and progression of tumors. Some studies have pointed out that more than 15% of cancers may be triggered by chronic inflammation (De Visser et al., 2006). Previous research has also clearly established that persistent low-grade inflammation plays an important role in the occurrence and development of tumors, and its impact may even exceed that of genetic factors in the evolution of tumors. Therefore an increasing number of researchers are focusing on inflammation-related tumor responses, dedicated to exploring the relationship between inflammation and tumors to provide more effective strategies for cancer prevention and treatment.

Cancer is a disease caused by cellular gene mutations and abnormalities in signaling pathways. Its essence lies in the acquisition of unlimited cell proliferation, resistance to apoptosis, and the ability to invade and metastasize. Cancers can be classified according to their tissue origins into carcinomas derived from epithelial cells (such as lung cancer), sarcomas derived from mesenchymal tissues (such as osteosarcoma), and hematological malignancies (such as lymphoma and leukemia) (Zyromski & White, 2011).

The process of carcinogenesis involves mutations in multiple driver genes, such as the activation of oncogenes (e.g., KRAS and MYC) and the inactivation of tumor suppressor genes (e.g., TP53 and RB1), as well as the disruption of DNA repair mechanisms (e.g., BRCA1/2 mutations). Epigenetic mechanisms, including abnormal DNA methylation and dysregulation of noncoding RNAs, also play a key role in tumorigenesis. Multiple cellular signaling pathways, such as PI3K/AKT/mTOR, MAPK/extracellular signal-regulated kinase (ERK), Wnt/β-catenin, and JAK/STAT, are often continuously activated due to genetic mutations. This promotes malignant cell transformation, the development of drug resistance, and immune evasion (Lee et al., 2020).

Inflammation and cancer have a profound intersection in pathophysiology. A large number of studies have confirmed that chronic inflammation is a key precursor state for the development of many types of tumors. For example, gastritis caused by *H. pylori* can develop into gastric cancer, chronic hepatitis caused by hepatitis B virus (HBV) infection can progress to hepatocellular carcinoma, and long-term ulcerative colitis can increase the risk of colorectal cancer. In these processes, inflammatory factors such as TNFα and IL-6 promote the proliferation of tumor cells and angiogenesis by activating signaling pathways such as STAT3 and NF-κB, while also enhancing the ability of immune evasion. In addition, oxidative stress caused by chronic inflammation can increase the risk of gene mutation. Changes in the tissue microenvironment, such as the remodeling of tumor-associated macrophages (TAMs) and fibroblasts, also further support tumor growth. The staging of cancer is mainly based on the TNM system, which includes the size of the primary tumor (T), regional lymph node involvement (N), and distant metastasis (M). It is not only used to assess disease progression but also to guide individualized treatment strategies (Wu et al., 2022).

1.2 Historical connections and modern understanding of inflammation and cancer

The association between inflammation and cancer was noted as early as the 19th century. The German pathologist Rudolf Virchow was one of the first scholars to propose the idea that "cancer originates from chronic inflammation" (Virchow, 1871). He observed the frequent infiltration of inflammatory cells in tumor tissues and suggested that tumors might arise from persistent inflammatory responses. Although this hypothesis was not widely confirmed at the time, it laid the foundation for subsequent research. Subsequently, with the development of immunology, pathology, and molecular biology, it has gradually been recognized that chronic inflammation is not only closely related to tissue repair and immune responses but can also directly affect the occurrence, development, and malignant progression of tumors through various signaling pathways and cytokines. This transition from clinical pathological phenomena to molecular mechanisms marks the modern transformation of research on inflammation and cancer.

From the mid-20th century to the present, systematic research on inflammation and cancer has gradually deepened. In the field of virology, it has been found that oncogenic viruses such as HBV and HPV often promote carcinogenesis against the backdrop of chronic inflammation. For example, persistent infection with HBV leads to chronic inflammation and fibrosis of liver tissue, which then progresses to hepatocellular carcinoma (Vyas et al., 1975). Similarly, chronic inflammation of cervical epithelial cells caused by HPV is closely related to the occurrence of cervical cancer. In addition, the correlation between autoimmune diseases (such as Crohn's disease and ulcerative colitis) and certain tumors (such as colorectal cancer) has also prompted researchers to further explore how chronic inflammation promotes the occurrence of cancer through systemic mechanisms. After the 1970s research on immune-related pathways was in full swing. Studies have shown that the inflammatory process not only involves the participation of immune cells but also involves a variety of cytokines, chemokines, oxidative stress products, and matrix remodeling enzymes, forming a complex tumor microenvironment (TME) that ultimately promotes tumor formation ("Experimental, and Microscopic Researches upon Inflammation, Tuberculisation, Tumours, the Formation of Callus, &c," n.d.).

Entering the 21st century, research on the relationship between inflammation and cancer has entered a stage of deep molecular-pathway analysis. Several signaling pathways have been definitively identified as key mechanisms by which inflammation promotes tumorigenesis. Among them, the NF-κB pathway is one of the most extensively studied. Under chronic inflammatory conditions, inflammatory factors such as TNFα and IL-1β activate the NF-κB signal via the IκB kinase (IKK) complex, thereby initiating the expression of numerous genes related to cell survival, proliferation, and inflammatory modulation (Zyuz'kov et al., 2023). Sustained activation of NF-κB enhances the antiapoptotic capacity of tumor cells and increases their resistance to chemotherapy and radiotherapy. In addition, the JAK/STAT3 pathway is activated in various inflammatory contexts; in particular, IL-6 family cytokines can induce STAT3 phosphorylation and nuclear translocation, thereby upregulating proproliferative and antiapoptotic molecules such as cyclin D1 and Bcl-xL (Zuo, Wang, et al., 2024, Zuo, Li, et al., 2024). STAT3 also participates in shaping the immunosuppressive microenvironment by promoting the recruitment of TAMs and regulatory T cells (Tregs).

The Wnt/β-catenin signaling pathway can function as a connection between inflammatory responses and cancer, as chronic inflammation can alter Wnt pathway activity via oxidative stress or cytokines that cause the accumulation of β-catenin within the nucleus and drive the expression of gene products that confer stem-like properties and invasive potential. In both inflammation-associated hepatocellular carcinomas and colorectal cancer, this pathway is often aberrantly activated, and the NLRP3 inflammasome also plays a critical role in tumor development. NLRP3 mediates the maturation of IL-1β and IL-18 via caspase-1, thereby enhancing immune evasion and microenvironment remodeling (Zu et al., 2019). Meanwhile, transforming growth factor-β (TGF-β) also functions as a dual factor of cancer development: It inhibits cell proliferation in an early stage but promotes cancer epithelial–mesenchymal transition (EMT), cell migration, and metastasis at a late stage of chronic inflammatory responses.

At key research milestones, Grivennikov et al. (2009) demonstrated that IL-6 promotes tumor formation in a colorectal cancer model via the STAT3 pathway, providing animal experimental evidence for the direct role of inflammatory factors in tumor driving. In 2010 Coussens and Werb (2002) systematically proposed in a Nature Review that "inflammation is the seventh hallmark of cancer," establishing that inflammation is not merely an accompanying phenomenon but an intrinsic driver of tumorigenesis and progression. Subsequently, the introduction of the TME concept placed the bidirectional interaction between inflammatory cells and tumor cells at the center of research. For example, TAMs promote angiogenesis and tissue invasion by secreting factors such as vascular endothelial growth factor (VEGF) and matrix metalloproteinases (MMPs), while simultaneously suppressing antitumor immune responses, thereby providing an "immune-privileged" protective umbrella for the tumor (Lin et al., 2006).

Today, inflammation is recognized as a fundamental component of cancer development, with molecular mechanisms spanning multiple dimensions, including the accumulation of gene mutations, defects in immune surveillance, and remodeling of the TME. Targeting inflammation-related molecular pathways has become an emerging anticancer strategy, with agents such as anti-IL-6 antibodies, JAK inhibitors, and NF-κB pathway blockers—some of which have already entered clinical trials.

1.3 Tumor microenvironment and inflammatory factors

The concept of the TME was first proposed by Lord et al. (1979). After implanting spheroids of 700–900 μm in diameter into the peritoneal cavity of mice, researchers observed that large numbers of lymphocytes and macrophages infiltrated the spheroids and formed close membrane connections with tumor cells. Although these in vivo multicellular spheroids lacked the stroma and vascular systems found in solid tumors, they exhibited many similarities to tumors in vivo and were suitable for studying interactions between tumor cells and host cells (Lord et al., 1979). The TME primarily comprises various cellular components—including tumor cells, tumor-associated fibroblasts, immune cells, and vascular endothelial cells—as well as molecular components such as the extracellular matrix, degrading enzymes, cytokines, chemokines, and immunosuppressive factors. It also exhibits unique physicochemical characteristics, such as hypoxia and acidity.

In recent years, the TME has become one of the fastest-growing areas in cancer research and is closely linked to tumor initiation and progression. Within this environment, infiltrating immune cells—including neutrophils, macrophages, B cells, T cells, Tregs, and myeloid-derived suppressor cells (MDSCs)—along with secreted cytokines, chemokines, and growth factors, interact with tumor cells to create a sustained inflammatory milieu that promotes tumor immune evasion, growth, invasion, and metastasis (Tan et al., 2021).

A variety of infiltrating molecules can modulate the chronic inflammatory milieu within tumors, inducing transformation of malignant epithelial cells, suppressing immune surveillance, and driving metastasis. The expression of these factors is often upregulated in both tumor and inflammatory cells. Among them, IL-6 plays a crucial role in stress responses and antiinfection processes, and the IL-6–STAT3 signaling pathway serves a key function in multiple tumor types (Yao et al., 2014). Studies have shown that aberrant STAT3 activation is important for MDSC development and inflammation-induced tumorigenesis. IL-6 can also induce tumor formation by enhancing ribosome biogenesis and down-regulating p53 expression and activity (Brighenti et al., 2014). Overexpression of the proinflammatory enzyme cyclo-oxygenase-2 (COX-2) is a major driver within the tumor inflammatory microenvironment; it not only regulates EMT in tumor cells, promoting invasion and metastasis, but also significantly influences proliferation, apoptosis, and immune evasion (Gómez-Valenzuela et al., 2021).

TNFα, as a key inflammatory factor, promotes the invasive capacity of mutant p53-expressing tumor cells and synergizes with NF-κB and JNK signaling pathways to drive tumor progression. Studies have shown that TNFα-induced chronic inflammation can further potentiate the oncogenic role of mutant p53 by enhancing the transcriptional activity of NF-κB and can even activate the NF-κB pathway through interaction with the tumor suppressor DAB2IP (Cooks et al., 2013). Although some studies indicate that TNFα-mediated chronic inflammation has a limited influence on p53-deficient tumors, its synergistic effect remains nonnegligible in certain contexts (Weisz et al., 2007). In addition, certain long intergenic noncoding RNAs (lincRNAs), such as lincRNA-p21, also play important regulatory roles within the TME (Jin et al., 2019). This molecule exerts tumor-suppressive effects by inducing G1 arrest and apoptosis, and its low expression in head and neck cancer is often associated with poor prognosis. lincRNA-p21 can directly bind to STAT3, inhibit its phosphorylation, and block the JAK2/STAT3 pathway, thereby suppressing STAT3-mediated tumor transformation. Both wild-type and mutant p53 can regulate the expression of lincRNA-p21, but the mechanisms differ (Tan et al., 2021). Ultimately, various protumorigenic factors, oxidative metabolites, proteases, and inflammatory factors within the TME—such as IL-6 and TNFα—can induce DNA damage and mutations through the activation of the NF-κB and STAT3 pathways, thereby initiating tumorigenesis. These activated signaling pathways can, in turn, enhance the expression of inflammatory factors, forming a positive feedback loop of "inflammation–tumor–inflammation" that sustains a chronic inflammatory microenvironment within the tumor and promotes malignant transformation.

TME consists of many kinds of molecules and various types of cells, such as fibroblasts, endothelial cells, pericytes, and mesenchymal stem cells, that all participate in initiating and

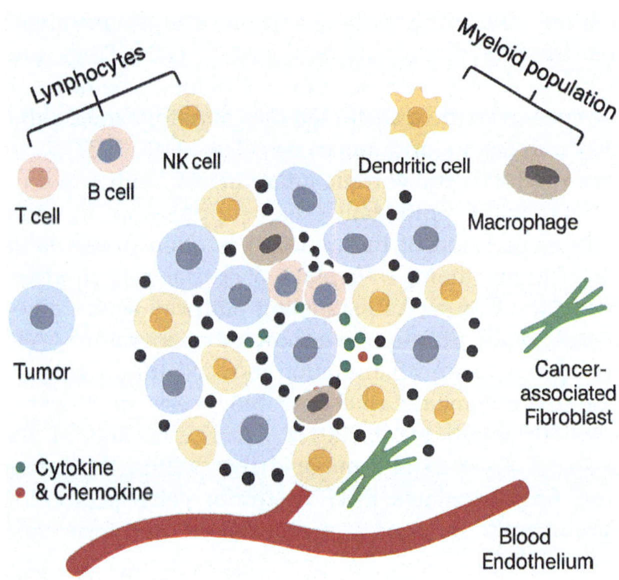

FIGURE 1.1 Infiltrating cellular components in the tumor microenvironment (TME). The various cells recruited by the TME play an important role in the occurrence and development of tumors.

progressing tumors (Fig. 1.1). Surrounding tumor cells, different kinds of stromal cells like fibroblasts, endothelial cells, pericytes, and mesenchymal stem cells usually get into action, constituting the tumor stroma collectively, during the tumor formation. These cells secrete numerous cytokines and chemokines, attracting immune cells into the tumor and forming the TME. These immune cells include T lymphocytes, B lymphocytes, monocytes/macrophages, neutrophils, dendritic cells, and natural killer cells and may account for up to 50% of the tumor mass. Within the TME, cells interact and influence each other through direct contact or secreted regulatory factors. These inflammation-associated cells often exhibit tumor-promoting properties, facilitating tumor cell survival and proliferation (Dymicka-Piekarska et al., 2021).

Fibroblasts occupy a prominent position within the TME. In particular, the interaction between tumor cells and stromal tissues activates fibroblasts, inducing their transformation into cancer-associated fibroblasts (CAFs). CAFs exhibit abnormal proliferation, secretion, and migratory characteristics, maintaining the environment required for EMT and promoting solid tumor progression. CAFs can secrete factors such as TGF-β, ILs, and VEGF to modulate tumor growth and inflammatory responses, further enhancing tumor cell survival and migration (Rihawi et al., 2021). Furthermore, CAFs can activate the NF-κB/COX-2/prostaglandin E2 (PGE2) proinflammatory signaling pathway and the hypoxia-inducible factor 1 (HIF1) signaling pathway. Studies have shown that CAFs promote the recruitment of myeloid-derived cells, activate MDSCs, and induce polarization of intratumoral macrophages toward the protumorigenic M2 phenotype, thereby creating an immune-evasive tumor environment (Giannoni et al., 2011).

Tumor-infiltrating immune cell populations, such as B cells, T cells, and natural killer cells, on the one hand, upregulate inflammatory responses through the secretion of chemokines and cytokines to exert antitumor effects; on the other hand, they can also assist tumor immune evasion by promoting a chronic inflammatory tumor environment, thereby playing a protumor role. Effector T cells—especially $CD8^+$ cytotoxic T cells and $CD4^+$ helper T cells—participate in antitumor immune responses. Tregs, a special subset of $CD4^+$ T cells expressing the transcription factor FOXP3, exert immunosuppressive and chronic inflammation-regulating functions (Monteran & Erez, 2019). In many solid tumors, high infiltration of Tregs usually predicts poor prognosis. Tregs suppress the function of effector T cells through direct contact or secretion of soluble factors. In addition, MDSCs, as immunosuppressive cells within the TME, can secrete immunosuppressive factors to promote tumor progression and inhibit antitumor immune responses (Cinier et al., 2021). Moreover, tumor-associated neutrophils are also present in the TME, and depending on their phenotype, they may exhibit either antitumor or protumor effects. For example, N1-type neutrophils inhibit tumor growth by expressing MMP8, whereas N2-type neutrophils promote tumor progression by upregulating MMP9 and secreting protumor factors such as CXCL1 and CXCL6 (Sangaletti et al., 2016). Tumor-associated platelets induce coagulation activation through tissue factor secreted by tumor cells, affecting angiogenesis in the TME and promoting tumor metastasis. Platelets help tumor cells survive and proliferate through interactions with them, especially by promoting platelet aggregation and adhesion to tumor cells.

1.4 Macrophage function and its role in tumor progression

Macrophages, as a class of innate immune cells, are generally derived from circulating monocytes that migrate into tissues and differentiate into mature macrophages (Fig. 1.2). They not only mount immune responses against invading agents such as cells, bacteria, or viruses, but also participate in tissue repair upon injury, serving as an essential component in maintaining organismal homeostasis. In the course of tumor development, macrophages constitute the largest cellular subpopulation. The large numbers of macrophages recruited into the TME are commonly defined as TAMs. TAMs can modulate tumor cell death, angiogenesis, secretion of growth factors, and extracellular MMPs, thereby regulating the inflammatory state of the TME and the initiation and progression of tumors (Dymicka-Piekarska et al., 2021).

A critical feature of macrophages is their ability to respond differently according to environmental stimuli. Typically, after stimulation by Th1-type factors such as interferon-γ (IFNγ), lipopolysaccharide, or TLRs, macrophages express proinflammatory factors IL-1, IL-6, and TNFα, exerting antimicrobial and immune-activating roles as an important line of defense against external stimuli; these are termed classically activated macrophages (M1 type). In contrast, Th2-type factors, such as IL-4, IL-13, and IL-10, can induce macrophages to express IL-10, arginase-1 (Arg-1), CD206, and others, exerting antiinflammatory, wound-healing, and tissue-repair functions while suppressing Th1 cell responses; these are termed alternatively activated macrophages (M2 type) (Sica & Mantovani, 2012). Further, depending on the stimulus, alternatively activated macrophages can be subdivided into M2a, M2b, and M2c subtypes, each exerting distinct functions. In addition, myeloid cell growth factors play important roles in monocyte recruitment and differentiation;

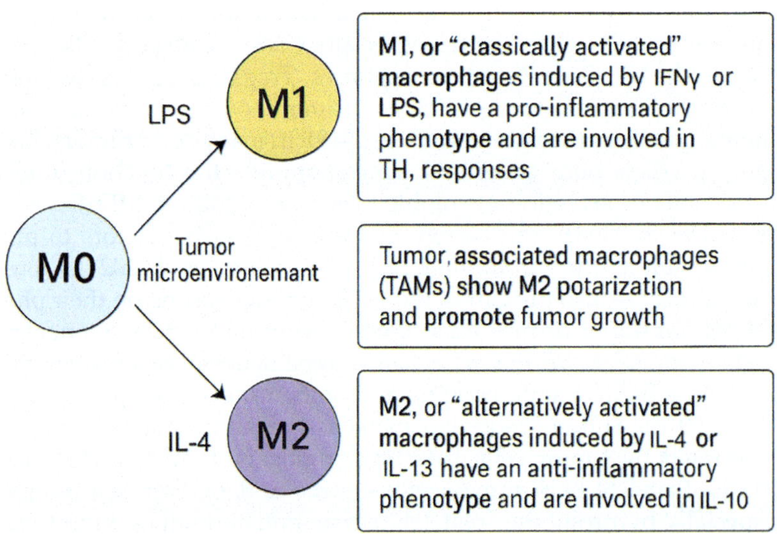

FIGURE 1.2 Macrophage polarization and its regulatory role in inflammation. Macrophages exhibit different functions under various stimuli. M1 type is primarily involved in inflammation and immune defense, while M2 type plays a role in antiinflammation and promoting tumor growth. *LPS*, Lipopolysaccharide.

macrophages cultured in CSF2 have been defined as M1 type, whereas those cultured in CSF1 have been defined as M2 type (Martinez & Gordon, 2014). Generally, the proinflammatory M1 phenotype and the antiinflammatory M2 phenotype represent two extremes of macrophage differentiation; however, the surrounding signals for macrophages are diverse and dynamically changing. Studies have further revealed that macrophages can switch from one phenotype to another in response to different stimuli, adapting to changes in environmental signals. The diversity and plasticity of phenotype and function are unique characteristics of macrophages (Tarique et al., 2015).

Among the various immune cells infiltrating the TME, macrophages are a major component and play a dominant role in tumor-associated inflammation. Research has shown that the development and differentiation of macrophages within tumors are highly complex; macrophages in the TME may exhibit an M1/M2 mixed phenotype (Martinez & Gordon, 2014). By analyzing tumor samples from patients with squamous cell carcinoma, researchers found high enrichment of both M1 marker CD127 and M2 markers CCL18 and CD209, confirming the high heterogeneity of TAMs (Pettersen et al., 2011). Using paraffin-embedded nonsmall cell lung cancer patient samples and dual staining for M1 markers CD68/HLA-DR and M2 markers CD68/CD163, researchers also observed that TAMs displayed approximately 70% M2 phenotype and 30% M1 phenotype, and high M1 macrophage infiltration correlated positively with prolonged patient survival. In ovarian cancer patient paraffin tissues, colocalization of iNOS/CD163 was detected, and an increased M2/M1 macrophage ratio was further shown to correlate with worsened ovarian cancer progression. TAMs isolated from primary renal cell carcinoma patient tissues and cultured in vitro also exhibited a hybrid phenotype, expressing both M2 markers CD163 and CD206 and proinflammatory factors TNFα, IL-1β, IL-6, and MCP-1 (Kovaleva et al., n.d.). These findings indicate that macrophage evolution is conserved across species. Although TAMs in tumors are heterogeneous and display an M1/M2 mixed phenotype, the prevailing view holds that tumor cells within the TME secrete M2-inducing factors such as IL-10 and VEGF, recruit monocyte-derived macrophages to infiltrate tumor tissues, and drive their differentiation toward the M2 phenotype. These M2-polarized macrophages subsequently play critical roles in disrupting adaptive immune responses and fostering protumor inflammatory environments (Qian & Pollard, 2010).

In the tumor milieu, numerous factors participate in the polarization regulation of TAMs. For example, tumor initiation and progression typically create a hypoxic microenvironment within the lesion; insufficient oxygen supply not only facilitates tumor invasion and metastasis but also aberrantly regulates angiogenesis. Studies have shown that tumor hypoxia can influence TAM differentiation and function, and TAMs residing in hypoxic regions secrete proangiogenic factors that in turn accelerate tumor proliferation (Mantovani et al., 2002). Tumor hypoxia downregulates expression of the M1 macrophage markers CD86 and CD40 but does not affect expression of the M2 markers CD206 and transferrin receptor; macrophages under such control promote tumor growth and migration (Almendros et al., 2014). Moreover, hypoxia results in inadequate oxygen and nutrient supply and delayed clearance of metabolic products, further altering cellular metabolism, and metabolites play crucial roles in TAM polarization. For instance, lactate generated by tumor metabolism can upregulate VEGF expression via HIF1α, inducing M2 polarization of TAMs. Lactate can also induce expression of the M2 marker Arg1 in macrophages, thereby promoting tumor growth (Colegio et al., 2014). During lactate-mediated signaling, ERK/STAT3 acts as a key regulator, driving M2 polarization of TAMs and accelerating breast cancer progression.

During TAM polarization, several transcription factors participate and play important roles. HIFs govern macrophage responses to hypoxia; HIF1α induces M1 polarization by activating NF-κB signaling and increasing iNOS expression, whereas HIF2α enhances Arg1 activity and suppresses nitric oxide production, thereby promoting M2 polarization (Liu et al., 2025). In tumor development, transcription factor STAT3 is commonly activated and exerts critical functions in inflammation. Studies demonstrate that STAT3 regulates the expression of cytokines IL-6 and IL-10, induces M2 macrophage polarization, and maintains an immunosuppressive intratumoral environment that further drives tumor progression. STAT3 can also bind the Arg1 promoter to modulate expression of M2-related genes, thereby facilitating M2 polarization (Fu et al., 2017). Certain interferon regulatory factors (IRFs) likewise participate in TAM polarization. Research shows that IRF4 regulates M2 macrophage polarization and promotes gastric cancer development via the IL-6/STAT3 pathway, correlating with poor patient prognosis. Additionally, nanoparticles carrying IRF5 combined with an IKKβ inhibitor can reverse the protumor M2 phenotype of TAMs into the antitumor M1 phenotype (Larionova et al., 2020).

In addition, oncogenes such as c-MYC can modulate the expression of M2 macrophage activation–related genes, including SCARB1, ALOX15, and MRC1, upregulate IL-4 signaling regulators STAT6 and PPARγ, and thereby induce M2 macrophage differentiation (Pello et al., 2012). Malignant fibrous histiocytoma amplified sequence 1 (MFHAS1) is a predicted oncoprotein that has been confirmed to exert tumor-promoting activity in vivo. Studies show that colon cancer cells can activate MFHAS1 to drive TAMs toward an M2 phenotype and activate STAT6 and KLF4, accelerating colon cancer progression (Zhong et al., 2019). Activation of PPARγ can also induce M2 polarization of Raw264.7 cells in an MFHAS1-dependent manner. Angiopoietin-like protein 2 (Angptl2) is aberrantly overexpressed in nonsmall cell lung cancer; studies reveal that Angptl2 recruits TAMs into tumors via the NF-κB signaling pathway and induces M2 polarization, enhancing tumor cell proliferation, invasion, and metastasis while correlating with poor patient survival (Zuo et al., 2023) (Fig. 1.3).

1.5 Targeting inflammatory pathways in cancer therapy

The TME brims with all types of immunological cells and factors, and an inflammatory response is an indispensable portion. Multiple proinflammatory cytokines like TNFα and IL-6 serve major functions in carcinogenesis and metastasis. These cytokines not only promote tumor-cell proliferation but also inhibit apoptosis and enhance tumor angiogenesis by activating relevant signaling pathways (e.g., NF-κB and JAK/STAT), or antiinflammatory signals (tumor immune escape). Some studies show that there is a relationship between continuous chronic inflammation and tumor initiation; particularly, the cancer risk in people with chronic inflammatory diseases is much higher compared to those without the same condition. Clinical trials show an increased risk of gastric cancer and colon cancer among people with chronic gastritis, Crohn's disease, and HBV-related chronic liver disease

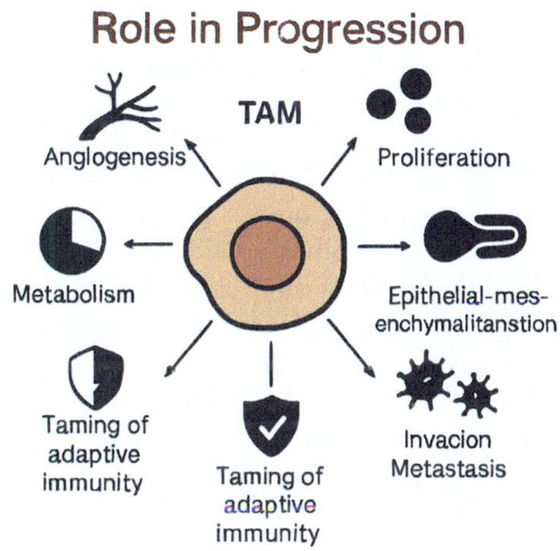

FIGURE 1.3 Role of TAMs in tumor progression. TAMs (tumor-associated macrophages) can promote the formation of tumor blood vessels, support the proliferation of tumor cells, and influence the metabolic processes of tumor cells, all of which collectively contribute to the progression and worsening of the tumor.

(Landskron et al., 2014). Thus inflammatory pathways have been put forward as potentially efficacious therapeutic targets. The prime objective behind employing these targeted treatments is to impede or prevent the proinflammatory actions found in TME via inactivating or blocking the inflammatory-inducing components as well as their signaling transduction cascades, leading to tumor growth arrest and metastasis suppression.

The NF-κB signal transduction cascade, one of the earliest discovered inflammatory cascades, is reportedly abnormally active in many types of tumors. NF-κB can drive tumorigenesis, stimulate tumor cell proliferation, metastasis, and chemoresistance by upregulating proinflammatory cytokines such as IL-8 and TNFα. NF-κB can also mediate tumor immune evasion by orchestrating the recruitment of immune-suppressive cells (e.g., Treg cells) and dampening antitumor immunity. Some researchers have tried to target the NF-κB pathway and found out that many small-molecule drugs (e.g., BAY 11–7082, and JSH-23) have antitumor effects in the clinical study (Yu et al., 2020). However, the clinical use of NF-κB inhibitors might still meet a few challenges, such as side-effects and insufficiency. Thus researchers need to carry on their efforts on NF-κB inhibitors.

The JAK/STAT signaling pathway is another inflammatory axis that exerts critical functions within the TME. IL-6, a key proinflammatory cytokine in this pathway, activates STAT3 to foster tumor-cell growth, migration, and immune evasion. Additionally, JAK/STAT activation induces drug resistance and accelerates disease progression. Targeted agents against the JAK/STAT axis have advanced rapidly in recent years. The JAK inhibitor ruxolitinib—originally approved for myeloproliferative neoplasms and certain leukemias—has demonstrated antitumor activity across multiple malignancies. Correspondingly, STAT3 inhibitors (e.g., Stattic) have shown significant antitumor efficacy in preclinical models (Berkley et al., 2025).

COX-2 is a typical proinflammatory enzyme that is usually upregulated in tumor cells, especially in colorectal cancer, breast cancer, and other tumors. COX-2 promotes tumor growth and metastasis by generating PGE2 and activating a series of proinflammatory pathways. PGE2 binds to EP receptors and activates multiple downstream signaling pathways (such as cAMP/PKA and PI3K/Akt), thereby promoting tumor cell proliferation and antiapoptosis. COX-2 inhibitors, such as celecoxib, are widely used in clinical practice, particularly for patients with colon cancer. Studies have shown that COX-2 inhibitors can reduce tumor incidence and improve patient prognosis (Eftekhari & Fardid, 2020). However, the use of COX-2 inhibitors still faces side-effect issues, especially an increased risk of cardiovascular events, which limits their clinical application.

IL-1β plays an important role in the TME, including promoting tumor cell proliferation, metastasis, and resistance to therapy. Inflammasomes are intracellular multiprotein complexes that can promote the secretion of proinflammatory cytokines such as IL-1β by activating caspase-1. Inhibitors targeting inflammasomes or IL-1β, such as anakinra (IL-1 receptor antagonist) and canakinumab (anti-IL-1β antibody), have been evaluated in multiple clinical trials and have shown certain efficacy. In a recent study, canakinumab was confirmed to significantly reduce mortality in lung cancer patients by inhibiting inflammatory responses, providing new evidence for IL-1β pathway-targeted therapy (Ridker et al., 2017). However, because the role of IL-1β involves multiple aspects of the immune system, comprehensive inhibition of IL-1β may lead to adverse immune reactions, so caution is needed in practical application.

1.6 Current status and challenges of research

Research focusing on the relationship between inflammation and cancer is moving toward clinical applications and, thus, its area of research is shifting accordingly. One prevailing area is Immunometabolism—changes in the environment of TME modulate immune cells in this area, such as T-cells, dendritic cells, and macrophages. Metabolic modifications change not only immune cells' functions but also how they respond. Recent findings show that immune cells might undergo immunological avoidance as their metabolism changes during tumorigenesis: Changes such as hypoxia and acidity in the TME lead to the change of immune cell metabolic programs to regulate their function and effector capacity (Zhao et al., n.d.; Clay et al., 2025). Thus immunometabolism provides novel insights into cancer immunotherapy as well as for understanding tumors. Moreover, with metabolic modulation and targeted therapy, cancer can also be treated. On the other hand, immune checkpoint inhibitors such as PD-1/PD-L1 inhibitors have made great achievements in anticancer therapy in recent years. However, despite the positive therapeutic response seen in many patients, we see widely varied efficacy among the others, which could very well stem from the complex inflammatory microenvironment that exists around cancer. This tumor milieu could play an important role in helping tumor cells avoid immune surveillance through inflammatory cell modulation.

Although substantial advances have been made in understanding the link between inflammation and cancer, many questions remain to be answered. Tissue inflammation and carcinogenesis are interrelated processes. However, tissue inflammation might facilitate or prevent cancer occurrence and development based on the specific context. Some kinds of inflammation promote an antitumor immune response, whereas other forms can lead to immune escape of cancer cells. Tumor cells induce immune modulation by secreting different types of immunosuppressive molecules to subvert host immune responses; therefore outcomes of the crosstalk between inflammation and the immune system depend on the complex interplays between multiple factors. Thus a simple dichotomous view that all inflammation is either tumorigenic or nontumorigenic would be inappropriate.

Individual patient variances can present significant challenges: Cancers are different types, patients' immune status is highly diverse, as well as their inflammatory response can be strong or weak, all of which mean that even when exactly the same protocol is followed for treatment across patients, the outcome might be very different. The pro- and antitumor inflammatory responses are modulated by factors such as genetic background, immune tolerance, microbiome composition, and tumor heterogeneity, furthermore, the role of inflammation in cancer immunotherapy. Although inflammatory reactions may produce new antigens and modulate T cell crosstalk in the tumor environment, and thereby shape checkpoint expression, antigen presentation, and escape from immune recognition remain to be established in most tumor entities; also including those typically recognized as highly inflamed ones. The inherent heterogeneity in host–microenvironment interactions is highly context-dependent and variously timed in any given tumors, posing a significant challenge for accurate forecasting of what type of inflammatory responses can or should be expected to influence what sort of immune therapeutic outcome.

Technical hurdles also persist. Although genomics, proteomics, and other omics technologies have provided abundant molecular data, the inflammation–cancer relationship cannot be fully elucidated by any single technological approach. Likewise, despite substantial advances in basic research, translating these discoveries into practical therapeutic strategies remains difficult. Antiinflammatory agents and immunomodulators have yet to achieve broad clinical application, partly because of the dual nature of inflammatory responses. Precisely modulating the degree and character of inflammation while avoiding adverse effects is an urgent problem that remains to be solved.

References

Abbasifarid, E., Bolhassani, A., Irani, S., Sotoodehnejadnematalahi, F., & Balalaeva, I. V. (2021). Synergistic effects of exosomal crocin or curcumin compounds and HPV L1-E7 polypeptide vaccine construct on tumor eradication in C57BL/6 mouse model. *PLoS One, 16*(10), e0258599. https://doi.org/10.1371/journal.pone.0258599.

Almendros, I., Wang, Y., Becker, L., Lennon, F. E., Zheng, J., Coats, B. R., Schoenfelt, K. S., Carreras, A., Hakim, F., Zhang, S. X., Farré, R., & Gozal, D. (2014). Intermittent hypoxia-induced changes in tumor-associated macrophages and tumor malignancy in a mouse model of sleep apnea. *American Journal of Respiratory and Critical Care Medicine, 189*(5), 593–601. https://doi.org/10.1164/rccm.201310-1830OC, http://www.atsjournals.org/doi/pdf/10.1164/rccm.201310-1830OC.

Berkley, K., Zalejski, J., & Sharma, A. (2025). Targeting STAT3 for Cancer Therapy: Focusing on Y705, S727, or Dual Inhibition? *Cancers, 17*(5), 755. https://doi.org/10.3390/cancers17050755.

Brighenti, E., Calabrese, C., Liguori, G., Giannone, F. A., Trerè, D., Montanaro, L., & Derenzini, M. (2014). Interleukin 6 downregulates p53 expression and activity by stimulating ribosome biogenesis: a new pathway connecting inflammation to cancer. *Oncogene, 33*(35), 4396–4406. https://doi.org/10.1038/onc.2014.1.

Chen, L., Deng, H., Cui, H., Fang, J., Zuo, Z., Deng, J., Li, Y., Wang, X., & Zhao, L. (2018). Inflammatory responses and inflammation-associated diseases in organs. *Oncotarget, 9*(6), 7204–7218. https://doi.org/10.18632/oncotarget.23208.

Cinier, J., Hubert, M., Besson, L., Di Roio, A., Rodriguez, C., Lombardi, V., Caux, C., & Ménétrier-Caux, C. (2021). Recruitment and expansion of tregs cells in the tumor environment—how to target them? *Cancers, 13*(8). https://doi.org/10.3390/cancers13081850, https://www.mdpi.com/2072-6694/13/8/1850/pdf.

Clay, R., Li, K., & Jin, L. (2025). Metabolic Signaling in the Tumor Microenvironment. *Cancers, 17*(1). https://doi.org/10.3390/cancers17010155, http://www.mdpi.com/journal/cancers/.

Colegio, O. R., Chu, N. Q., Szabo, A. L., Chu, T., Rhebergen, A. M., Jairam, V., Cyrus, N., Brokowski, C. E., Eisenbarth, S. C., Phillips, G. M., Cline, G. W., Phillips, A. J., & Medzhitov, R. (2014). Functional polarization of tumour-associated macrophages by tumour-derived lactic acid. *Nature, 513*(7519), 559–563. https://doi.org/10.1038/nature13490, http://www.nature.com/nature/index.html.

Cooks, T., Pateras, I. S., Tarcic, O., Solomon, H., Schetter, A. J., Wilder, S., Lozano, G., Pikarsky, E., Forshew, T., Rozenfeld, N., Harpaz, N., Itzkowitz, S., Harris, C. C., Rotter, V., Gorgoulis, V. G., & Oren, M. (2013). Mutant p53 Prolongs NF-κB Activation and Promotes Chronic Inflammation and Inflammation-Associated Colorectal Cancer. *Cancer Cell, 23*(5), 634–646. https://doi.org/10.1016/j.ccr.2013.03.022, https://www.journals.elsevier.com/cancer-cell.

Coussens, L. M., & Werb, Z. (2002). Inflammation and cancer. *Nature, 420*(6917), 860–867. https://doi.org/10.1038/nature01322.

De Visser, K. E., Eichten, A., & Coussens, L. M. (2006). Paradoxical roles of the immune system during cancer development. *Nature Reviews. Cancer, 6*(1), 24–37. https://doi.org/10.1038/nrc1782.

Dymicka-Piekarska, V., Koper-Lenkiewicz, O. M., Zińczuk, J., Kratz, E., & Kamińska, J. (2021). Inflammatory cell-associated tumors. Not only macrophages (TAMs), fibroblasts (TAFs) and neutrophils (TANs) can infiltrate the tumor microenvironment. The unique role of tumor associated platelets (TAPs). *Cancer Immunology, Immunotherapy, 70*(6), 1497–1510. https://doi.org/10.1007/s00262-020-02758-7, link.springer.de/link/service/journals/00262/index.htm.

Eftekhari, Z., & Fardid, R. (2020). The bystander effect of ultraviolet radiation and mediators. *Journal of Biomedical Physics and Engineering, 10*(1), 111–118. https://doi.org/10.31661/jbpe.v0i0.956, http://jbpe.sums.ac.ir/article_44588_eb1327922e0eb49264b1c58968ebdc0e.pdf.

Experimental, and Microscopic Researches upon Inflammation, Tuberculisation, Tumours, the Formation of Callus, &c. Med Chir Rev. 1846 (5).235–247. (n.d.).

Fu, X. L., Duan, W., Su, C. Y., Mao, F. Y., Lv, Y. P., Teng, Y. S., Yu, P. W., Zhuang, Y., & Zhao, Y. L. (2017). Interleukin 6 induces M2 macrophage differentiation by STAT3 activation that correlates with gastric cancer progression. *Cancer Immunology, Immunotherapy, 66*(12), 1597–1608. https://doi.org/10.1007/s00262-017-2052-5, link.springer.de/link/service/journals/00262/index.htm.

Furman, D., Campisi, J., Verdin, E., Carrera-Bastos, P., Targ, S., Franceschi, C., Ferrucci, L., Gilroy, D. W., Fasano, A., Miller, G. W., Miller, A. H., Mantovani, A., Weyand, C. M., Barzilai, N., Goronzy, J. J., Rando, T. A., Effros, R. B., Lucia, A., Kleinstreuer, N., & Slavich, G. M. (2019). Chronic inflammation in the etiology of disease across the life span. *Nature Medicine, 25*(12), 1822–1832. https://doi.org/10.1038/s41591-019-0675-0, http://www.nature.com/nm/index.html.

Gelfand, M., Weinberg, R. W., & Castle, W. M. (1967). Relation between carcinoma of the bladder and infestation with Schistosoma haematobium. *Lancet, 1*(7502), 1249–1251. https://doi.org/10.1016/s0140-6736(67)92714-6.

Giannoni, E., Bianchini, F., Calorini, L., & Chiarugi, P. (2011). Cancer Associated Fibroblasts Exploit Reactive Oxygen Species Through a Proinflammatory Signature Leading to Epithelial Mesenchymal Transition and Stemness. *Antioxidants & Redox Signaling, 14*(12), 2361–2371. https://doi.org/10.1089/ars.2010.3727.

Goldstein, I., Marcel, V., Olivier, M., Oren, M., Rotter, V., & Hainaut, P. (2011). Understanding wild-type and mutant p53 activities in human cancer: new landmarks on the way to targeted therapies. *Cancer Gene Therapy, 18*(1), 2–11. https://doi.org/10.1038/cgt.2010.63.

Grivennikov, S., Karin, E., Terzic, J., Mucida, D., Yu, G. Y., Vallabhapurapu, S., Scheller, J., Rose-John, S., Cheroutre, H., Eckmann, L., & Karin, M. (2009). IL-6 and Stat3 Are Required for Survival of Intestinal Epithelial Cells and Development of Colitis-Associated Cancer. *Cancer Cell, 15*(2), 103–113. https://doi.org/10.1016/j.ccr.2009.01.001, https://www.journals.elsevier.com/cancer-cell.

Gudkov, A. V., Gurova, K. V., & Komarova, E. A. (2011). Inflammation and p53: A tale of two stresses. *Genes and Cancer, 2*(4), 503–516. https://doi.org/10.1177/1947601911409747.

Gómez-Valenzuela, F., Escobar, E., Pérez-Tomás, R., & Montecinos, V. P. (2021). The Inflammatory Profile of the Tumor Microenvironment, Orchestrated by Cyclooxygenase-2, Promotes Epithelial-Mesenchymal Transition. *Frontiers in Oncology, 11*. https://doi.org/10.3389/fonc.2021.686792, http://www.frontiersin.org/Oncology/about.

Jin, S., Yang, X., Li, J., Yang, W., Zhang, Z., & Ma, H. (2019). 53-targetedlinc RNA-p21actsasatumor suppressorbyinhibitingJAK2/STAT3signalingpathwaysinheadandnecksquamouscell carcinoma[J]. *Molecular Cancer, 18*(1).

O.V. Kovaleva, D.V. Samoilova, M.S. Shitova, A. Gratchev. (n.d.).

Landskron, G., De La Fuente, M., Thuwajit, P., Thuwajit, C., & Hermoso, M. A. (2014). Chronic inflammation and cytokines in the tumor microenvironment. *Journal of Immunology Research, 2014*. https://doi.org/10.1155/2014/149185, http://www.hindawi.com/journals/jir/.

Larionova, I., Kazakova, E., Patysheva, M., & Kzhyshkowska, J. (2020). Transcriptional, Epigenetic and Metabolic Programming of Tumor-Associated Macrophages. *Cancers (Basel), 29*.

Lee, S., Rauch, J., & Kolch, W. (2020). Targeting MAPK Signaling in Cancer: Mechanisms of Drug Resistance and Sensitivity. *International Journal of Molecular Sciences, 21*(3), 1102. https://doi.org/10.3390/ijms21031102.

Lin, E. Y., Li, J. F., Gnatovskiy, L., Deng, Y., Zhu, L., Grzesik, D. A., Qian, H., Xue, X. N., & Pollard, J. W. (2006). Macrophages regulate the angiogenic switch in a mouse model of breast cancer. *Cancer Research, 66*(23), 11238–11246. https://doi.org/10.1158/0008-5472.CAN-06-1278.

Liu, J., Wang, M., & Zhao, Y. (2025). The Regulatory Network of Transcription Factors in Macrophage Polarization. *ImmunoTargets and Therapy, 14*, 555–575. https://doi.org/10.2147/ITT.S494550, https://www.dovepress.com/article/download/103632.

Lord, E. M., Penney, D. P., Sutherland, R. M., & Cooper, R. A. (1979). Morphological and functional characteristics of cells infiltrating and destroying tumor multicellular spheroids in vivo. *Virchows Archiv B, Cell Pathology Including Molecular Pathology, 31*(1), 103–116. https://doi.org/10.1007/BF02889928.

Mantovani, A., Sozzani, S., Locati, M., Allavena, P., & Sica, A. (2002). Macrophage polarization: tumor-associated macrophages as a paradigm for polarized M2 mononuclear phagocytes. *Trends in Immunology, 23*(11), 549–555. https://doi.org/10.1016/s1471-4906(02)02302-5.

Mantovani, A., Allavena, P., Sica, A., & Balkwill, F. (2008). Cancer-related inflammation. *Nature, 454*(7203), 436–444. https://doi.org/10.1038/nature07205.

Martinez, F. O., & Gordon, S. (2014). The M1 and M2 paradigm of macrophage activation: Time for reassessment. *F1000Prime Reports, 6*. https://doi.org/10.12703/P6-13, http://f1000.com/prime/reports/b/6/13/pdf.

Monteran, L., & Erez, N. (2019). The Dark Side ofFibroblasts: Cancer-Associated Fibroblasts as Mediators of Immunosuppression in the Tumor Microenvironment [J]. *Frontiers in Immunology, 10*.

Mossman, B. T., Lounsbury, K. M., & Reddy, S. P. (2006). Oxidants and signaling by mitogen-activated protein kinases in lung epithelium[J]. *American Journal of Respiratory Cell and Molecular Biology, 34*(6), 666–669.

Pello, Pizzol, D., Mirolo, M., Soucek, Zammataro, L., Amabile, L., DoniA, A., Nebuloni, Swigart, L. B., Evan, G. I., MantovaniA, & Locati, M. (2012). Role ofc-MYC in alternative activation of human macrophages and tumor-associated macrophage biology. *Blood, 12*(2).

Pettersen, J. S., Fuentes-Duculan, J., Suárez-Fariñas, M., Pierson, K. C., Pitts-Kiefer, A., Fan, L., Belkin, D. A., Wang, C. Q. F., Bhuvanendran, S., Johnson-Huang, L. M., Bluth, M. J., Krueger, J. G., Lowes, M. A., & Carucci, J. A. (2011). Tumor-associated macrophages in the cutaneous SCC microenvironment are heterogeneously activated. *Journal of Investigative Dermatology, 131*(6), 1322–1330. https://doi.org/10.1038/jid.2011.9, https://www.sciencedirect.com/science/journal/0022202X.

Qian, B. Z., & Pollard, J. W. (2010). Macrophage Diversity Enhances Tumor Progression and Metastasis. *Cell, 141*(1), 39–51. https://doi.org/10.1016/j.cell.2010.03.014, https://www.sciencedirect.com/journal/cell.

Ridker, P. M., MacFadyen, J. G., Thuren, T., Everett, B., Libby, P., Glynn, R. J., Lorenzatti, A., Krum, H., Varigos, J., Siostrzonek, P., Sinnaeve, P., Fonseca, F., Nicolau, J., Gotcheva, N., Genest, J., Yong, H., Urina-Triana, M., Milicic, D., Cifkova, R., ... Gersh, B. (2017). Effect of interleukin-1β inhibition with canakinumab on incident lung cancer in patients with atherosclerosis: exploratory results from a randomised, double-blind, placebo-controlled trial. *The Lancet, 390*(10105), 1833–1842. https://doi.org/10.1016/S0140-6736(17)32247-X, http://www.journals.elsevier.com/the-lancet/.

Rihawi, K., Ricci, A. D., Rizzo, A., Brocchi, S., Marasco, G., Pastore, L. V., Llimpe, F. L. R., Golfieri, R., & Renzulli, M. (2021). Tumor-associated macrophages and inflammatory microenvironment in gastric cancer: Novel translational implications. *International Journal of Molecular Sciences, 22*(8). https://doi.org/10.3390/ijms22083805, https://www.mdpi.com/1422-0067/22/8/3805/pdf.

Rook, G. A. W., & Dalgleish, A. (2011). Infection, immunoregulation, and cancer. *Immunological Reviews, 240*(1), 141–159. https://doi.org/10.1111/j.1600-065x.2010.00987.x.

Sangaletti, S., Tripodo, C., Santangelo, A., Castioni, N., Portararo, P., Gulino, A., Botti, L., Parenza, M., Cappetti, B., Orlandi, R., Tagliabue, E., Chiodoni, C., & Colombo, M. P. (2016). Mesenchymal Transition of High-Grade Breast Carcinomas

Depends on Extracellular Matrix Control of Myeloid Suppressor Cell Activity. *Cell Reports, 17*(1), 233–248. https://doi.org/10.1016/j.celrep.2016.08.075, http://www.sciencedirect.com/science/journal/22111247.

Sica, A., & Mantovani, A. (2012). Macrophage plasticity and polarization: in vivo veritas. *Journal of Clinical Investigation, 122*(3), 787–795. https://doi.org/10.1172/jci59643.

Stolte, M. (1992). Helicobacter pylori gastritis and gastric MALT-lymphoma. *The Lancet, 339*(8795), 745–746. https://doi.org/10.1016/0140-6736(92)90645-j.

Tan, Z., Xue, H., Sun, Y., Zhang, C., Song, Y., & Qi, Y. (2021). The Role of Tumor Inflammatory Microenvironment in Lung Cancer. *Frontiers in Pharmacology, 12*. https://doi.org/10.3389/fphar.2021.688625.

Tarique, A. A., Logan, J., Thomas, E., Holt, P. G., Sly, P. D., & Fantino, E. (2015). Phenotypic, functional, and plasticity features of classical and alternatively activated human macrophages. *American Journal of Respiratory Cell and Molecular Biology, 53*(5), 676–688. https://doi.org/10.1165/rcmb.2015-0012OC, http://www.atsjournals.org/doi/pdf/10.1165/rcmb.2015-0012OC.

Virchow, R. (1871). War Typhus and Dysentery. *Chic Med Exam, 7*, 432–445.

Vyas, G. N., Roberts, I., Mackay, I. R., & Gust, I. D. (1975). Immunologic mechanisms in hepatitis B assayed by antigen-binding lymphocytes. *The American Journal of the Medical Sciences, 270*(2), 241–246. https://doi.org/10.1097/00000441-197509000-00003.

Weisz, L., Damalas, A., Liontos, M., Karakaidos, P., Fontemaggi, G., Maor-Aloni, R., Kalis, M., Levrero, M., Strano, S., Gorgoulis, V. G., Rotter, V., Blandino, G., & Oren, M. (2007). Mutant p53 enhances nuclear factor κB activation by tumor necrosis factor α in cancer cells. *Cancer Research, 67*(6), 2396–2401. https://doi.org/10.1158/0008-5472.CAN-06-2425.

Wu, M., Shi, Y., Zhu, L., Chen, L., Zhao, X., & Xu, C. (2022). Macrophages in Glioblastoma Development and Therapy: A Double-Edged Sword. *Life (Chicago, Ill. 1978), 12*(8), 1225. https://doi.org/10.3390/life12081225.

Yao, X., Huang, J., Zhong, H., Shen, N., Faggioni, R., Fung, M., & Yao, Y. (2014). Targeting interleukin-6 in inflammatory autoimmune diseases and cancers. *Pharmacology & Therapeutics, 141*(2), 125–139. https://doi.org/10.1016/j.pharmthera.2013.09.004.

Yu, H., Lin, L., Zhang, Z., Zhang, H., & Hu, H. (2020). Targeting NF-κB pathway for the therapy of diseases: mechanism and clinical study. *Signal Transduction and Targeted Therapy, 5*(1). https://doi.org/10.1038/s41392-020-00312-6.

Zhao, L. Liu, Y. Zhang, S. Wei, L. Cheng, H. Wang, J. Wang, Impacts and mechanisms of metabolic reprogramming of tumor microenvironment for immunotherapy in gastric cancer. Cell Death Dis. 13 (4). (n.d.).

Zhong, J., Guo, C., Hou, W., Shen, N., & Miao, C. (2019). Effects of MFHAS1 on cognitive impairment and dendritic pathology in the hippocampus of septic rats. *Life Sciences, 235*, 116822. https://doi.org/10.1016/j.lfs.2019.116822.

Zu, Y., Mu, Y., Li, Q., Zhang, S.-T., & Yan, H.-J. (2019). Icariin alleviates osteoarthritis by inhibiting NLRP3-mediated pyroptosis. *Journal of Orthopaedic Surgery and Research, 14*(1). https://doi.org/10.1186/s13018-019-1307-6.

Zuo, B. W., Yao, W. X., Fang, M. D., Ren, J., Tu, L. L., Fan, R. J., & Zhang, Y. M. (2023). Boris knockout eliminates AOM/DSS-induced in situ colorectal cancer by suppressing DNA damage repair and inflammation. *Cancer Science, 114*(5), 1972–1985. https://doi.org/10.1111/cas.15732, http://onlinelibrary.wiley.com/journal/10.1111/(ISSN)1349-7006.

Zuo, X., Wang, X., Ma, T., Chen, S., Cao, P., Cheng, H., Yang, N., Han, X., Gao, W., Liu, X., & Sun, Y. (2024). TNFRSF19 within the 13q12. 12 Risk Locus Functions as a Lung Cancer Suppressor by Binding Wnt3a to Inhibit Wnt/β-Catenin Signaling. *Molecular Cancer Research MCR, 22*(3), 227–239 1.

Zuo, Y., Li, H., Wang, X., Liang, Y., Huang, C., Nai, G., Ruan, J., Dong, W., & Lu, X. (2024). Inhibition of JAK/STAT3 Expression by Acute Myeloid Leukemia-Targeted Nanoliposome for Chemotherapy Enhancement. *ACS Omega, 9*(36), 37901–37909. https://doi.org/10.1021/acsomega.4c00710.

Zyromski, N. J., & White, P. B. (2011). Pancreatic cancer in obesity: Epidemiology, clinical observations, and basic mechanisms. *Anti-cancer Agents in Medicinal Chemistry, 11*(5), 470–478. https://doi.org/10.2174/187152011795677445, http://www.eurekaselect.com/578/journal/anti-cancer-agents-medicinal-chemistry.

Zyuz'kov, G. N., Miroshnichenko, L. A.'evna, Chayikovskyi, A. V.'evich, & Kotlovskaya, L. Y.'evna (2023). Nf-κb: A Target for Synchronizing the Functioning Nervous Tissue Progenitors of Different Types in Alzheimer's Disease. *Current Molecular Pharmacology, 16*(2), 234–241. https://doi.org/10.2174/1874467215666220601144727.

CHAPTER

2

Emerging technologies and future research directions in inflammation and cancer research

Xingwei Zhao and Yang Yu

Department of Cardiology, The Affiliated Hospital of Southwest Medical University, Luzhou, Sichuan Province, P.R. China

2.1 Introduction

The tumor microenvironment (TME) is an important biological signaling pathway that regulates tissue homeostasis and organizes the processes of tissue repair. Increasing evidence has shown that information is involved in the occurrence and development of cancer, especially its early phase and progression phase. The TME includes neoplastic cells, immune cells, blood vessels, and lymphatic vessels, as well as the extracellular matrix. Among these factors, chronic low-grade inflammation with sustained cytokine levels is considered the dominant driver of the TME. It stimulates innate and chemokine release and recruits immune cells, which then activate key canonical pathways, such as the NF-κB and JAK/STAT pathways, which rewire tumor metabolism and epigenetic landscapes, accelerating the malignant process (Basheer et al., 2021; Noy & Pollard, 2014; Xu et al., 2025). Tumor-Associated Macrophages (TAMs) promote angiogenesis and metastasis while setting up an immunosuppressive environment, allowing cancer cells to avoid immune surveillance. In principle, there is a correlation between inflammation and cancer: an intrinsic pathway activated directly by oncogenic mutations in cancer cells, an extrinsic pathway activated by persistent infections, or autoimmune insults that both lead to the activation of transcription factors such as NF-κB, STAT3, and HIF-1α, thus generating a protumorigenic inflammatory network (Grivennikov & Karin, 2010). Inflammation is, therefore, a double-edged weapon that is able to kill the seeds of tumors via immunosurveillance but is equally able to increase tumor growth via immunosuppression and protumorigenic signaling (Yang & Lin, 2017; Zhao et al., 2024).

Recent advances in single-cell sequencing, high-throughput gene editing, and big-data analytics have led to revolutionary methods for elucidating how inflammatory signals

Inflammation in Tumorigenesis and Cancer Treatment
DOI: https://doi.org/10.1016/B978-0-443-36649-9.00010-4

orchestrate immune evasion and therapeutic resistance; new approaches targeting inflammatory circuitries with increased accuracy and precision may become possible via improved understanding of the underlying mechanisms. Moreover, major molecular elements in the inflammation-cancer continuum are depicted schematically (Fig. 2.1).

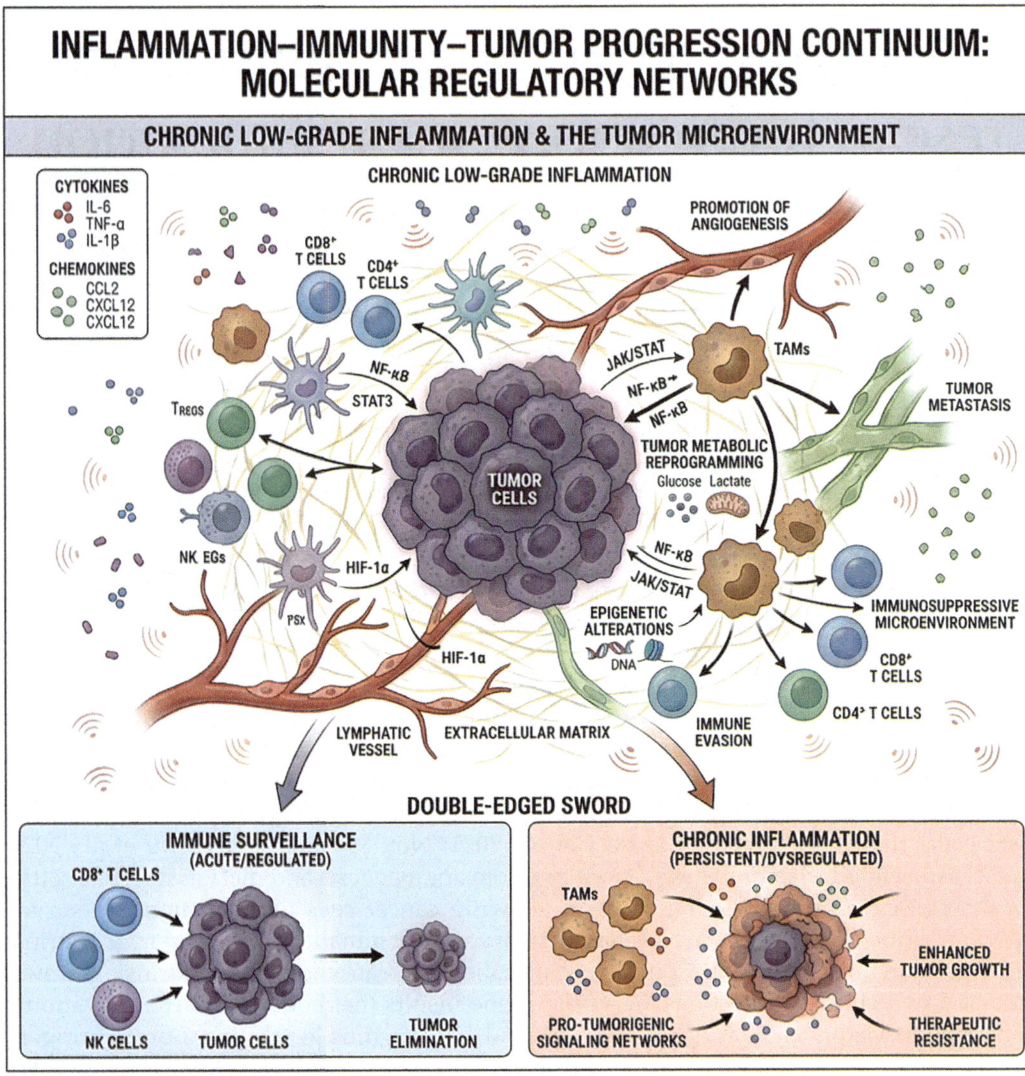

FIGURE 2.1 Three-dimensional cellular overview of the inflammation–cancer axis. The figure shows how inflammation and cancer interact at the cellular level. External factors, such as exogenous infections and mutations, directly or indirectly drive immune monitoring of the tumor microenvironment as well as immune suppression; TAMs/CAMs constitute the cytokine network that mediates T-cell exhaustion, whereas cancer-associated fibroblasts constitute profibrogenic cues. Furthermore, three signaling pathways (NF-κB, STAT3, and HIF-1α) are closely related to the inflammation–◯ ◯ △ ƒ ∮ ⩕cancer axis.

2.2 Transformative impact of emerging technologies on inflammation and cancer research

2.2.1 Clustered regularly interspaced short palindromic repeats gene-editing technology

Clustered regularly interspaced short palindromic repeats (CRISPR)/CRISPR-associated protein 9 endonuclease (Cas9) gene editing technology allows researchers to dissect cancer mechanisms, including those involved in inflammation and neoplastic progression, with unparalleled accuracy and speed. Inflammation, which has been known for years to be involved in many cancer types, has recently been shown to promote tumor initiation, progression, and metastasis across all solid cancers. Inflammation initiates and promotes tumorigenesis by reprogramming gene expression, secreting cytokines, evading the immune response, and stimulating blood vessel growth. Using CRISPR-based tools, investigators can specifically target genes within the inflammatory response axis both in vitro and in vivo, which allows them to generate causal insights into the disease process and identify new therapeutic targets for intervention.

By targeting important regulators of inflammatory signaling pathways (such as NF-κB, IL-6, STAT3, and COX-2) via CRISPR/Cas9, it is possible to remodel a chronic inflammatory TME (Kanarek et al., 2010). By deleting the p65 subunit of NF-κB, IκB degradation and nuclear translocation are inhibited, suppressing the downstream expression of IL-1β, TNF-α, and IL-8 and resulting in decreased cancer cell proliferation and migration (Mace et al., 2018).

CRISPR-mediated disruption of IL-6 or its downstream transcription factor STAT3 stops the canonical JAK/STAT3 axis to interrupt the activation of cancer-associated fibroblasts, reinvigorate exhausted T cells, and thus prevent tumor-mediated immunosuppression. These approaches can be applied in the clinic to explain how inflammatory cytokines shape the immune landscape and reveal their potential as targets for clinical treatment. Epithelial–mesenchymal transition (EMT) has been used to induce some inflammation-related tumor mutations in human cancers; for example, inserting activating mutations into COX-2 promoters elevates transcription, resulting in increased levels of PGE_2. An excess of prostaglandin E_2 (PGE_2) engages with EP receptors to activate the AKT/MAPK signaling pathway, which stimulates angiogenesis and the EMT process and leads to increased invasiveness and metastatic potential. Furthermore, CRISPR-engineered orthotopic mouse models can be employed for dynamic in vivo investigations of inflammation-induced tumorigenesis.

Sustained NF-κB activity functions as a molecular link between chronic inflammation and cancer formation (tumorigenesis). Recent studies have shown that CRISPR targeting of IKKβ, the main kinase involved in IκBα phosphorylation, leads to a reduction in downstream proinflammatory gene expression and a significant decrease in tumor development and metastasis in both breast and hepatocellular carcinoma model systems, reinforcing the potential of CRISPR-based antiinflammatory interventions.

In addition to defining the tumorigenic pathway, CRISPR/Cas9 was successfully applied to clarify other tumor-related mechanisms, such as immune evasion mechanisms. Tumor cells can upregulate immune checkpoint molecules, such as PD-L1 or CTLA-4, which induce paralysis of cytotoxic T lymphocytes (Ishizuka et al., 2019). CRISPR/Cas9-mediated knockout (KO) of PD-1 in CD8+ T cells removes the brakes of effector function, increasing the ability of CD8+ T cells to recognize and kill tumor cells (Hu et al., 2019). Research from the Department of Medicine at the University of Geneva's College of Medicine revealed that PD-1−/− CAR-T cells have better antitumor efficacy both in vitro and in vivo than WT CAR-T cells do and thus exhibit enhanced tumor suppression activities (Jia et al., 2022). Furthermore, the combination of PD-1-KO CAR-T cells with PD-1/PD-L1 blockade has been shown to act synergistically against solid tumors in murine models (Jia et al., 2022). Thus the combination of PD-1-KO CAR-T cells with PD-L1 blockade may advance the clinical and preclinical therapeutic strategies associated with immunotherapy and the genomic editing technique.

Overall, CRISPR gene editing enables the identification of the individual roles that inflammatory genes play in tumor initiation and immune escape. In this way, both conceptual and technical frameworks for precise targeting of the inflammation–cancer axis have been established, and integration with single-cell and spatial omics will enable next-generation individualized therapeutic designs. Application pathways of CRISPR/Cas9 gene-editing technology (Fig. 2.2).

Gene KO schematic showing the procedure of CRISPR/Cas9-guided genome editing of tumors. First, the DNA is delivered via electroporation of single-guide RNAs. Specific targets include all tumor-relevant genes, also known as key oncogenic regulators, such as NF-κB (nuclear factor kappa-light-chain-enhancer of activated B cells), which are genetically knocked out or repressed at the transcription level via gRNAs (guide RNAs).

Tumor-infiltrating lymphocyte (TIL) signal transducer and activator of transcription 3 and cyclooxygenase-2 (COX-2) have been specifically identified via CRISPR. The edited cells were confirmed in an orthotopic tumor model to evaluate their downstream effects on the immune system. In the tumor immune microenvironment, we observed improved T-cell (T lymphocyte) activity and modified programmed cell death protein 1 (PD-1) expression in TILs, confirming the synergy between CRISPR-based genome engineering and immune regulation.

2.2.2 Single-cell sequencing methods

TME-cell RNA sequencing (scRNA-seq) fundamentally reshapes our knowledge of the TME and its inflammatory nature; however, given that bulk sequencing approaches involve only average expression patterns, which ignore the diversity between cells and the exact pattern of cell changes over time. Through scRNA-seq, the transcriptomes can be resolved in an unbiased manner with the intent of cataloging various immune and stromal subpopulations (Trehan et al., 2025). Furthermore, in combination with spatial transcriptomics/proteomics information, scRNA-seq links specific cellular states to their respective cell-specific local tissue niches, providing fundamental mechanisms underlying immune evasion, inflammatory reprogramming, and intrapatient heterogeneity of immunotherapy responses.

Recent investigations have revealed the intricate circuitry linking inflammation to immune evasion at the level of cells and molecules. TAMs bearing SPP1 constitute a major immunosuppressive hub along the myeloid axis. These TAMs actively interact physically

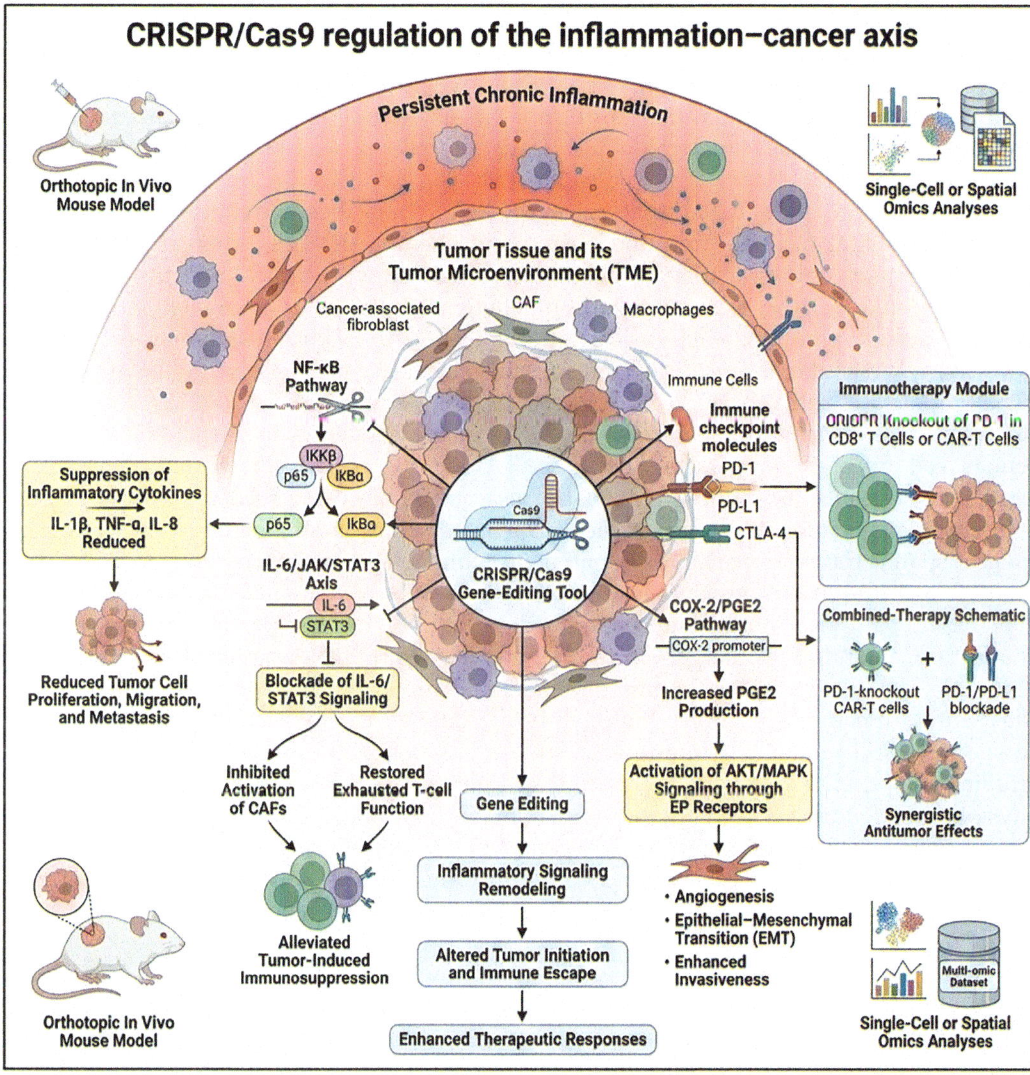

FIGURE 2.2 Clustered regularly interspaced short palindromic repeats (CRISPR)/CRISPR-associated protein 9 endonuclease (Cas9) application pipeline in oncological research and immune therapy development. Application pathways of CRISPR/Cas9 gene-editing technology.

and/or molecularly with terminally exhausted CD8+ T cells and remodel chemokine gradients and metabolic landscapes for survival and establishment of an immune-privileged niche (Y. Liu et al., 2025). The transcription factor ZEB2 operates as a master switch to orchestrate these functions, cosuppressing type I IFN and antigen presentation signaling to lock down TAMs into a fixed antiimmune state (Helmink et al., 2020; Sheban et al., 2025).

The lymphoid compartment is where B-cell maturation pathways drive the development and function of tertiary lymphoid structures (TLSs). In turn, mature follicular TLSs correlate with an increased immunotherapy response, whereas metabolic dysregulation (e.g., glutamine restriction) impairs their antitumor efficacy (Quail et al., 2022). The diversity of neutrophils was further untangled, and a distinct subset was shown to have antigen-presenting capacity.

Chromatin regulators (CRs) that release CXCL8 have been identified as oncogene-inducing cells that facilitate immune escape and chemoresistance, whereas other groups expressing antioncogenic factors are positively associated with clinical benefits (Peng et al., 2015). CRs—like EZH2/PRC2-mediated epigenetic silencing of chemokines, which down-regulates tumor immunogenicity—RSF affects the cGAS-STING inflammatory signaling pathway, whereas the absence of p53 results in the release of IL-34 to rewire the myeloid niche (Papalexi & Satija, 2018).

Rapid advances in technology have enabled many discoveries; in particular, scRNA-seq defines cell lineages and states, while scATAC-seq visualizes inflammation-associated regulatory elements, and multiomics platforms such as CITE-seq record all these together with chromatin accessibility and surface proteomes within a single cell (Liu et al., 2020). Finally, spatial transcriptomics and spatial proteomics add position information to these coordinates through linkage back to histology.

Signaling pathways that dictate tissue-resident immune-evasion programs were revealed. In addition, emerging spatial genomics methods (e.g., slide-DNA-seq and ExIGS) associate genotypic alterations with inflammatory niches to move the field away from the "static atlas" into "dynamic causality" (Frangieh et al., 2021). In vivo perturb-seq harnesses the power of CRISPR-mediated interference in combination with single-cell gene expression profiling to provide functional screening for genes that allow immune evasion under physiological conditions (Zedao Liu, Yang, et al., 2025). Longitudinal single-cell multiomics is now being used in the clinic, with recent reports following nonsmall cell lung cancer patients indicating that it can be used to identify therapy-response trajectories that allow biomarkers of early efficacy and adaptive treatment switching to be defined (Yuan et al., 2025).

Convergent data permit actionable directions toward (1) pharmacological reprogramming of SPP1-positive TAMs; (2) TLS maturity-based stratification for immunotherapy; (3) combination of epigenetic drugs and immune checkpoint blockade in a rational manner; and (4) incorporation of spatial omics measures into the design and response evaluation of clinical trials to close the loop from mechanistic discovery to therapeutic use.

Single-cell and spatial multiomics facilitate the depiction of the fundamental mechanisms behind inflammatory events leading to cancer and its clinical translation process. With respect to SPP1-induced TAM and TLS formation, along with multiple other discoveries within this landscape up to CRs, novel inflammation-driven targets are constantly being identified, and platform innovation has progressed from scRNA-seq/scATAC-seq/space-genome to in vivo Perturb-seq technology development. With the integration of existing diagnosable platforms or intervention protocols, single-cell or spatial-multiomic technologies can assist us in "observationally" learning about inflammation or directly executing "engineering inflammation" and boosting precision oncology. Single-cell spatial multiomics also revealed immune regulatory mechanisms in the TME caused by inflammation (Fig. 2.3).

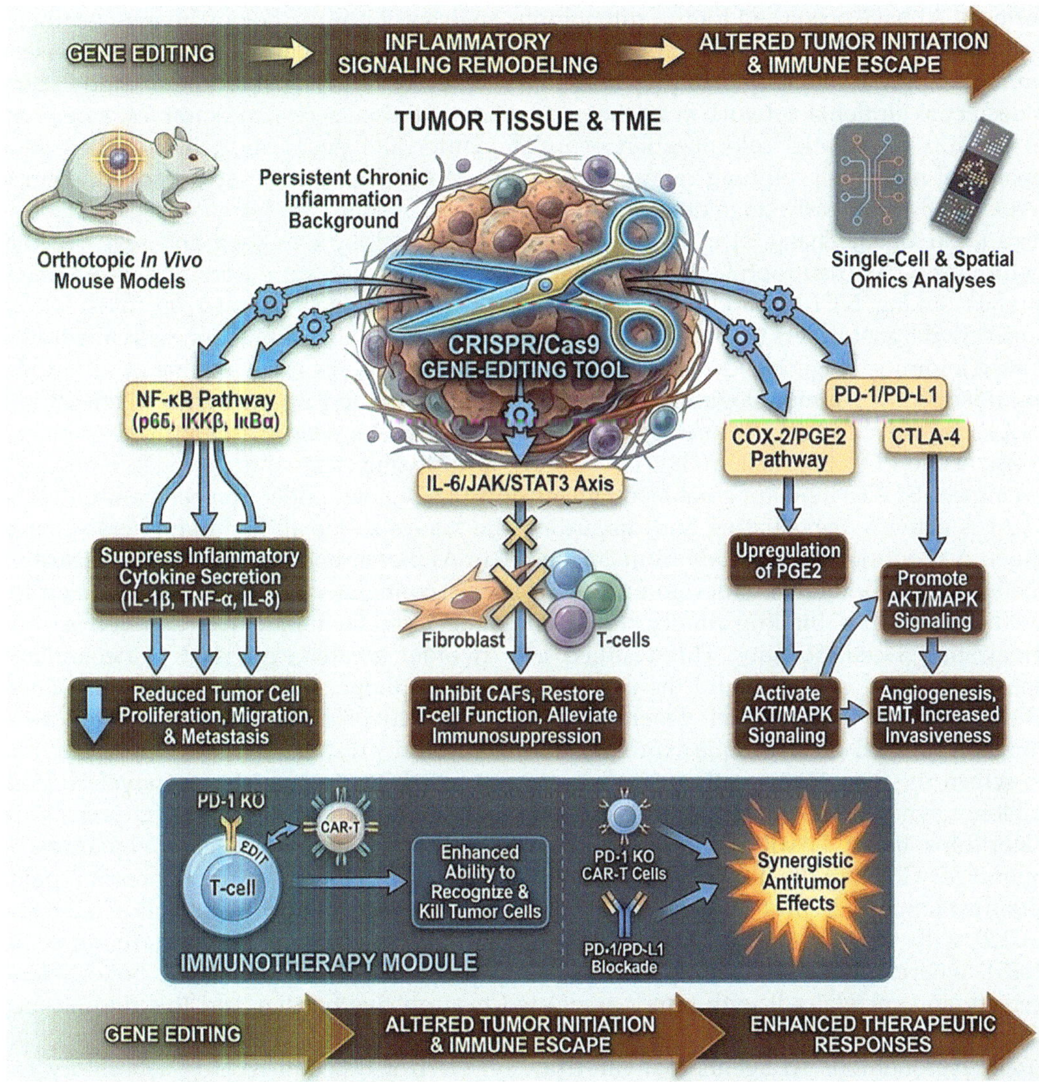

FIGURE 2.3 Inflammation–tertiary lymphoid structure (TLS) axis shapes the tumor immune microenvironment. Condensed paragraph: Single-cell and spatial multiomics show that inflammatory signals in the tumor microenvironment drive TLS maturation via IRF7/CIITA, while TAM-derived SPP1 boosts PD-L1 to silence cytotoxic T cells; clustered regularly interspaced short palindromic repeats deletion of ZEB2 validates the axis as a druggable immune modulator. *Cas9*, CRISPR-associated protein 9 endonuclease.

2.2.3 Artificial intelligence in cancer and inflammation research

In recent years, artificial intelligence (AI) has offered great opportunities to reveal the role of cancer biology, especially with respect to how cancer progresses through inflammation. Convolutional neural networks (CNNs), graph-based deep learning methods, and other forms of AI have been used for the autonomous analysis of histopathology images, genomics profiles, and inflammatory biomarkers, deciphering the obscure associations between immune infiltration and cancer progression (Wang et al., 2024). A multicenter study using a deep convolutional network in 2024 could be one of those successful examples: a network to quantify the spatial colocalization of inflammatory and neoplastic cells in whole-slide images of non-small cell lung cancer (NSCLC) patients to achieve an area under the curve (AUC) of 0.94 for early-stage detection and surpass pathologists in intraobserver variability tests (Sixu Chen, Zhang, et al., 2024). Explainable AI overlay was used and revealed that peritumor NETs (neutrophil extracellular traps) were the key feature leading to mechanistic studies linking NETosis and EMT. In addition to those analyses based on images, self-supervised transformers trained on more than 10,000 tumors, in combination with integrative transcriptomics, epigenomics, and proteomics, stratified patients into "inflamed," "immune-excluded," and "immunologically cold" subgroups, associated with distinctive NF-kB and STAT3 activity patterns (Morel et al., 2021), with transfer learning predicting de novo resistance to PD-1 blockade in 83% of cases and prioritizing rational drug combinations, for example, a STAT3 inhibitor combined with an anti-PD-L1, both under prospective validation.

AI is actively reevaluating and discarding the "one-size-fits-all" immunotherapy paradigm. A proof-of-concept study from 2025 used an AI that applied a reinforcement learning methodology to iteratively design patient-specific neoantigen vaccines while balancing the prediction of MHC binding affinity, the inflammatory cytokine milieu (IL-6 and TNF-α), and preexisting T-cell clonality. This resulted in a twofold greater expansion of neoantigen-specific CD8+ T cells than did the use of a standard epitope selection method (R.J. Chen, Ding, et al., 2024). In parallel, generative adversarial networks were used to create virtual tumor cells, such as the unique expression and interferon-γ response of patients' PD-L1, and to screen in silico 1500 small-molecule compounds, which revealed that a novel HDAC3 inhibitor synergized with anti–CTLA-4 therapy in patient-derived organoids. Radiogenomic algorithms link CT/MRI/PET radiomic features with inflammatory gene signatures: a hybrid 3D-CNN/gradient-boosting model is trained on combined feature-expression pairs. Contrast-enhanced CT of HCC predicts PTEN-loss-driven inflammatory signaling (IL-8 and CCL2) with 91% sensitivity to select PI3K-targeted therapy noninvasively (Huang et al., 2025), whereas FDG-PET-based deep learning quantifies intratumoral metabolic heterogeneity and correlates it with tumor-associated macrophage burden, and this finding may serve as an imaging biomarker to predict the response of CSF-1R inhibitors (Pelka et al., 2021). Autonomous AI agents that can draw on electronic health records, laboratory test results, and imaging are able to provide real-time therapeutic recommendations. A prospective pilot study in 2025 suggested that an oncology decision-support system cut the time taken for time-to-treatment decisions by 38% and raised concordance with multidisciplinary tumor board suggestions for advanced melanoma complicated by immune-related adverse events from 78% to 94% (Prakash, 2023).

In parallel with its surge, AI is changing almost all of the inflammation–cancer continuum, from early diagnosis and molecular subclassification to virtual drug screening and adaptive therapy optimization. As algorithms become more interpretable and datasets richer in multiomics content, AI fundamentally redefines how AI-generated heatmaps decode tumor–inflammation cross-talk in the future, diagnostics and treatment of inflammation-driven cancer (Fig. 2.4).

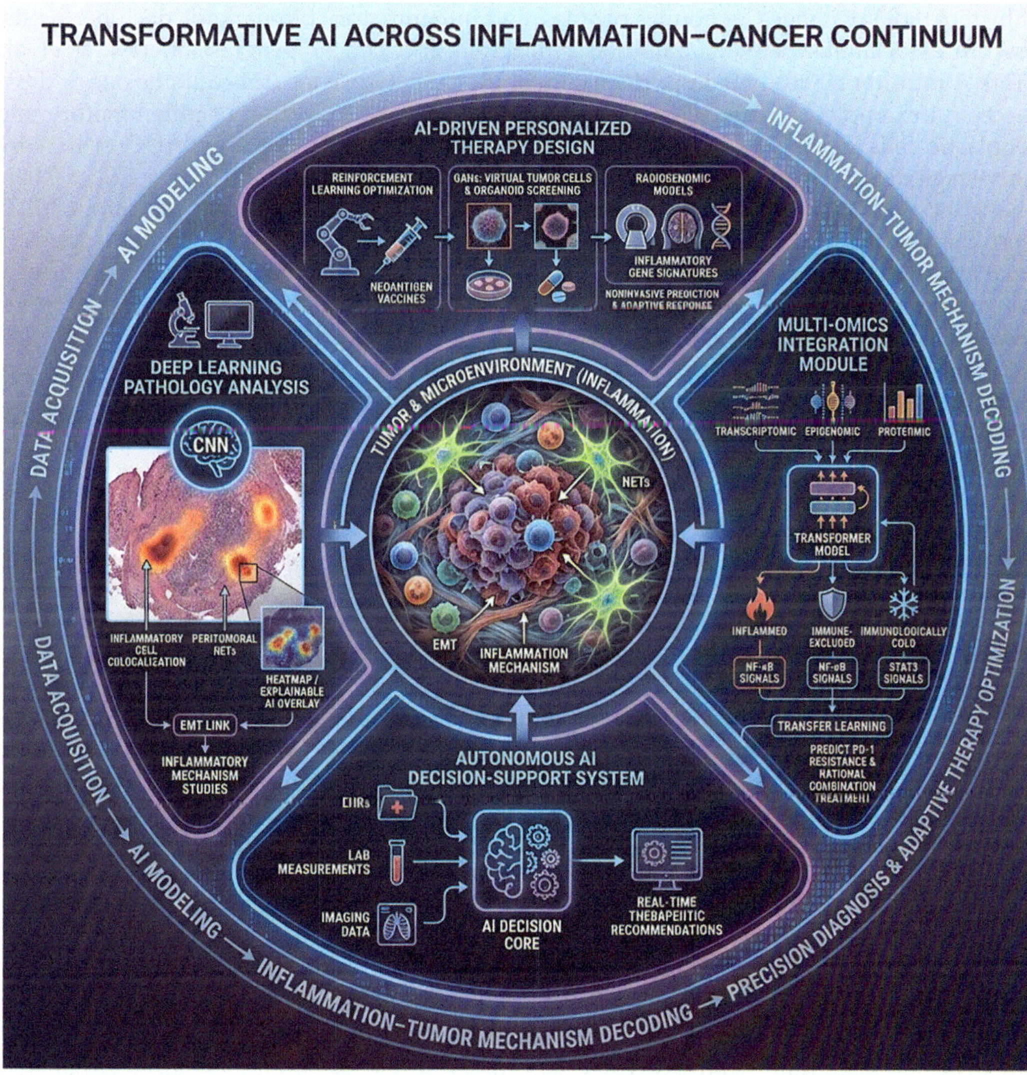

FIGURE 2.4 Tumor–inflammation interplay to pinpoint precision therapies for lung cancer and melanoma. The artificial intelligence (AI) model produces outputs that correctly distinguish types of lung cancer from melanoma via multimodal inputs, including imaging, genomics, and clinical data. Then, personalized therapeutic strategies are determined according to these results. The effectiveness of the whole process is assessed by comparing the AI model outputs with the outcomes of the clinicians' decision-making.

2.2.4 Nanomedicine technologies in inflammation and cancer research

In recent years, AI has offered great opportunities to reveal the role of cancer biology, especially with respect to how cancer progresses through inflammation. CNNs, graph-based deep learning methods, and other forms of AI have been used for the autonomous analysis of histopathology images, genomics profiles, and inflammatory biomarkers, deciphering the obscure associations between immune infiltration and cancer progression (Wang et al., 2024). A multicenter study using a deep convolutional network in 2024 could be one of those successful examples: a network to quantify the spatial colocalization of inflammatory and neoplastic cells in whole-slide images of NSCLC patients to achieve an AUC of 0.94 for early-stage detection and surpass pathologists in intraobserver variability tests (Sixu Chen, Zhang, et al., 2024). Explainable AI overlay was used and revealed that peritumor NETs were the key feature leading to mechanistic studies linking NETosis. Epithelial–mesenchymal transition. In addition to those analyses based on images, self-supervised transformers trained on more than 10,000 tumors, in combination with integrative transcriptomics, epigenomics, and proteomics, stratified patients into "inflamed," "immune-excluded," and "immunologically cold" subgroups, associated with distinctive NF-kB and STAT3 activity patterns (Morel et al., 2021), with transfer learning predicting de novo resistance to PD-1 blockade in 83% of cases and prioritizing rational drug combinations, for example, a STAT3 inhibitor combined with an anti-PD-L1, both under prospective validation.

AI is actively reevaluating and discarding the "one-size-fits-all" immunotherapy paradigm. A proof-of-concept study from 2025 used an AI that applied a reinforcement learning methodology to iteratively design patient-specific neoantigen vaccines while balancing the prediction of MHC binding affinity, the inflammatory cytokine milieu (IL-6 and TNF-α), and preexisting T-cell clonality. This resulted in a twofold greater expansion of neoantigen-specific CD8+ T cells than did the use of a standard epitope selection method (R.J. Chen, Ding, et al., 2024). In parallel, generative adversarial networks were used to create virtual tumor cells, such as the unique expression and interferon-γ response of patients' PD-L1, and to screen in silico 1500 small-molecule compounds, which revealed that a novel HDAC3 inhibitor synergized with anti–CTLA-4 therapy in patient-derived organoids. Radiogenomic algorithms link CT/MRI/PET radiomic features with inflammatory gene signatures: a hybrid 3D-CNN/gradient-boosting model is trained on combined feature-expression pairs. Contrast-enhanced CT of HCC predicts PTEN-loss-driven inflammatory signaling (IL-8 and CCL2) with 91% sensitivity to select PI3K-targeted therapy noninvasively (Huang et al., 2025), whereas FDG-PET-based deep learning quantifies intratumoral metabolic heterogeneity and correlates it with tumor-associated macrophage burden, and this finding may serve as an imaging biomarker to predict the response of CSF-1R inhibitors (Pelka et al., 2021). Autonomous AI agents that can draw on electronic health records, laboratory test results, and imaging are able to provide real-time therapeutic recommendations. A prospective pilot study in 2025 suggested that an oncology decision-support system cut the time taken for time-to-treatment decisions by 38% and raised concordance with multidisciplinary tumor board suggestions for advanced melanoma complicated by immune-related adverse events from 78% to 94% (Prakash, 2023).

2.2.5 Nanomedicine technologies in inflammation and cancer research

Nanomedicine will enable future clinical advancements in the revolutionizing of traditional oncology and antiinflammatory therapies through an extremely high degree of drug biodistribution, release kinetics, and target selectivity. Through the proper design of delivery nanocarriers (such as liposomes, polymeric nanoparticles, inorganic nanoshells, and biomimetic vesicles), targeted cancer cells or diseased tissue can be effectively targeted with a sufficient therapeutic payload to reduce off-target toxicity.

Nanotechnology has changed the landscape of both cancer diagnosis and treatment through dual functions, both delivering precision drugs to the correct location in the body and working as a highly sensitive early warning system. As surface-functionalized nanoparticles loaded with antibodies, peptides, or small molecules specifically bind to tumor- or inflammation-related markers (folate receptors, VCAM-1, or PD-L1), fine-tuning their size (20–200 nm), shape, and zeta potential allows for optimized vascular permeability and intratumoral penetration. For example, pH-sensitive liposomes loaded with the STAT3 inhibitor napabucasin release the drug only in the acidic microenvironment of the tumor, leading to an increase in intratumoral drug concentrations of more than 5.7 times relative to those of free drug as well as strong suppression of IL-6-mediated inflammatory signaling (Vendrell et al., 2013). Parallel nanodiagnostic platforms leverage gold nanoparticle-based surface-enhanced Raman scattering (SERS) to detect ctDNA with femtomolar-level sensitivity. MicroRNAs and cytokines were detected by a multiplexed SERS assay that also measured IL-8, TNF-α, and miR-21, achieving greater than 92% sensitivity and 88% specificity in the detection of early-stage pancreatic cancer, outperforming the CA19-9 marker (Wells et al., 2024). Likewise, magnetic nanowires functionalized with anti-CD64 antibodies capture circulating proinflammatory neutrophils, providing a snapshot of a patient's systemic inflammation and accelerating response monitoring when used in conjunction with checkpoint inhibitors (Jang et al., 2025).

In addition to just sensing and delivering therapeutics, nanomaterials can be used as potent immunomodulatory agents to remodel the TME. A novel hybrid nanolipid-polymer scaffold that codelivered anti-PD-L1 siRNA and the TLR7/8 agonist resiquimod was able to reverse T-cell exhaustion present in tumors in a triple-negative mouse model of breast cancer (Lin et al., 2025), increasing CD8+IFN-γ+infiltration to 4.3-fold and achieving complete regression in 60% of the treated group, whereas mannose-decorated nanoparticles delivering IL-12 mRNA were effective in only 10%–15% of the mice. Specifically, M2-polarized TAMs were converted into the M1 proinflammatory phenotype, and the treatment sensitized tumors to subsequent anti–CTLA-4 therapy (Liu et al., 2023). A reactive oxygen species (ROS)-scavenging polymeric nanosphere containing a CXCR4 antagonist was able to neutralize tumor-derived ROS and block the recruitment of immunosuppressive cells via CXCL12 for the treatment of chronic inflammatory disorders that drive resistance and metastasis.

It significantly reduced radiation-induced pulmonary fibrosis and increased the survival of mice (Greten & Grivennikov, 2019). Similarly, biocompatible manganese-doped nanoclusters activate the cGAS-STING signaling pathway specifically at tumor sites to enhance type I interferon signaling and antitumor immunity without affecting healthy tissues or nearby cells (Oliveira et al., 2025). In the future, clinical translation would most likely revolve around so-called "zero-burden" designs, such as PLGA or porous silicon cores that could be tuned to degrade. Traditional methods for TIS, including the use of immune-camouflage coatings (CD47 or autologous cell membranes) and tumor-selective triggers (pH, enzymes, or ROS) for the release of the drug and limited off-target toxicity, will become common (Peng et al., 2025). TIS, by integrating combinatorial nanoregimens loaded with CRISPR-Cas9 mRNA, real-time imaging reporters, and AI-guided dosing, could produce closed-loop therapeutic systems that dynamically respond to inflammatory and neoplastic cues.

Nanomedicine combines targeting, immunomodulation, and ultrasensitive detection for simultaneous blockade of oncogenic signal transduction and inflammatory amplification. This has led to rapid advances in precision therapy for both cancer and inflammation. Nanomedicine enables precise antiinflammatory and anticancer control (Fig. 2.5).

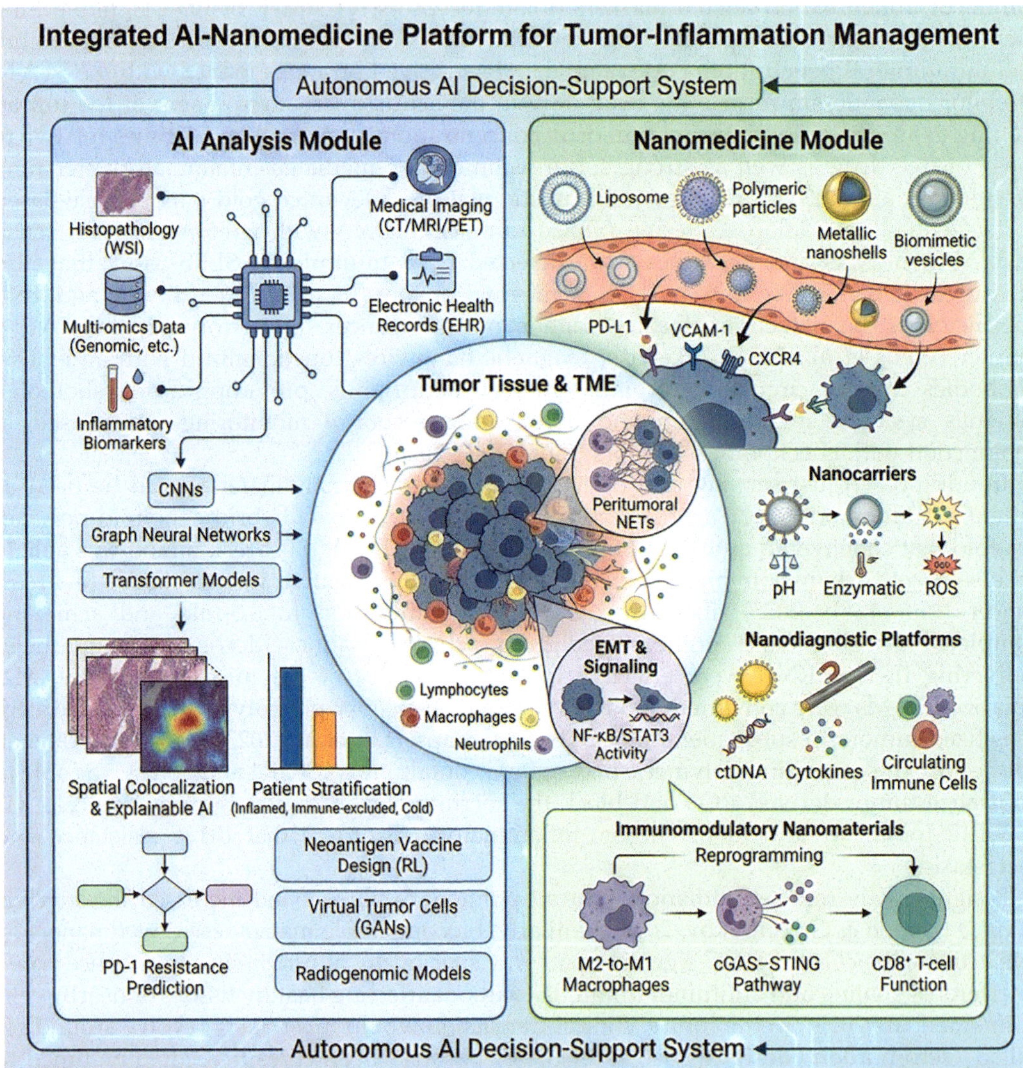

FIGURE 2.5 Nanomedicine enables precise antiinflammatory and anticancer control. Nanomedicine combines gene editing, single-cell sequencing and artificial intelligence (AI) for the earliest possible diagnosis of cancer, personalized treatment of cancer, and modulation of the precision immune response in inflamed cancers. *EMT*, Epithelial–mesenchymal transition; *TME*, tumor microenvironment.

2.2.6 Spatial-CITE-seq 2.0 in inflammation and cancer research

Spatial-CITE-seq 2.0 provides high-plex spatial multiomics data for the acquisition of whole-transcriptome information combined with 30–300 surface proteins localized in tissue sections with an imaging resolution of ≤500 nm by cohybridizing spatially barcoded mRNAs and DNA-barcoded antibodies (ADTs). It also generates a three-dimensional map containing RNA expression, protein abundance, and subcellular coordinates. By providing a more comprehensive understanding of the intercellular associations, immune escape, and resistance networks present in inflamed or neoplastic tissue, this innovative technology can be used to develop new methods for studying disease-related changes between cell types (Oliveira et al., 2025; Peng et al., 2025).

Spatial-CITE-seq 2.0 uses a 2.5-μm-pixel-printed bead that carries an individual barcode to capture transcribed mRNAs and AB-tag complexes inside a 200-nm diffusion radius and uses a 12-h in situ workflow to profile 100 protein species and 25,000 genes from a single 6 mm^2 section, increasing the efficiency of mRNA capture 3.4-fold and reducing the rate of antibody cross-talk by 45%, thereby enabling the discovery of some rare checkpoints, such as LAG-3 and TIGIT (Liu et al., 2021). With this resolution, human colorectal cancers exhibit a 12 μm IL-6-driven STAT3-activation zone (B–C and D–G) (Liu et al., 2024), whereas thyroid carcinomas harbor IL-23$^+$ CD86$^+$ DCs in TLSs, which amplify Th17 expansion (Yunhe Liu, Sinjab, et al., 2025). Moreover, another type of cancer with a 28 μm "immune-exclusion radius," namely, melanoma, presents PD-L1$^+$ nests surrounded by a local IFN-γ exhaustion-dependent immune exclusion area that generates PD-L1-dependent anti-PD-1 resistance (AUC=0.89) via JAK2 amplification.

Vertical HER2+ breast biopsies taken under surveillance under trastuzumab–docetaxel treatment showed a threefold increase in CXCL10+ APCs and PTEN loss emerging 18 μm from such cells, connecting local inflammatory gradients with PI3K pathway mutation selection (g) (Yu et al., 2025). Fusing this platform with CRISPR-LNP delivery led to 64% phospho-STAT3 suppression exclusively in F4/80+ macrophages 5–25 μm from pancreatic tumor glands (G), confirming that macrophage-directed STAT3 disruption dampens paracrine inflammation while sparing direct antitumor immunity. The members of the spatial-CITE-consortium have made their analyses and validations of spatial platforms publicly available through a shared GitHub repository of protocols and pipelines; a panmarket tri-county study revealed that a 22-fingerprint "inflammatory-cold" signature predicts a lack of response to PD-1 blockade in MSI-high CRC with 94% negative predictive value .

Spatial-CITE-seq 2.0 combines single-cell multiomics and intact tissue architecture to visualize and manipulate inflammation in the TME, which, together with CRISPR, AI, and nanomedicine, will support and strengthen future precision-oncology trials.

2.3 Challenges and future directions in inflammation–cancer research

While breakthroughs in AI, big data, and blockchain can revolutionize humanity, implementing inflammation–cancer research findings into noninvasive, safe, effective, accessible, and equitable clinical practices is challenging, as it can yield positive results for patients and healthcare providers. To achieve this progress, there are a few points of action that we can take over the next 10 years.

Most preclinical models miss human relevancy due to distortion of the real-world "supertumor" balance due to murine immunity and the creation of engineered "supertumor" models, whereas single-cell and spatial omics models must address subcellular resolution, throughput, and lab-batch effects and lack noninvasive longitudinal proxies, whereas AI tools are also limited by bias from datasets, an in-text black-box causality gap, and a lack of an FDA/EMA benchmarking atlas. Furthermore, CRISPR technologies leave out trailing off-target chromosomal alterations and controversies concerning global equity and justice issues. In addition, nanomedicines face batch-to-batch variance in LNPs, the immunogenicity of PEG linkages, and an unclear long-term metabolic destiny for inorganic nanoparticles.

To advance, we introduce the "6C" convergent roadmap: cross-disciplinary teams, FAIR common data ecosystems, causal hybrid-AI models, standardized CRISPR safety/surveillance, clinical grade scalable nanomanufacturing incorporating QbD metrics, and cost-effective global deployment embedding health economic models in LMICs—allowing concurrent technological innovation, biological validation, ethical oversight, and equitable access to translate descriptive precision to interventional precision for all inflammatory-driven cancers worldwide.

2.4 Conclusion

Inflammation and cancer used to be considered separate phenomena, but we now understand them to be inherently linked in the tumorigenesis process, as well as immune evasion and therapy resistance. This transition is largely due to the confluence of five techniques: CRISPR editing delivers precise nucleotide-level modulation of inflammatory oncogenic circuits, and single-cell or spatial multiomics illuminates cellular heterogeneity and immune-privileged niches.

AI that combines gigapixel images, multiomic profiles, and clinical metadata can predict biomarkers and personalize immunotherapy. Nanomedicine delivers both antiinflammatory and antineoplastic agents together into the tumor bed. With Spatial-CITE-seq 2.0, the high-resolution, subcellular "GPS" guidance now spans the entire inflammatory tumor ecosystem. All three technologies work on precision inflammation-oncology treatment tailored to both a patient's genome and the spatial distribution of inflammation in his/her tumor.

However, species-specific immunity, AI bias, manufacturing limits, and global equity gaps require collaborative efforts from cross-disciplines, open-science data ecosystem creation, and adaptive regulations. The next grand challenge will be to transmute the current descriptive explosion into closed-loop therapeutics wherein a sensory organism detects and responds in real time to inflammatory or oncogenic stimuli with AI-guided digital twin-made decisions, intervenes with edited CRISPR cells or nanoencapsulated drugs, learns from outcomes and recalibrates its cycle for each, and views inflammation as the two-edged sword of turning control to precision tuning levers for the prevention, control, and cure of cancer. Emerging technologies in the field of inflammation-cancer research are summarized in Table 2.1

TABLE 2.1 Summary of emerging technologies and advances in inflammation–cancer research.

Section	Main focus	Key technologies/ mechanisms	Major findings/advances	Future directions and challenges	References
CRISPR gene editing	Dissecting inflammation-driven tumor progression and immune evasion	CRISPR/Cas9, NF-κB, IL-6, STAT3, COX-2	CRISPR gene editing blocks inflammatory signaling (e.g., STAT3 and NF-κB), inhibiting tumor growth and enhancing immune response	Combining CRISPR with single-cell and spatial-omics for more precise therapies	Kanarek et al. (2010), Mace et al. (2018), Ishizuka et al. (2019), Hu et al. (2019)
Single-cell sequencing	Mapping immune and stromal cell dynamics in the TME	scRNA-seq, CITE-seq, scATAC-seq	Identified SPP1^{+} TAMs as immunosuppressive hubs and discovered ZEB2 as a master regulator in inflammation	Integrating multiomics with clinical trials to personalize immunotherapy	Trehan et al. (2025), Y. Liu, Yang, et al. (2025), Sheban et al. (2025), Quail et al. (2022)
AI	AI to integrate imaging, genomic, and inflammatory data for cancer diagnosis and therapy	Deep learning, Transformers, GANs, reinforcement learning	AI detects early-stage tumors (AUC=0.94) and predicts immune evasion; AI-designed vaccines boost T-cell expansion	Overcoming data bias, improving model explainability, and creating real-time clinical AI tools	Wang et al. (2024), Sixu Chen, Zhang et al. (2024), Morel et al. (2021), R.J. Chen, Ding, et al. (2024)
Nanomedicine	Targeted drug delivery and immune modulation in the TME	Nanoparticles, pH-sensitive liposomes, SERS sensors	Nanomedicine delivers drugs directly to tumors, reprograms TAMs, and detects biomarkers (e.g., IL-8 and TNF-α) at femtomolar levels	Enhancing biodegradability, reducing immunogenicity, and combining nanomedicine with CRISPR and AI	Vendrell et al. (2013), Wells et al. (2024), Jang et al. (2025), Liu et al. (2023)
Spatial-CITE-seq 2.0	High-resolution spatial profiling of gene and protein interactions in TME	Spatial RNA–protein comapping, barcoded antibodies	Revealed inflammation zones linked to immune evasion and therapy resistance (e.g., PD-1/ PD-L1 resistance)	Standardizing data pipelines and increasing throughput for clinical applications	Oliveira et al. (2025), Peng et al. (2025), Liu et al. (2021)

AI, Artificial intelligence; *Cas9*, CRISPR-associated protein 9 endonuclease; *CRISPR*, clustered regularly interspaced short palindromic repeats; *SERS*, surface-enhanced Raman scattering; *TME*, tumor microenvironment.

References

Basheer, A. S., Abas, F., Othman, I., & Naidu, R. (2021). Role of inflammatory mediators, macrophages, and neutrophils in glioma maintenance and progression: Mechanistic understanding and potential therapeutic applications. *Cancers, 13*(16), 4226. https://doi.org/10.3390/cancers13164226.

Chen, R. J., Ding, T., Lu, M. Y., Williamson, D. F. K., Jaume, G., Song, A. H., Chen, B., Zhang, A., Shao, D., Shaban, M., Williams, M., Oldenburg, L., Weishaupt, L. L., Wang, J. J., Vaidya, A., Le, L. P., Gerber, G., Sahai, S., Williams, W., & Mahmood, F. (2024). Towards a general-purpose foundation model for computational pathology. *Nature Medicine, 30*(3), 850–862. https://doi.org/10.1038/s41591-024-02857-3, https://www.nature.com/nm/.

Chen, S., Zhang, P., Duan, X., Bao, A., Wang, B., Zhang, Y., Li, H., Zhang, L., & Liu, S. (2024). Lesion localization and pathological diagnosis of ovine pulmonary adenocarcinoma based on MASK R-CNN. *Animals: An Open Access Journal from MDPI, 14*(17), 2488. https://doi.org/10.3390/ani14172488.

Frangieh, C. J., Melms, J. C., Thakore, P. I., Geiger-Schuller, K. R., Ho, P., Luoma, A. M., Cleary, B., Jerby-Arnon, L., Malu, S., Cuoco, M. S., Zhao, M., Ager, C. R., Rogava, M., Hovey, L., Rotem, A., Bernatchez, C., Wucherpfennig, K. W., Johnson, B. E., Rozenblatt-Rosen, O., ... Izar, B. (2021). Multimodal pooled Perturb-CITE-seq screens in patient models define mechanisms of cancer immune evasion. *Genetics, 53*(3), 332–341. https://doi.org/10.1038/s41588-021-00779-1, http://www.nature.com/ng/index.html.

Greten, F. R., & Grivennikov, S. I. (2019). Inflammation and cancer: Triggers, mechanisms, and consequences. *Immunity, 51*(1), 27–41. https://doi.org/10.1016/j.immuni.2019.06.025, www.immunity.com.

Grivennikov, S. I., & Karin, M. (2010). Dangerous liaisons: STAT3 and NF-κB collaboration and crosstalk in cancer. *Cytokine and Growth Factor Reviews, 21*(1), 11–19. https://doi.org/10.1016/j.cytogfr.2009.11.005.

Helmink, B. A., Reddy, S. M., Gao, J., Zhang, S., Basar, R., Thakur, R., Yizhak, K., Sade-Feldman, M., Blando, J., Han, G., Gopalakrishnan, V., Xi, Y., Zhao, H., Amaria, R. N., Tawbi, H. A., Cogdill, A. P., Liu, W., LeBleu, V. S., Kugeratski, F. G., ... Wargo, J. A. (2020). B cells and tertiary lymphoid structures promote immunotherapy response. *Nature, 577*(7791), 549–555. https://doi.org/10.1038/s41586-019-1922-8, http://www.nature.com/nature/index.html.

Hu, W., Zi, Z., Jin, Y., Li, G., Shao, K., Cai, Q., Ma, X., & Wei, F. (2019). CRISPR/Cas9-mediated PD-1 disruption enhances human mesothelin-targeted CAR T cell effector functions. *Cancer Immunology, Immunotherapy, 68*(3), 365–377. https://doi.org/10.1007/s00262-018-2281-2.

Huang, L., Wu, X., You, J., Jin, Z., He, W., Sun, J., Shen, H., Liu, X., Yue, X., Cai, W., Zhang, S., & Zhang, B. (2025). Artificial intelligence can predict personalized immunotherapy outcomes in cancer. *Cancer Immunology Research, 13*(7), 964–977. https://doi.org/10.1158/2326-6066.cir-24-1270.

Ishizuka, J. J., Manguso, R. T., Cheruiyot, C. K., Bi, K., Panda, A., Iracheta-Vellve, A., Miller, B. C., Du, P. P., Yates, K. B., Dubrot, J., Buchumenski, I., Comstock, D. E., Brown, F. D., Ayer, A., Kohnle, I. C., Pope, H. W., Zimmer, M. D., Sen, D. R., Lane-Reticker, S. K., ... Haining, W. N. (2019). Loss of ADAR1 in tumours overcomes resistance to immune checkpoint blockade. *Nature, 565*(7737), 43–48. https://doi.org/10.1038/s41586-018-0768-9 Available from: http://www.nature.com/nature/index.html.

Jang, D., Choi, H., Lee, J., Chun, Y., Heo, Y.-H., Lee, L. P., Ahn, D. J., Shin, I.-S., Kim, D. H., Seo, Y. H., & Kim, S. (2025). Inflamed tissue-targeting polyphenol-condensed antioxidant nanoparticles with therapeutic potential. *Advanced Healthcare Materials, 14*(11). https://doi.org/10.1002/adhm.202500495.

Jia, Q., Chu, H., Jin, Z., Long, H., & Zhu, B. (2022). High-throughput single-cell sequencing in cancer research. *Signal Transduction and Targeted Therapy, 7*(1). https://doi.org/10.1038/s41392-022-00990-4.

Kanarek, N., London, N., Schueler-Furman, O., & Ben-Neriah, Y. (2010). Ubiquitination and degradation of the inhibitors of NF-kappaB. *Cold Spring Harbor Perspectives in Biology, 2*(2), a000166. https://doi.org/10.1101/cshperspect.a000166.

Lin, Y. H., Chen, C. W., Chen, M. Y., Xu, L., Tian, X., Cheung, S. H., Wu, Y. L., Siriwon, N., Wu, S. H., & Mou, K. Y. (2025). The bacterial outer membrane vesicle-cloaked immunostimulatory nanoplatform reinvigorates T cell function and reprograms tumor immunity. *ACS Nano, 19*(21), 19866–19889. https://doi.org/10.1021/acsnano.5c02541, http://pubs.acs.org/journal/ancac3.

Liu, J., Geng, X., Hou, J., & Wu, G. (2021). New insights into M1/M2 macrophages: Key modulators in cancer progression. *Cancer Cell International, 21*(1). https://doi.org/10.1186/s12935-021-02089-2.

Liu, X., Peng, T., Xu, M., Lin, S., Hu, B., Chu, T., Liu, B., Xu, Y., Ding, W., Li, L., Cao, C., & Wu, P. (2024). Spatial multi-omics: Deciphering technological landscape of integration of multi-omics and its applications. *Journal of Hematology & Oncology, 17*(1). https://doi.org/10.1186/s13045-024-01596-9.

Liu, Y., Yu, Y., Hu, C., Jiang, M., Zhao, C., Li, X., Cheng, L., & Zhou, C. (2025). ZEB2 upregulation modulates the polarization of TAMs toward the immunosuppressive state in EGFR-TKI-resistant NSCLC. *Journal of Cancer Metastasis and Treatment, 8*. https://doi.org/10.20517/cdr.2024.206, jcmtjournal.com/.

Liu, Y., Yang, M., Deng, Y., Su, G., Enninful, A., Guo, C. C., Tebaldi, T., Zhang, D., Kim, D., Bai, Z., Norris, E., Pan, A., Li, J., Xiao, Y., Halene, S., & Fan, R. (2020). High-spatial-resolution multi-omics sequencing via deterministic barcoding in tissue. *Cell, 183*(6), 1665. https://doi.org/10.1016/j.cell.2020.10.026.

Liu, Y., DiStasio, M., Su, G., Asashima, H., Enninful, A., Qin, X., Deng, Y., Nam, J., Gao, F., Bordignon, P., Cassano, M., Tomayko, M., Xu, M., Halene, S., Craft, J. E., Hafler, D., & Fan, R. (2023). High-plex protein and whole transcriptome co-mapping at cellular resolution with spatial CITE-seq. *Nature Biotechnology, 41*(10), 1405–1409. https://doi.org/10.1038/s41587-023-01676-0.

Liu, Y., Sinjab, A., Min, J., Han, G., Paradiso, F., Zhang, Y., Wang, R., Pei, G., Dai, Y., Liu, Y., Cho, K. S., Dai, E., Basi, A., Burks, J. K., Rajapakshe, K. I., Chu, Y., Jiang, J., Zhang, D., Yan, X., ... Wang, L. (2025). Conserved spatial subtypes and cellular neighborhoods of cancer-associated fibroblasts revealed by single-cell spatial multi-omics. *Cancer cell, 43*(5), 905. https://doi.org/10.1016/j.ccell.2025.03.004.

Liu, Z., Yang, Z., Wu, J., Zhang, W., Sun, Y., Zhang, C., Bai, G., Yang, L., Fan, H., Chen, Y., Zhang, L., Jiang, B., Liu, X., Ma, X., Tang, W., Liu, C., Qu, Y., Yan, L., Zhao, D., ... Zhang, Z. (2025). A single-cell atlas reveals immune heterogeneity in anti-PD-1-treated non-small cell lung cancer. *Cell, 188*(11), 3081. https://doi.org/10.1016/j.cell.2025.03.018.

Mace, T. A., Shakya, R., Pitarresi, J. R., Swanson, B., McQuinn, C. W., Loftus, S., Nordquist, E., Cruz-Monserrate, Z., Yu, L., Young, G., Zhong, X., Zimmers, T. A., Ostrowski, M. C., Ludwig, T., Bloomston, M., Bekaii-Saab, T., & Lesinski, G. B. (2018). IL-6 and PD-L1 antibody blockade combination therapy reduces tumour progression in murine models of pancreatic cancer. *Gut, 67*(2), 320–332. https://doi.org/10.1136/gutjnl-2016-311585.

Morel, K. L., Sheahan, A. V., Burkhart, D. L., Baca, S. C., Boufaied, N., Liu, Y., Qiu, X., Cañadas, I., Roehle, K., Heckler, M., Calagua, C., Ye, H., Pantelidou, C., Galbo, P., Panja, S., Mitrofanova, A., Wilkinson, S., Whitlock, N. C., Trostel, S. Y., ... Ellis, L. (2021). EZH2 inhibition activates a dsRNA–STING–interferon stress axis that potentiates response to PD-1 checkpoint blockade in prostate cancer. *Nature Cancer, 2*(4), 444–456. https://doi.org/10.1038/s43018-021-00185-w, https://www.nature.com/natcancer/.

Noy, R., & Pollard, J. W. (2014). Tumor-associated macrophages: From mechanisms to therapy. *Cell Press, United States Immunity, 41*(1), 49–61. https://doi.org/10.1016/j.immuni.2014.06.010, www.immunity.com.

Oliveira, M. Fd, Romero, J. P., Chung, M., Williams, S. R., Gottscho, A. D., Gupta, A., Pilipauskas, S. E., Mohabbat, S., Raman, N., Sukovich, D. J., Patterson, D. M., Taylor, S. E. B., Romero, J. P., de Oliveira, M. F., & Taylor, S. E. B. (2025). High-definition spatial transcriptomic profiling of immune cell populations in colorectal cancer. *Nature Genetics, 57*(6), 1512–1523. https://doi.org/10.1038/s41588-025-02193-3, https://www.nature.com/ng/.

Papalexi, E., & Satija, R. (2018). Single-cell RNA sequencing to explore immune cell heterogeneity. *Nature Reviews. Immunology, 18*(1), 35–45. https://doi.org/10.1038/nri.2017.76.

Pelka, K., Hofree, M., Chen, J. H., Sarkizova, S., Pirl, J. D., Jorgji, V., Bejnood, A., Dionne, D., Ge, W. H., Xu, K. H., Chao, S. X., Zollinger, D. R., Lieb, D. J., Reeves, J. W., Fuhrman, C. A., Hoang, M. L., Delorey, T., Nguyen, L. T., Waldman, J., ... Su, Mj (2021). Spatially organized multicellular immune hubs in human colorectal cancer. *Cell, 184*(18), 4734. https://doi.org/10.1016/j.cell.2021.08.003, https://www.sciencedirect.com/journal/cell.

Peng, D., Kryczek, I., Nagarsheth, N., Zhao, L., Wei, S., Wang, W., Sun, Y., Zhao, E., Vatan, L., Szeliga, W., Kotarski, J., Tarkowski, R., Dou, Y., Cho, K., Hensley-Alford, S., Munkarah, A., Liu, R., & Zou, W. (2015). Epigenetic silencing of TH1-type chemokines shapes tumour immunity and immunotherapy. *Nature, 527*(7577), 249–253. https://doi.org/10.1038/nature15520.

Peng, M., Zhu, Y., Hu, Y., Wen, J., & Huang, W. (2025). Advances in the regulation of macrophage polarization by the tumor microenvironment. *Discover Oncology, 16*(1). https://doi.org/10.1007/s12672-025-03258-9.

Prakash, S. (2023). Nano-based drug delivery system for therapeutics: A comprehensive review. *Biomedical Physics & Engineering Express, 9*(5), 052002. https://doi.org/10.1088/2057-1976/acedb2.

Quail, D. F., Amulic, B., Aziz, M., Barnes, B. J., Eruslanov, E., Fridlender, Z. G., Goodridge, H. S., Granot, Z., Hidalgo, A., Huttenlocher, A., Kaplan, M. J., Malanchi, I., Merghoub, T., Meylan, E., Mittal, V., Pittet, M. J., Rubio-Ponce, A., Udalova, I. A., van den Berg, T. K., ... Kubes, P. (2022). Neutrophil phenotypes and functions in cancer: A consensus statement. *Journal of Experimental Medicine, 219*(6). https://doi.org/10.1084/jem.20220011.

Sheban, F., Phan, T. S., Xie, K., Ingelfinger, F., Gur, C., Shapir Itai, Y., Blecher-Gonen, R., Yu, C., Avellino, R., Chalan, P., Freitag, K., Yofe, I., Yutkin, V., Boyeau, P., Ergen, C., Hong, J., Mazuz, K., Liu, Y., Chen, K., ... Amit, I.

(2025). ZEB2 is a master switch controlling the tumor-associated macrophage program. *Cancer Cell, 43*(7), 1227. https://doi.org/10.1016/j.ccell.2025.03.021, https://www.sciencedirect.com/science/journal/15356108.

Trehan, R., Huang, P., Zhu, X. B., Wang, X., Soliman, M., Strepay, D., Nur, A., Kedei, N., Arhin, M., Ghabra, S., Rodríguez-Matos, F., Benmebarek, M. R., Ma, C., Korangy, F., & Greten, T. F. (2025). SPP1 + macrophages cause exhaustion of tumor-specific T cells in liver metastases. *Nature Communications, 16*(1). https://doi.org/10.1038/s41467-025-59529-0, https://www.nature.com/ncomms/.

Vendrell, M., Maiti, K. K., Dhaliwal, K., & Chang, Y. T. (2013). Surface-enhanced Raman scattering in cancer detection and imaging. *Trends in Biotechnology, 31*(4), 249–257. https://doi.org/10.1016/j.tibtech.2013.01.013.

Wang, X., Zhao, J., Marostica, E., Yuan, W., Jin, J., Zhang, J., Li, R., Tang, H., Wang, K., Li, Y., Wang, F., Peng, Y., Zhu, J., Zhang, J., Jackson, C. R., Zhang, J., Dillon, D., Lin, N. U., Sholl, L., ... Yang, S. (2024). A pathology foundation model for cancer diagnosis and prognosis prediction. *Nature, 634*(8035), 970–978. https://doi.org/10.1038/s41586-024-07894-z.

Wells, K., Liu, T., Zhu, L., & Yang, L. (2024). Immunomodulatory nanoparticles activate cytotoxic T cells for enhancement of the effect of cancer immunotherapy. *Nanoscale, 16*(38), 17699–17722. https://doi.org/10.1039/d4nr01780c.

Xu, J., Ding, L., Mei, J., Hu, Y., Kong, X., Dai, S., Bu, T., Xiao, Q., & Ding, K. (2025). Dual roles and therapeutic targeting of tumor-associated macrophages in tumor microenvironments. *Signal Transduction and Targeted Therapy, 10*(1). https://doi.org/10.1038/s41392-025-02325-5.

Yang, L., & Lin, P. C. (2017). Mechanisms that drive inflammatory tumor microenvironment, tumor heterogeneity, and metastatic progression. *Seminars in Cancer Biology, 47*, 185–195. https://doi.org/10.1016/j.semcancer.2017.08.001, http://www.elsevier.com/inca/publications/store/6/2/2/9/4/3/index.htt.

Yu, L., Liebenberg, K., Shen, Y., Liu, F., Xu, Z., Hao, X., Wu, L., Zhang, W., Chan, H. L., Wei, B., Lorenzi, P. L., Gao, Y., Bado, I., Becerra-Dominguez, L., Rivas, C. H., Aguirre, S., Pingel, B. C., Wu, Y.-H., Ding, Y., ... Zhang, X. H.-F. (2025). Tumor-derived arachidonic acid reprograms neutrophils to promote immune suppression and therapy resistance in triple-negative breast cancer. *Immunity, 58*(4), 909. https://doi.org/10.1016/j.immuni.2025.03.002.

Yuan, L., Wang, Q., Sun, F., & Shi, H. (2025). Deep learning and inflammatory markers predict early response to immunotherapy in unresectable NSCLC: A multicenter study. *Biomolecules and Biomedicine, 25*(10), 2252–2268. https://doi.org/10.17305/bb.2025.12324.

Zhao, M., Cheng, X., Shao, P., Dong, Y., Wu, Y., Xiao, L., Cui, Z., Sun, X., Gao, C., Chen, J., Huang, Z., & Zhang, J. (2024). Bacterial protoplast-derived nanovesicles carrying CRISPR-Cas9 tools re-educate tumor-associated macrophages for enhanced cancer immunotherapy. *Nature Communications, 15*(1). https://doi.org/10.1038/s41467-024-44941-9.

SECTION II

Micro/nano-modulation of cancer inflammation and immunometabolism

CHAPTER

3

Recent advances and future research directions in the crosstalk between inflammation and tumors

Shuai Shao

Department of Cardiology, The Affiliated Hospital of Southwest Medical University, Luzhou, Sichuan, P.R. China

3.1 Introduction

The conceptual connection between inflammation and tumors can be traced back to Rudolf Virchow's classic observation in 1863 (Antonucci & Karin, 2024). Virchow was found to have a great deal of leukocyte infiltration in tumor tissues and stated that tumors often appear in chronic inflammatory sites. Thus it implies that inflammation may contribute to tumor formation. This early concept held that continuous inflammatory stimulation can create a microenvironment favorable for tumor development, which laid the foundation for modern tumor immunology and tumor inflammation research. Subsequently, a large number of epidemiological research and experimental investigations have confirmed this view, for example, the obvious association between inflammatory bowel disease and colorectal cancer, the association between chronic hepatitis and hepatocellular carcinoma (HCC), and the association between Helicobacter pylori infection and gastric cancer (Dunleavy et al., 2023; Palatianou et al., 2023). Over the past two decades, the progress of molecular biology and immunology has gradually transformed Virchow's hypothesis into a theoretical framework that has distinct molecular mechanisms. At present, everyone generally feels that inflammation through the complex interactions among immune cells, stromal cells, and tumor cells influences several stages of tumorigenesis and development. The key inflammatory signaling pathways, such as the NF–κB–STAT3, Mitogen-Activated Protein Kinase(MAPK), and PI3K–AKT signaling pathways, play a core role in regulating gene expression related to cell proliferation, survival, angiogenesis, and immune escape, thus integrating the inflammatory stimulation into the biological processes promoting tumor (Zhang et al., 2024). Meanwhile, the development of tumor immunology and immunotherapy further reveals the dual roles of inflammation in cancer: on the one

Inflammation in Tumorigenesis and Cancer Treatment
DOI: https://doi.org/10.1016/B978-0-443-36649-9.00004-9

hand, specific immune responses that can inhibit the occurrence of tumors, and on the other hand, persistent or dysregulated inflammatory responses that may drive the progression and metastasis of tumors (Mao et al., 2022).

In recent years, the development of single-cell sequencing, spatial transcriptomics, and multiomics integration analysis has further deepened our understanding of the mechanism by which inflammation drives tumor occurrence. These studies make it clear that the inflammatory signals are by no means simple linear pathways but are in fact dynamic regulatory networks composed of multiple cell populations and complex feedback loops (Ravari et al., 2023). A large amount of evidence indicates that cancer-related inflammation has been regarded as one of the important signs of cancer and plays a key role in the occurrence, development, and metastasis of tumors (Coussens & Werb, 2002; Singh et al., 2019). The chronic inflammation and the acute inflammatory response are indeed fundamentally different. Acute inflammation is usually of short duration and protective, while chronic inflammation is marked by the continuous activation of immune cells and the long-term production of inflammatory mediators, thereby causing a microenvironment that is conducive to the occurrence and development of tumors.

One of the important mechanisms through which chronic inflammation promotes tumorigenesis is the induction of genomic instability conditions. During the inflammatory period, the generated reactive oxygen species (ROS) and reactive nitrogen species (RNS) can directly damage the DNA, causing chromosomal mutations, chromosomal instability, and epigenetic changes. Meanwhile, the inflammatory signaling pathways can also activate the transcriptional programs that drive cell survival and proliferation, making the damaged cells evade apoptosis and gradually accumulate carcinogenic mutations. Moreover, chronic inflammation can indeed significantly alter the tumor microenvironment. Inflammatory cytokines such as interleukin-6 (IL-6), interleukin-1β (IL-1β), and tumor necrosis factor-α (TNF-α) can activate key transcription factors like nuclear factor-κB (NF-κB) and signal transducer and activator of transcription 3 (STAT3), and then regulate the expression of angiogenesis, metabolic reprogramming as well as immunosuppressive genes (Neurath, 2024). These signaling pathways that can promote tumor angiogenesis, change cell metabolism, and also inhibit antitumor immune responses are the ones that provide support for tumor growth. At the same time, chronic inflammation can recruit and activate various immunosuppressive cells, including tumor-associated macrophages (TAMs), myeloid-derived suppressor cells (MDSCs), and regulatory T cells (Tregs), further enhancing tumor-promoting inflammation and weakening effective antitumor immune responses (Fig. 3.1).

In this chapter, we systematically summarize the important research progress in the field of inflammation and tumor interaction in recent years, focusing on the key molecular signaling pathways, inflammatory mediators, and cell interactions that regulate the inflammatory–tumor microenvironment (iTME). Additionally, this chapter will particularly focus on the emerging roles of metabolic reprogramming, epigenetic regulation, and microbiota-related inflammation in tumor progression. At the same time, we will discuss the rapidly developing research techniques, including single-cell multiomics, spatial transcriptomics, and systems biology methods, which are reshaping our understanding of the inflammation–tumor interaction mechanism.

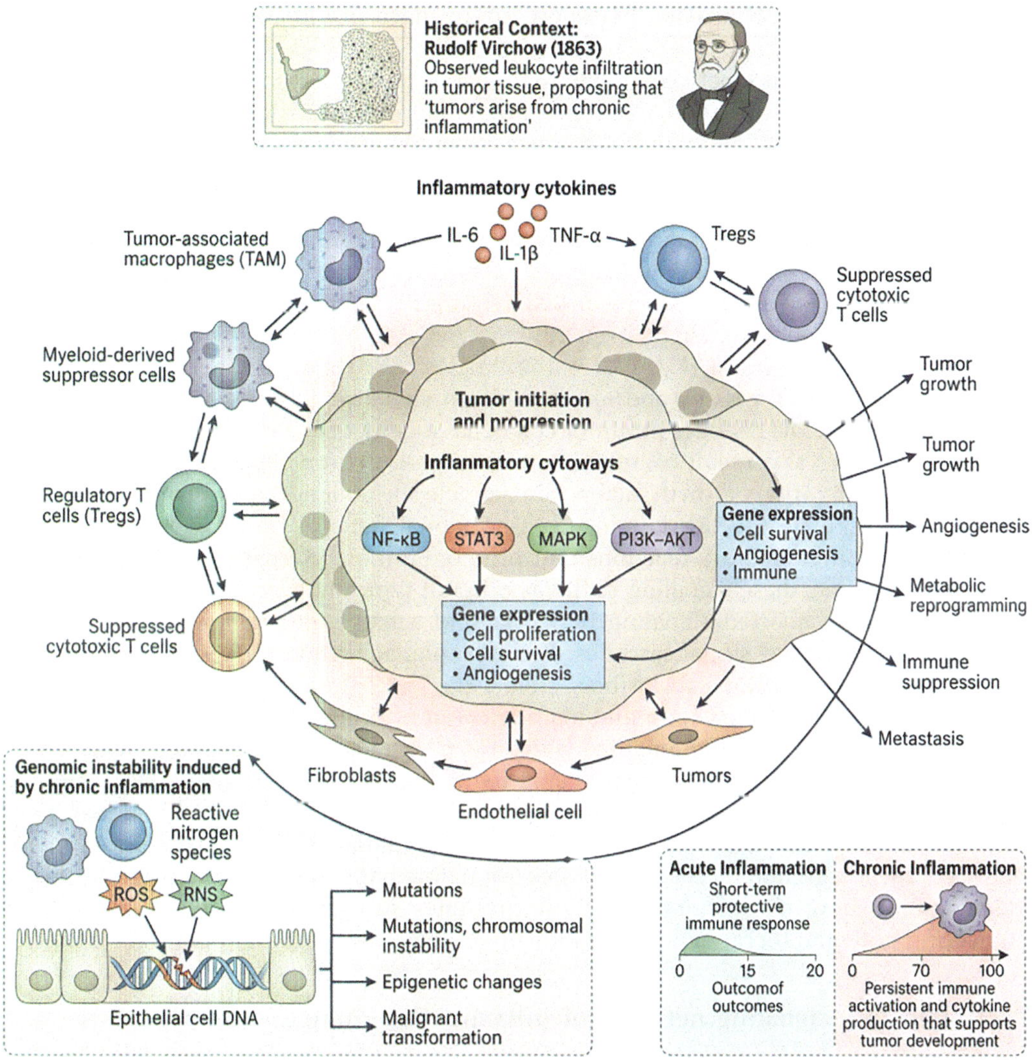

FIGURE 3.1 Inflammation-driven mechanisms linking chronic inflammation to tumor initiation and progression. Chronic inflammation promotes tumor development through interconnected molecular and cellular mechanisms. Inflammatory cytokines such as IL-6, IL-1β, and TNF-α activate key signaling pathways, including NF-κB, STAT3, MAPK, and PI3K–AKT in tumor cells, driving transcriptional programs that regulate proliferation, survival, angiogenesis, and immune evasion. Persistent inflammatory responses also generate reactive oxygen and nitrogen species (ROS/RNS), leading to DNA damage, genomic instability, and oncogenic transformation. In the tumor microenvironment, interactions among tumor cells, stromal cells, and immune populations—such as tumor-associated macrophages (TAMs), myeloid-derived suppressor cells (MDSCs), and regulatory T cells (Tregs)—create an immunosuppressive and tumor-promoting network. Together, these processes integrate inflammatory signaling, genomic instability, and microenvironmental remodeling to support tumor growth, metabolic reprogramming, and metastasis.

3.2 Molecular mechanisms between inflammation and tumor development

The molecular interface between inflammation and tumor development is regulated by a complex signaling network that integrates inflammatory signals and tumor-related transcriptional programs. Inflammatory cytokines, chemokines, and damage-associated molecular patterns (DAMPs) can activate multiple intracellular signaling cascades, thereby reshaping the gene expression, cell metabolism, and immune responses in the tumor microenvironment. These signals not only trigger the initial transformation of tumors but also continuously promote tumor progression by facilitating cell proliferation, survival, angiogenesis, immune escape, and metastasis. In this regulatory network, there are a great number of highly conserved signaling pathways in evolution that play a key central role, including the NF-κB, the JAK/STAT3, the MAPK/ERK(Extracellular Signal-Regulated Kinase), the PI3K–AKT–mTOR, and also the Notch signaling pathway (Chen et al., 2023). The occurrences are the changes in tumor cell behaviors that can be brought about by these signaling pathways as a result of inflammatory stimuli. Inflammatory mediators like IL-6, TNF-α, IL-1β, and various growth factors can activate these signaling pathways, and in this manner, they regulate the overlapping transcriptional networks and also synergistically bring about the inflammatory reactions that promote tumors (Rzeszotarska et al., 2022).

At the same time, these signaling pathways do not typically function independently but form highly interconnected signaling networks and achieve integration through complex feedback regulation and signal cascades. For example, activation of NF-κB can induce the expression of IL-6, and IL-6 can further activate the JAK/STAT3 signaling axis, forming a self-reinforcing inflammatory loop that maintains tumor cell survival and immunosuppression (Jeong et al., 2025). Inflammatory signaling pathways also participate in regulating tumor metabolic reprogramming, epigenetic regulation, and cell plasticity. This suggests that inflammation is not only an accompanying phenomenon in the tumor microenvironment but also a systemic driving factor in regulating tumor evolution. Therefore in-depth analysis of the integration mechanism of these signaling pathways is of great significance for understanding how chronic inflammation promotes malignant transformation and for discovering potential therapeutic targets for inflammation-related tumors (Fig. 3.2).

3.2.1 The core signaling network of inflammation-induced tumorigenesis

In the molecular network of inflammation and tumor development, multiple key signaling pathways jointly form the core regulatory axis that governs tumor occurrence and progression. Among them, the NF-κB signaling pathway is regarded as the most crucial transcriptional regulatory hub connecting chronic inflammation and tumor occurrence (Powers et al., 2024). NF-κB belongs to the Rel family of transcription factor complexes (including p65/RelA, RelB, c-Rel, p50, and p52) (Zhou et al., 2025). In a resting state, it binds to the inhibitory protein IκB and remains in the cytoplasm. When cells are stimulated by inflammatory factors such as TNF-α, IL-1β, pathogen-associated molecular patterns, DAMPs, or ROS, the upstream IKK complex (IKKα/IKKβ/NEMO) is activated and induces IκB phosphorylation and degradation, thereby releasing NF-κB and allowing it to translocate to the nucleus (Xu et al., 2025). Once in the nucleus, NF-κB can directly bind to κB DNA elements and drive the expression of various proinflammatory and protumor

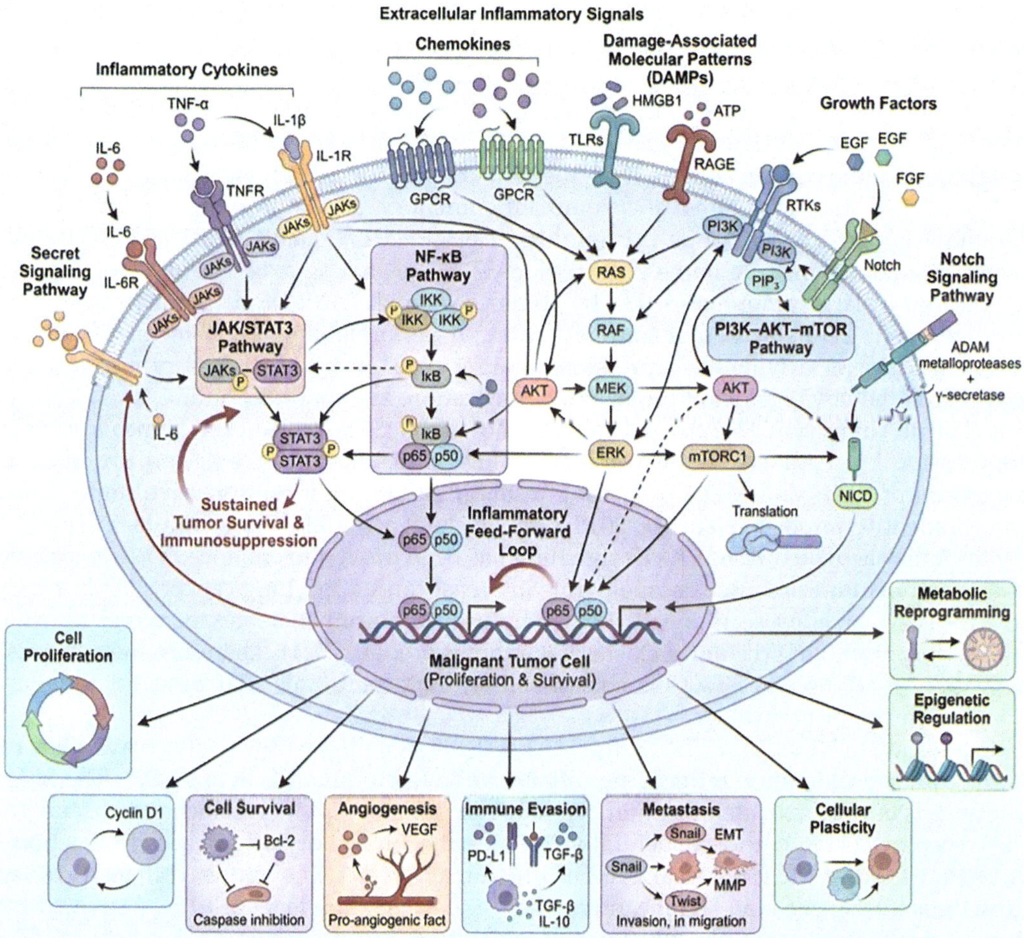

FIGURE 3.2 Inflammatory signaling networks driving tumor progression. Inflammatory stimuli—including cytokines (IL-6, TNF-α, IL-1β), chemokines, DAMPs, and growth factors—activate interconnected intracellular signaling pathways in tumor cells, including NF-κB, JAK/STAT3, MAPK/ERK, PI3K-AKT–mTOR, and Notch. These pathways form an integrated signaling network with feedback loops (such as the NF-κB–IL-6–STAT3 axis) that convert inflammatory signals into tumor-promoting programs, regulating proliferation, survival, angiogenesis, immune evasion, metastasis, and cellular metabolic and epigenetic reprogramming within the tumor microenvironment. *RTK*, Receptor tyrosine kinase; TLR, toll-like receptor.

genes, including interleukin-6（IL-6）, tumor necrosis factor-alph（TNF-α）, C-X-C motif chemokine ligand 8（CXCL8）, vascular endothelial growth factor（VEGF）, B-cell lymphoma-extra large（BCL-XL）, and cellular FLICE-like inhibitory protein（c-FLIP）, thereby maintaining a persistent inflammatory state in the tumor microenvironment and promoting tumor cell survival, angiogenesis, and immune cell recruitment. Recent studies have further shown that NF-κB is continuously activated in various inflammation-related cancers, such as gastric cancer associated with Helicobacter pylori infection, HCC associated with chronic hepatitis, and colorectal cancer associated with inflammatory bowel disease (Kennel et al., 2023; Zhang et al., 2025). In these disease models, NF-κB not only drives the expression of inflammatory factors but also promotes immune escape and tumor invasion by inducing the expression of PD-L1, COX-2, and matrix metalloproteinase (MMP) family proteins.

Further studies have shown that the NF-κB signaling pathway does not function independently but maintains a chronic inflammatory state through the formation of complex signal feedback loops (Abu-Sultanah et al., 2025; Zhang et al., 2025). The most typical regulatory module is the NF–κB–IL-6–STAT3 signaling axis. NF-κB can induce the production of large amounts of IL-6 by tumor cells and TAMs, and IL-6 activates STAT3 through the gp130-JAK receptor complex. After phosphorylation, STAT3 forms a dimer and enters the nucleus, driving the expression of target genes such as BCL-2, survivin, cyclin D1, and VEGF, thereby enhancing tumor cell proliferation, antiapoptotic ability, and angiogenesis (Patritti Cram et al., 2022). Studies have shown that STAT3 also participates in immune suppression by regulating the expression of PD-L1, IL-10, and TGF-β, and promotes the expansion of Tregs and MDSCs, thereby reshaping the immunosuppressive tumor microenvironment (Campbell & Turner, 2018; Grabowski et al., 2021). For example, in HCC, the continuously activated IL-6/STAT3 signaling has been proven to enhance PD-L1 expression and promote tumor immune escape, while in breast cancer and lung cancer, TAMs activate STAT3–TGM2 axis by secreting IL-6, thereby inducing epithelial–mesenchymal transition (EMT) and promoting distant metastasis (Grabowski et al., 2021). Therefore the synergistic activation of NF-κB and STAT3 is considered an important molecular basis for inflammation-driven tumor occurrence.

In addition to NF-κB and STAT3, the MAPK/ERK signaling pathway also plays a key role in the tumor proliferation induced by inflammation (Abu-Sultanah et al., 2025). The MAPK pathway is usually activated through cytokine receptors, receptor tyrosine kinases, and Toll-like receptors (TLRs), and sequentially initiates the phosphorylation cascade reaction of RAS–RAF–MEK–ERK (Sun et al., 2025). Inflammatory factors such as TNF-α, IL-1β, and growth factors such as can significantly enhance the activation level of ERK. Activated ERK can enter the nucleus and phosphorylate transcription factors such as AP-1, c-Fos, and ELK-1, thereby promoting the expression of cell cycle-related genes (such as cyclin D1, MYC) and driving tumor cell proliferation(Anastasaki et al., 2022). Moreover, there is also a wide-ranging cross-regulatory relationship between the MAPK pathway and the NF-κB as well as STAT3. For example, in colorectal cancer, chronic intestinal inflammation can enhance the EMT and invasive ability of tumor cells via the TLR–MAPK–NF-κB signaling axis; while in melanoma and lung cancer, it is found that the activation of the MAPK signaling can maintain the tumor stem-cell-like characteristics through a STAT3-dependent transcriptional network (He et al., 2024). These studies show that the MAPK signaling not only takes part in the regulation of cell proliferation but also plays a crucial role in inflammation-driven tumor plasticity and metastasis.

Meanwhile, the PI3K–AKT–mTOR signaling pathway plays a central role in the metabolic adaptation of inflammatory-related tumors. Inflammatory factors and growth factors activate PI3K to convert PIP2 into PIP3, thereby recruiting and activating protein Kinase B (AKT) (Feng et al., 2022). AKT further activates the mTORC1 and mTORC2 signaling complexes, thereby driving the metabolic reprogramming of tumor cells (Lin, Rao, et al., 2024). This pathway not only enhances cell survival by regulating downstream target proteins such as BAD, FOXO, and GSK3β, but also supports rapid tumor growth by promoting glycolysis, lipid synthesis, and nucleotide metabolism (Yang & Moss, 2023). Recent studies have shown that inflammatory factors IL-6 and TNF-α can promote mTOR-dependent metabolic programs through the PI3K–AKT signaling and induce tumor cells to produce large amounts of lactic acid, thereby inhibiting the antitumor activity of $CD8^+$ T cells and NK cells (Bennour et al., 2022; Drougard et al., 2024). For example, in inflammatory liver cancer and colorectal cancer, the metabolic reprogramming driven by the PI3K–AKT–mTOR pathway is considered an important source of immune suppression in the tumor microenvironment, and this discovery has also promoted clinical research on the combination of PI3K and mTOR inhibitors with immunotherapy.

In addition, the Notch signaling pathway mainly functions in the occurrence of inflammatory-related tumors by regulating cell fate determination and cell plasticity. Notch signaling is activated through direct cell-to-cell contact(Roeck et al., 2025). When Notch receptors bind to ligands Delta-like or Jagged, the γ-secretase-mediated proteolytic reaction releases the intracellular domain of Notch (NICD), which enters the nucleus and binds to the CSL/RBP-Jκ transcriptional complex to induce the expression of HES and HEY family genes (Francette & Arndt, 2024). In the iTME, Notch signaling not only regulates tumor cell behavior but also participates in the regulation of immune cell functions. For example, in pancreatic cancer and colorectal cancer, Notch signaling can promote the maintenance of tumor stem cells and the EMT process; in immune cells, Notch signaling alters the tumor immune ecology by regulating macrophage polarization and T cell differentiation (Boutilier & Elsawa, 2021).

3.2.2 Inflammatory mediators as drivers of tumor progression

In the iTME, multiple inflammatory mediators jointly form a key molecular network that drives tumor occurrence and progression. These soluble signaling molecules not only regulate the recruitment and activation of immune cells but also directly promote tumor development by reshaping the signal transduction, metabolic state, and intercellular communication of tumor cells. Recently, research shows that proinflammatory cytokines, chemokines, lipid inflammatory mediators, ROS, and DAMPs jointly constitute the core signal modules that propel tumor progression (Yu et al., 2023). These molecules that are integrated into the NF-κB, STAT3, MAPK, and PI3K–AKT signaling networks will form continuous inflammatory circuits within the tumor microenvironment, thus promoting the proliferation, immune evasion, and metastasis of tumor cells.

Recent studies have further demonstrated that STAT3 can also reconfigure the immunosuppressive tumor microenvironment by regulating immune regulatory factors such as PD-L1, IL-10, and TGF-β (Fan et al., 2023; Pang et al., 2023). For example, in HCC, the IL-6/STAT3 signal induced by chronic hepatitis has been proven to drive tumor stem-cell-like characteristics and promote tumor recurrence. Additionally, IL-1β induces the expression of various inflammatory and angiogenesis-related genes through the IL-1R–MyD88–IRAK–NF-κB signaling axis, including VEGF and MMP family proteins, thereby promoting angiogenesis and matrix degradation (Li, Zeng, et al., 2025). In melanoma and colorectal cancer, the IL-1β-mediated inflammatory network has been found to enhance EMT and promote metastasis and spread (Sloan & Chang, 2025). At the same time, TNF-α continuously activates the NF-κB and MAPK signaling pathways in the chronic inflammatory environment, induces the expression of antiapoptotic molecules, and maintains the protumor inflammatory state (Valentini et al., 2022). In inflammatory bowel disease–related colorectal cancer, TNF-α and IL-6 synergistically activate the NF-κB–STAT3 signaling module, which is considered an important mechanism for inflammation-driven tumor occurrence.

Moreover, CXCL8 can promote the formation of tumor-associated neutrophils (TANs), thereby establishing an immunosuppressive inflammatory microenvironment. In non–small cell lung cancer and breast cancer, the CXCL8–CXCR2 signaling axis has been proven to promote angiogenesis and enhance the tumor metastasis potential (Chen et al., 2024). On the other hand, the CCL2–CCR2 signaling axis plays an important role in the recruitment of TAMs. For example, in pancreatic ductal adenocarcinoma (PDAC), the CCL2 secreted by tumor cells can recruit monocytes and induce their differentiation into immunosuppressive TAMs, thereby inhibiting the antitumor immune response mediated by $CD8^+$ T cells (Gu et al., 2024). Additionally, the CXCL12–CXCR4 signaling axis plays a key role in tumor metastasis. CXCL12 is mainly secreted by stromal cells and cancer-associated fibroblasts (CAFs), and its binding to CXCR4 can induce tumor cell migration and promote the formation of metastatic foci (Chen et al., 2024). For instance, in breast cancer bone metastasis and pancreatic cancer liver metastasis, this signaling axis is considered an important mechanism driving tumor cell chemotactic migration, and thus CXCR4 inhibitors have emerged as potential antimetastasis therapeutic strategies (Bhattacharjee et al., 2022).

In addition to protein-based inflammatory factors, lipid inflammatory mediators and oxidative stress signals also play significant roles in the iTME. Lipid mediators produced by the arachidonic acid metabolic pathway, such as prostaglandin E2 (PGE2) and leukotrienes, are regulated by the COX-2 and 5-LOX enzyme systems (Robinson et al., 2023). PGE2 can promote tumor cell proliferation by activating EP2/EP4 receptors and downstream cAMP–PKA and PI3K–AKT signaling pathways, and inhibit the maturation of dendritic cells and T cell activation, thereby forming an immunosuppressive microenvironment. In colorectal cancer and gastric cancer, COX-2 overexpression and PGE2 production are considered important molecular events driving tumor inflammation. At the same time, the large amount of ROS produced under chronic inflammation can not only induce DNA damage and gene mutations, but also activate NF-κB, MAPK, and HIF-1α signaling pathways through oxidative modification of signaling proteins, thereby promoting tumor cell metabolic reprogramming (Lin, Rao, et al., 2024). For example, in the process of liver fibrosis to HCC transformation, ROS has been proven to activate hepatic stellate cells and induce fibrosis and inflammatory responses, thereby providing a proinflammatory microenvironment for tumor occurrence (Zhang et al., 2021).

Recent studies have also revealed that DAMPs play a crucial role in the interaction between inflammation and tumors. DAMPs such as HMGB1, ATP, and extracellular DNA can be recognized by TLRs or NOD-like receptors, thereby triggering innate immune responses and activating the inflammatory signaling network (Kaur & Secord, 2021). Among them, the NLRP3 inflammasome is one of the most important inflammatory signaling complexes, and its activation can induce caspase-1-dependent maturation and release of IL-1β and IL-18, thereby amplifying the inflammatory response and shaping the tumor-promoting microenvironment (Daniel et al., 2023). In gastric cancer, colorectal cancer, and HCC, DAMP-mediated NLRP3 inflammasomes have been proven to promote tumor occurrence and immune escape (Greca & Magez, 2011).

Moreover, the activation of inflammasomes can also induce pyroptosis (a type of inflammatory cell death), which may exhibit both tumor-promoting and tumor-suppressing dual effects in different tumor environments. Overall, these inflammatory mediators form a continuous inflammatory circuit in the tumor microenvironment through complex signal integration, thereby playing a core regulatory role in tumor occurrence, progression, and metastasis, and providing an important theoretical basis for precise antitumor treatment targeting the inflammatory signaling network.

3.2.3 Epigenetic and transcriptional regulation

In the process of tumor development driven by chronic inflammation, epigenetic regulation and transcriptional network remodeling are increasingly regarded as important mechanisms connecting inflammatory signals with tumor gene expression programs. Inflammatory signals not only directly regulate gene transcription through classical signaling pathways (such as NF-κB, STAT3, and MAPK) but also can reprogram the transcriptional state of cells on a longer time scale by altering DNA methylation, histone modifications, and chromatin structure (Wang et al., 2022). Recent multiomics studies have shown that chronic inflammation can induce extensive epigenetic remodeling, forming a persistent and stable protumor transcriptional program (Chen et al., 2022). For example, in chronic hepatitis-related HCC, inflammatory factors (such as IL-6 and TNF-α) can activate STAT3 and NF-κB signaling, thereby recruiting histone acetyltransferase p300/CBP to the promoter regions of inflammation-related genes, enhancing H3K27ac modification and promoting the continuous expression of inflammatory genes (Tanwar et al., 2025). This inflammation-driven epigenetic reprogramming not only maintains the inflammatory response but also activates cell cycle and antiapoptotic-related genes, thereby promoting tumor development.

Chronic inflammation can also reprogram tumor-related transcriptional networks by altering chromatin accessibility. Recent studies based on ATAC-seq and single-cell epigenomics have shown that inflammatory signals can induce the formation of new enhancers genome-wide and reconfigure the binding sites of key transcription factors (Grandi et al., 2022; Li, Jiang, et al., 2025). In inflammatory bowel disease–related colorectal cancer, continuous NF-κB signaling can drive the formation of inflammation-induced enhancers, which are enriched with the binding sites of STAT3, AP-1, and IRF family transcription factors, thereby synergistically activating protumor gene expression (Wu et al., 2023). Similar mechanisms have also been observed in PDAC, where inflammatory signals can reprogram chromatin structure to activate kirsten rat sarcoma viral oncogene homolog (KRAS) -dependent transcription programs and enhance the plasticity and invasiveness of tumor cells (Theis & Harrison, 2023). Further studies have found that this chromatin reprogramming can form what is called "inflammatory memory," that is, cells maintain an open chromatin state after experiencing inflammatory stimulation, making them more sensitive to subsequent inflammatory signals, thereby promoting tumor development (Jovasevic et al., 2024).

In addition to the classical epigenetic modifications, noncoding RNAs (ncRNAs) also play a crucial role in the transcriptional regulatory network between inflammation and tumors. MicroRNAs (miRNAs) can regulate inflammatory signaling pathways by targeting mRNAs. For instance, miR-21 and miR-155 are highly expressed in various inflammation-related cancers and can enhance the activity of NF-κB and STAT3 signaling pathways by inhibiting negative regulatory molecules such as PTEN or SOCS1, thereby promoting tumor cell proliferation and immune evasion (Roerden & Spranger, 2025). In gastric cancer and colorectal cancer, the inflammation-induced miR-21 has been proven to enhance EMT and promote tumor metastasis (Chen et al., 2024). Meanwhile, long ncRNAs (lncRNAs) regulate the expression of inflammation-related genes by interacting with chromatin modification complexes or transcription factors. For example, lncRNAs HOTAIR and LINK-A can regulate the histone methylation status by recruiting the PRC2 complex, thereby promoting the inflammatory-driven tumor transcription program (Hou et al., 2023).

CircRNAs usually regulate the availability of miRNAs by acting as miRNA sponges, thereby indirectly regulating the inflammatory signaling pathways. In HCC and lung cancer, some circRNAs can enhance the activity of NF-κB and STAT3 signaling pathways by adsorbing tumor suppressor miRNAs such as miR-7 or miR-34, thereby promoting tumor cell proliferation and metastasis (Abu-Sultanah et al., 2025). Moreover, recent studies have shown that some circRNAs can directly interact with RNA-binding proteins or transcription complexes to regulate the transcription of inflammatory genes. These findings indicate that the ncRNA network constitutes an important transcriptional regulatory hierarchy in the inflammatory-driven tumor development process (Kondratyeva et al., 2024; Medina Ferrer & Nayak, 2025).

3.3 Cellular crosstalk in the inflammatory tumor microenvironment

3.3.1 Tumor-associated immune cells

The iTME, which is a particularly dynamic ecosystem, is composed of tumor cells, immune cells, and stromal cells. The complex interactions between immune cells and between immune cells and tumor cells form an important mechanism driving tumor progression. Recent research indicates that tumor-associated immune cells not only participate in antitumor immune responses but also have activities through the inflammatory signal network that promote tumor cell proliferation, metastasis, as well as immune escape (Mo et al., 2021). During this process, TAMs, neutrophils, MDSCs, and T cells of different subsets, which form the most important immune regulatory unit in the iTME, and achieve dynamic regulation through multilevel signal networks.

Among various immune cells, TAMs are one of the most abundant immune cells in the tumor microenvironment. Their functions highly depend on the polarization state. TAMs usually display a phenotype similar to M2 and possess the functions of promoting tumor growth and suppressing immunity. Tumor cells that secrete factors such as CSF-1, CCL2, IL-10, and TGF-β will cause mononuclear cells to differentiate into M2-type macrophages and also activate signaling pathways like STAT3, PI3K–AKT, NF-κB, and HIF-1α, thus creating a signal cycle that promotes tumor development (Lin, Rao, et al., 2024). Recently, single-cell transcriptome research has further discovered that the function of TAMs is not only dependent on the classic M1/M2 polarization mode but is also influenced by metabolic reprogramming and epigenetic regulation(Wang et al., 2022). In PDAC the lactic acid secreted by tumor cells can activate the HIF–1α–STAT3 axis, making TAMs express VEGF and ARG1, thus promoting angiogenesis and suppressing T cell activity (Jing et al., 2022). In

HCC and gastric cancer, a similar mechanism is also observed, in which TAMs and tumor cells form a positive feedback loop through the interleukin-6 (IL-6)–signal transducer and activator of transcription 3 (STAT3) signaling pathway, maintaining a chronic inflammatory state and promoting tumor progression.

Besides macrophages, neutrophil granulocytes, which are TANs, namely, TANs, have recently been quite a concern in the iTME. Neutrophils can promote tumor metastasis by forming neutrophil extracellular traps, which are reticular structures composed of DNA, histones, and granule proteins, and the formation process of them depends on PAD4-mediated histone citrullination and the ROS signaling pathway (Borrelli et al., 2024). The research shows that NETs can capture circulating tumor cells and can also prompt them to adhere to the vascular endothelium, thus promoting distant metastasis. For example, in pancreatic cancer and breast cancer, the NETs have been confirmed to be capable of inducing the formation of liver metastasis (Qin et al., 2023). Additionally, NETs can activate the TLR9 and NF-κB signaling pathways, which can enhance the invasive ability of tumor cells and also promote the formation of premetastatic niches by remodeling the extracellular matrix (ECM) (Grabowski et al., 2021).

Another crucial cell with immunomodulatory function is the MDSCs, which play an important part in inflammation-driven immune suppression. MDSCs mainly impede T cell activation through ways such as ARG1, iNOS, and ROS. And they bring about immunosuppressive microenvironments by releasing IL-10 and TGF-β. Recently, a researche find that tumor-generated granulocyte-macrophage colony-stimulating factor (GM–CSF), IL-6, and VEGF can make MDSCs expand and function actively through STAT3 and NF-κB signaling pathways Zhang et al., 2025). In lung cancer and HCC, the accumulation of MDSCs is regarded as an important cause of immune therapy resistance. In addition, MDSCs will also reshape the ECM by secreting S100A8/A9 protein and MMP9, and by doing this, it promotes tumor metastasis as well as angiogenesis (Feng et al., 2025).

The role of T-cell subsets in inflammation-related tumors is indeed quite complicated. Th17 cells that can secrete inflammatory factors such as IL-17 and IL-22 are going to promote chronic inflammation and also enhance tumor-related angiogenesis. In colorectal cancer and liver cancer, they are regarded as those that indeed have the function of promoting tumors. On the contrary, Tregs that express FOXP3, CTLA-4, and PD-1 do create an immunosuppressive environment by inhibiting the activation of effector T cells. Recent research indicates that the IL-6–STAT3 signaling pathway in the tumor microenvironment can cause the differentiation of Th17 cells and can also suppress the stability of Tregs, thus forming a newly created inflammation-driven immune regulatory network (Jones et al., 2021). Moreover, under long-term inflammatory stimulation, $CD8^+$ T cells often enter a state of functional exhaustion, a state that is characterized by the continuous expression of immune checkpoint molecules like PD-1, TIM-3, and LAG-3. This T cell exhaustion is especially prominent in chronic virus infection-related liver cancer and melanoma and has already become an important target of immune checkpoint inhibitor therapy.

3.3.2 Stromal and structural components

The inflamed tumor microenvironment is not only composed of immune cells but also consists of a series of key structural cells and stromal components as well. These elements together shape the spatial ecosystem in which tumor development takes place. In this system, the main structural framework of tumor tissue is constituted by CAFs, vascular endothelial cells, and ECM, and it takes part in tumor progression through mechanisms such as secreting inflammatory factors, remodeling tissue structures, and regulating cell migration signal gradients. Recent single-cell transcriptomic and spatial transcriptomic studies indicate that tumor stromal cells, which not only provide structural support but also regulate immune responses, angiogenesis, and tumor cell plasticity through complex paracrine signaling networks, do indeed play a core role in inflammation-driven tumor progression.

Among the tumor stromal cells, the CAFs, are important effector cells that can regulate the inflammatory microenvironment. CAFs that generally originate from local fibroblasts, bone marrow-derived mesenchymal cells, or tumor cells during the EMT process are activated because of inflammatory signals such as TGF-β, IL-1β, PDGF, and TNF-α (Wang et al., 2024). Activated CAFs, which can secrete various inflammatory factors and chemokines like IL-6, CXCL12, CCL2, and VEGF, then promote the recruitment of immune cells and make the proliferation of tumor cells more vigorous (Pea et al., 2025). Additionally, the cancer-related fibroblast regulates the tumor-associated inflammatory response through the NF-κB, STAT3, as well as the YAP/TAZ signaling pathways. For example, in PDAC, fibroblasts generate CXCL12, and then, via the CXCR4 signaling axis, $CD8^+$ T cells are stopped from entering the tumor core region, thereby forming an immunosuppressive microenvironment. In breast cancer and colorectal cancer the CAFs can also change the structure and tissue stiffness of the ECM by secreting MMPs and lysyl oxidase (LOX) family proteins, thus promoting the invasion and metastasis of tumor cells (Chakraborty et al., 2022). Recent research has also found that CAFs have a high degree of heterogeneity and different subpopulations (such as myofibroblast-like CAFs, inflammatory CAFs, and antigen-presenting CAFs) play distinct roles in inflammation regulation and immune escape (Tisch & Ruiz de Almodóvar, 2021).

The ECM, which is a crucial structural platform in the tumor microenvironment and plays an important role in the spatial propagation of inflammatory signals, is indeed like that. The ECM, which is composed of collagen, fibronectin, laminin, and various glycosaminoglycans, and the structure and mechanical properties of it constantly changes during tumor development. Inflammatory signals can promote the degradation and remodeling of the ECM by inducing the expression of MMPs and ADAM family proteins, thereby releasing growth factors and chemokines that are stored in the ECM. For example, in colorectal cancer and lung cancer, the degradation of the ECM mediated by MMP-9 can release VEGF and TGF-β, thus promoting the formation of vascular and immunosuppressive ones (Choi et al., 2024). Moreover, the remodeling of the ECM can bring about chemokine gradients and mechanical gradients, which can be regulated by integrin, FAK, and YAP/TAZ signaling pathways, thereby controlling the migration and invasion of tumor cells. Recently, the research has put forward that the ECM is not merely a structural scaffold but also a "signal reservoir," which regulates the spatial distribution of inflammatory factors and growth factors, thereby creating a stable signal network within the tumor microenvironment (Picard & Shirihai, 2022).

3.3.3 Intercellular communication networks

Within the iTME, cells do not exist on their own but form a highly dynamic interactive system through complex signal networks. Recent research indicates that the interactions among tumor cells, immune cells, and stromal cells depend on a multitiered information transfer mechanism, including such crucial communication modes as cytokine-mediated paracrine signaling loops, extracellular vesicles (EVs), and metabolic coupling (Gil-Henn et al., 2024). These mechanisms not only decide the intensity and duration of the inflammatory response but also play a core role in regulating tumor cell proliferation, immune escape, and metastasis. With the development of single-cell omics and spatial biology techniques, more and more evidence indicates that these communication networks constitute the important molecular basis driving the evolution of the tumor ecosystem.

Tumor cells and their surrounding immune cells can secrete various inflammatory cytokines, such as IL-6, IL-1β, TNF-α, TGF-β, and CXCL8, which form positive feedback signaling loops by activating NF-κB, STAT3, MAPK, and PI3K–AKT signaling pathways (Abu-Sultanah et al., 2025). For example, in colorectal cancer and HCC, the IL-6 secreted by tumor cells can activate the STAT3 signaling pathway, thereby promoting tumor cell proliferation and inducing more inflammatory factors from TAMs, forming an amplification signaling loop of IL-6–STAT3–NF-κB (Mikami & Kanai, 2023). Similar signaling networks have also been widely reported in pancreatic cancer, where tumor cells and CAFs form a continuous inflammatory signaling network through the IL-1–JAK/STAT3 signaling axis, thereby maintaining an immunosuppressive microenvironment (Tian et al., 2025). Additionally, recent spatial transcriptomics studies have found that cytokine signals are not uniformly distributed but form spatial cytokine gradients in tumor tissues, thereby driving the directional migration of immune cells and shaping the local immune ecology (Tian et al., 2021).

In addition to soluble cytokines, exosomes and EVs also play important roles in inflammatory-related cell communication. Exosomes are membrane-bound vesicles with a diameter of approximately 30–150 nm, which can carry various bioactive molecules, including miRNAs, lncRNAs, proteins, and lipid signaling molecules. Recent studies have shown that tumor-derived exosomes can promote tumor progression by reprogramming the function of immune cells. For example, in melanoma and lung cancer, exosomes released by tumor cells can carry the PD-L1 protein, thereby inhibiting the activity of $CD8^+$ T cells and enhancing immune escape (Tian et al., 2021). In gastric cancer and HCC, miR-21 and miR-155 in tumor-derived exosomes can induce macrophages to polarize toward the immunosuppressive M2 phenotype and enhance inflammation-related tumor growth (Mo et al., 2021). Moreover, exosomes are involved in the formation of premetastatic niches. For instance, in pancreatic cancer, MIF (macrophage migration inhibitory factor) in tumor-derived exosomes can induce the production of TGF-β by liver Kupffer cells, thereby promoting liver metastasis (Borrelli et al., 2024). These findings indicate that exosomes are not only important mediators of cell communication but also may serve as important molecular tools for driving tumor metastasis in response to inflammation.

In recent years, metabolic coupling between immune cells and tumor cells has been regarded as a key regulatory mechanism in the inflammatory–tumor interaction network. In iTMEs, different cell types form a complex metabolic network by exchanging metabolites. For example, tumor cells often produce a large amount of lactic acid through aerobic glycolysis (Warburg effect), and these lactic acids can be transported by MCT1/MCT4 transporter proteins and be taken up by macrophages and Tregs, thereby inducing an immunosuppressive phenotype (Li et al., 2020). Studies have shown that in melanoma and breast cancer, lactic acid can promote the M2 polarization of TAMs by activating HIF-1α and

STAT3 signaling pathways and inhibit the cytotoxic function of $CD8^+$ T cells (Chen et al., 2025; Mily et al., 2020). In addition, tumor cells can change the local metabolic environment by consuming glucose and amino acids (such as tryptophan and arginine). For example, the IDO1 (indoleamine 2,3-dioxygenase) expressed by tumor cells can convert tryptophan into kynurenine, thereby inhibiting T cell proliferation and promoting Treg differentiation. In lung cancer and glioblastoma, this metabolic competition is considered an important mechanism of immune suppression (Sribnick et al., 2022).

3.4 System-level dynamics of inflammation–tumor interactions

3.4.1 Inflammation-driven tumor evolution

Recent studies have shown that chronic inflammation not only plays a promoting role in the early stage of tumor occurrence, but also continuously shapes the genomic structure and cell population composition of tumors by influencing the tumor evolutionary trajectories (Liu et al., 2025). From the perspective of systems biology, the iTME provides a continuously selective pressure environment for tumor cells where cytokines, oxidative stress, and immune surveillance together bring about the dynamic evolution of tumor cell populations. Inflammation-related signals (such as NF-κB, STAT3, and HIF-1α) that can change the proliferation and survival ability of tumor cells, making cells with adaptive mutations gain a growth advantage, this inflammation-driven clonal selection will gradually cause an increase in the heterogeneity of the tumor cell population and also form cell subpopulations that are more invasive and resistant to treatment. For example, in the case of colitis-related colorectal cancer, the long-term inflammation will cause the clonal expansion of cells that have TP53 and KRAS mutations, thereby speeding up the progression of the tumor (Lin, Brittan, et al., 2024).

The chronic inflammatory environment can also generate genomic instability through various ways, and this is one of the important driving factors in tumor evolution. A large quantity of ROS and RNS generated by inflammatory cells will directly damage DNA, leading to situations like base oxidation, DNA double-strand breaks, and replication errors. Moreover, inflammatory signals can further amplify genomic instability by inhibiting the DNA repair system. For instance, NF-κB and STAT3 signals can downregulate the expression of mismatch repair and homologous recombination repair–related genes, thereby increasing mutation accumulation (Ferragut Cardoso et al., 2021). Recent studies have found that in hepatitis virus-related HCC, chronic inflammation leads to continuous ROS production, thereby inducing TERT promoter mutations and chromosomal instability (Richardson et al., 2022). Similar mechanisms have also been observed in Helicobacter pylori infection-related gastric cancer, where inflammation-induced DNA damage can promote TP53 mutations and chromosomal rearrangements, thereby promoting tumor occurrence (Qing et al., 2023).

The inflammatory environment not only increases the mutation frequency but also shapes the mutation landscape of tumors. Large-scale cancer genome studies in recent years have shown that certain mutation signatures are closely related to inflammation-related enzymes. For example, the apolipoprotein B mRNA editing enzyme, catalytic polypeptide-like family cytosine deaminase, is often upregulated in the inflammatory environment and can change the genomic structure of tumors by inducing C-to-T or C-to-G mutations (Beltran et al., 2025). In breast cancer, bladder cancer, and head and neck squamous cell carcinoma, APOBEC-related mutation signatures are considered to be closely related to chronic inflammation and immune signals. Additionally, the expression of inflammation-induced AID (activation-induced cytidine deaminase) can also induce somatic mutations in nonlymphocytes. For example, in the gastric cancer that is related to Helicobacter pylori, AID is abnormally activated, and then it causes the mutation of such key genes as TP53, CDKN2A, and PIK3CA (Ji et al., 2023). These findings show that inflammation not only prompts the occurrence of mutations but also may, through specific molecular mechanisms, form the tumor's specific genomic structure.

On the system level, the dynamic ecosystem that is brought about by the cumulative mutations driven by inflammation and clonal selection is employed for tumor evolution. As time goes by, the tumor cell population undergoes adaptation and change under the combined action of inflammatory stress and immune selection pressure thus giving rise to new subclones and forming complex tumor heterogeneity. For instance, in chronic hepatitis B–related liver cancer, the continuous inflammation not only drives the accumulation of gene mutations but also selects through immune pressure tumor clones with immune escape characteristics like PD-L1 upregulation or antigen presentation defects, and so on (Jena et al., 2024). This evolution process, which is driven by inflammation, is considered an important mechanism of tumor metastasis and treatment resistance. Future research needs to combine single-cell genomics, evolutionary modeling, and spatial multiomics technologies to systematically analyze how inflammatory pressure shapes the tumor evolution trajectory, thereby providing a theoretical basis for developing novel therapeutic strategies targeting the interplay between inflammation and tumors.

3.4.2 Metabolic reprogramming

Recent studies have shown that the interaction between inflammation and tumors is not only manifested at the level of classical cytokine signaling pathways, but also profoundly at the systemic reprogramming of metabolism (metabolic reprogramming). In the iTME, tumor cells, immune cells, and stromal cells form dynamic inflammatory metabolic circuits through complex metabolic interactions. These metabolic networks not only provide energy and biosynthetic raw materials for tumor cells but also promote tumor progression by regulating the function of immune cells and inflammatory signal transduction. Inflammatory factors such as IL-6, TNF-α, and IL-1β can activate key metabolic regulatory factors such as HIF-1α, mTOR, MYC, and NF-κB, thereby driving tumor cells to shift to a glycolytic state, known as the Warburg effect. For example, in inflammatory-related HCC and colorectal cancer, the IL-6–STAT3 signaling can upregulate the expression of key glycolytic enzymes such as GLUT1, HK2, and PFKFB3, enhancing the uptake and metabolic flux of glucose by tumor cells, thereby promoting cell proliferation and enhancing antiapoptotic ability.

In addition to glycolysis, inflammatory signals also regulate lipid metabolism to reprogram the metabolic state of tumor cells. Lipid metabolism has a dual function in the iTME: It provides membrane synthesis and energy reserves for tumor cells and participates in the generation of inflammatory signaling molecules. Inflammatory cytokines can activate the SREBP1, PPAR, and ACC/FASN axes to enhance fatty acid synthesis, thereby promoting tumor cell growth and migration. For example, in non–small cell lung cancer and pancreatic cancer, the NF-κB and STAT3 signaling can induce the expression of lipid synthesis-related enzymes and promote the dependence of tumor cells on fatty acids for metabolism. Moreover, lipid metabolism products in the inflammatory environment, such as prostaglandins and leukotrienes, can further enhance the inflammatory response and promote tumor angiogenesis by activating the COX-2–PGE2 signaling pathway. Recent metabolomics studies have also found that TAMs and MDSCs exhibit significant lipid accumulation in the inflammatory environment. This lipid metabolic reprogramming can enhance their immunosuppressive function, thereby promoting tumor immune escape.

During the inflammatory-driven metabolic reprogramming process, lactate has gradually been recognized as an important signaling molecule connecting tumor metabolism and immune regulation. The traditional view holds that lactate is merely a metabolic waste product of glycolysis, but recent studies have shown that lactate has significant signaling and regulatory functions in the tumor microenvironment. Tumor cells release large amounts of lactate through LDHA-mediated lactate production and MCT4 transporter proteins into the microenvironment, thereby forming a local acidic environment. This acidic environment not only inhibits the activity of effector T cells and natural killer cells (NK cells) but also induces functional changes in immunosuppressive cells by activating GPR81 and HIF-1α signaling pathways. For example, in melanoma and breast cancer, lactate can promote the polarization of TAMs to the M2 immunosuppressive phenotype and induce their expression of VEGF and ARG1, thereby promoting angiogenesis and inhibiting antitumor immune responses.

In addition, lactate has been found to regulate gene expression through new epigenetic mechanisms. The recently proposed histone lactylation modification provides a new perspective for understanding the connection between tumor metabolism and inflammatory regulation. Lactate can change chromatin structure by inducing histone lactylation and regulating the expression of inflammation-related genes. For example, in macrophages, lactate-induced histone lactylation can upregulate the expression of M2 polarization-related genes (such as ARG1 and MRC1), thereby enhancing the immunosuppressive function.

3.4.3 Spatial and temporal dynamics

The interaction between inflammation and tumors not only manifests as a molecular signaling network, but also exhibits distinct spatial and temporal organizational characteristics. In the iTME, the spatial distribution of different cell populations within the tissue structure and their dynamic changes over time jointly determine the nature of the inflammatory response and its impact on tumor progression. In recent years, with the development of single-cell sequencing (scRNA-seq) and spatial transcriptomics (spatial transcriptomics) technologies, researchers have been able to analyze the spatial organization patterns of cell populations and signaling pathways in the tumor microenvironment at the tissue scale. These studies have revealed that inflammatory signals are not uniformly distributed but form specific inflammatory microregions within the tumor tissue. These microregions are composed of immune cells, tumor cells, and stromal cells and are regulated by local cytokine networks to control tumor growth and immune responses.

Spatial transcriptomics research has found that there are multiple functionally specific spatial immune niches in iTMEs. For example, in PDAC and HCC, spatial omics analysis shows that the tumor edge regions often enrich in inflammatory factors such as IL-6, TNF-α, and CXCL chemokines, accompanied by the activation of STAT3 and NF-κB signaling pathways, thereby forming inflammatory regions that promote tumor proliferation and immunosuppression. At the same time, the core regions of the tumor often exhibit obvious hypoxia and metabolic stress signals, such as HIF-1α activation and lactate accumulation, which further affect the functional state of immune cells. Spatial multiomics research has also revealed that the distribution of TAMs, CAFs, and T cells in the tissue has highly structured characteristics and forms a stable cell interaction network through local cytokine gradients and chemotactic signals. For example, in colorectal cancer, spatial transcriptomics research has found that IL-6–STAT3 signaling-active TAMs often aggregate with CAFs to form inflammatory fibrotic regions, which are considered important microenvironmental structures promoting tumor invasion and immune escape.

In addition to the spatial structure, the temporal dynamic changes of the inflammatory response also play a vital role in the process of tumor development as well. The acute inflammation is usually a defensive reaction of the body to tissue injury or infection, characterized by the short-term recruitment of inflammatory cells as well as the release of cytokines. But when the inflammatory stimulation continues to exist, the inflammatory response will gradually change into chronic inflammation, thereby providing a favorable environment for tumor development. In this process, inflammatory signaling pathways like NF-κB, STAT3, COX-2, and NLRP3 inflammasomes are continuously activated, and then long-term functional alterations of immune cells and stromal cells will be triggered. For example, in the case of inflammatory bowel disease–related colorectal cancer, repeated acute inflammatory attacks can gradually transform into a sustained chronic inflammatory state and at the same time, as the IL-6–STAT3 signaling axis is continuously activated, this promotes the proliferation of epithelial cells as well as the development of tumors.

The chronic inflammation can also promote tumor development by gradually altering the tissue microenvironment as well. In the early stage the inflammatory response mainly shows as the recruitment of immune cells and tissue repair responses however when inflammation persists the microenvironment gradually changes into an immunosuppressive and tumor-promoting state for example in chronic hepatitis B–related HCC long-term inflammation can result in continuous immune cell infiltration and fibrosis in liver tissue and by activating signaling pathways like TGFβ STAT3 and YAP/TAZ it promotes hepatocyte transformation and tumor formation. In the gastric cancer that is related to Helicobacter pylori infection, a similar temporal evolution process is also observed, in which this chronic inflammation gradually leads to the atrophy of the gastric mucosa, intestinal metaplasia, and finally results in the appearance of tumors.

3.5 Future research directions

Recent studies have gradually expanded the inflammatory–tumor interaction from a single signaling pathway model to a complex "inflammatory cancer ecosystem." In this framework, tumor cells, immune cells, and stromal cells form dynamic interactions through multilevel signaling networks, with myeloid cells, T cell subsets, fibroblasts, and endothelial cells constituting key functional modules. Advances in single-cell sequencing and spatial multiomics techniques have enabled researchers to analyze the topological structure and functional coupling relationships of these multicell networks at the tissue scale. For instance, spatial transcriptomics studies have shown that in brain metastases and lung adenocarcinoma metastatic foci, different immune cell populations form local ecological niches with specific inflammatory signal characteristics, and maintain a stable inflammatory network structure through ligand-receptor signaling and metabolic exchange. These findings suggest that future research needs to understand the tumor microenvironment as a systemic ecological network driven by multicell interactions, and identify key regulatory nodes in the network using systems biology methods, thereby providing new therapeutic strategies targeting the inflammatory microenvironment.

In addition to the spatial structure, the temporal dynamic situation of the inflammatory response in the course of tumor development is also extremely important. Acute inflammation is usually eliminated through immune cell recruitment and tissue repair responses, while persistent inflammation will gradually transform into chronic inflammation, thus promoting tumor formation and immune escape. In this process, signal axes, like IL-1, IL-6/STAT3, NF-κB, and COX-2/PGE2, are continuously activated, forming a stable immune suppression network in the tumor microenvironment. An increasing number of studies indicate that inflammatory signals have different roles at different time points: Early inflammation often drives immune surveillance and tissue repair, while late chronic inflammation, through mechanisms like myeloid cell recruitment, immune metabolic suppression, and vascular remodeling, promotes tumor progression. Therefore, in future research, the longitudinal multiomics analysis and the dynamic model ought to be combined so as to systematically analyze the regulation patterns of inflammatory signals at different stages of tumor progression, and in such a way, the potential therapeutic time window can be identified.

In the context of precision medicine, the personalized targeting of the inflammatory pathways is gradually becoming a key direction in tumor treatment. Traditional antiinflammatory therapies usually focus on individual cytokines or signaling molecules, yet increasing evidence indicates that the inflammatory network has obvious diversity and redundancy. Therefore future treatment strategies need to classify and stratify patients through multidimensional biomarkers, for example, developing comprehensive predictive models based on such indicators as cytokine profiles, immune cell compositions, metabolic characteristics, and spatial immune structures, and the like. In recent years, clinical studies targeting inflammatory pathways such as IL-1β, IL-6, JAK–STAT3, and CCR2-mediated myeloid cell recruitment have provided important evidence for this strategy. By integrating spatialomics, bioinformatics, and clinical data, it is hoped to establish an inflammation-related biomarker system that can predict treatment responses and risk of resistance, thereby promoting the development of precision targeted inflammation therapy.

Furthermore, more and more studies have shown that tumor-associated inflammatory responses are closely linked to the microbiome and immunometabolism. The microbiota in the gut and within the tumor can regulate the host immune system through metabolites (such as short-chain fatty acids, bile acid derivatives, and tryptophan metabolites), thereby influencing tumor immune responses and inflammatory states. For example, some microbial metabolites can regulate the functions of myeloid cells and T cells by activating AhR, TLR, or NLRP3 inflammasome signaling pathways, and play an important role in immune treatment responses. Therefore integrating microbiome research with the immunometabolic

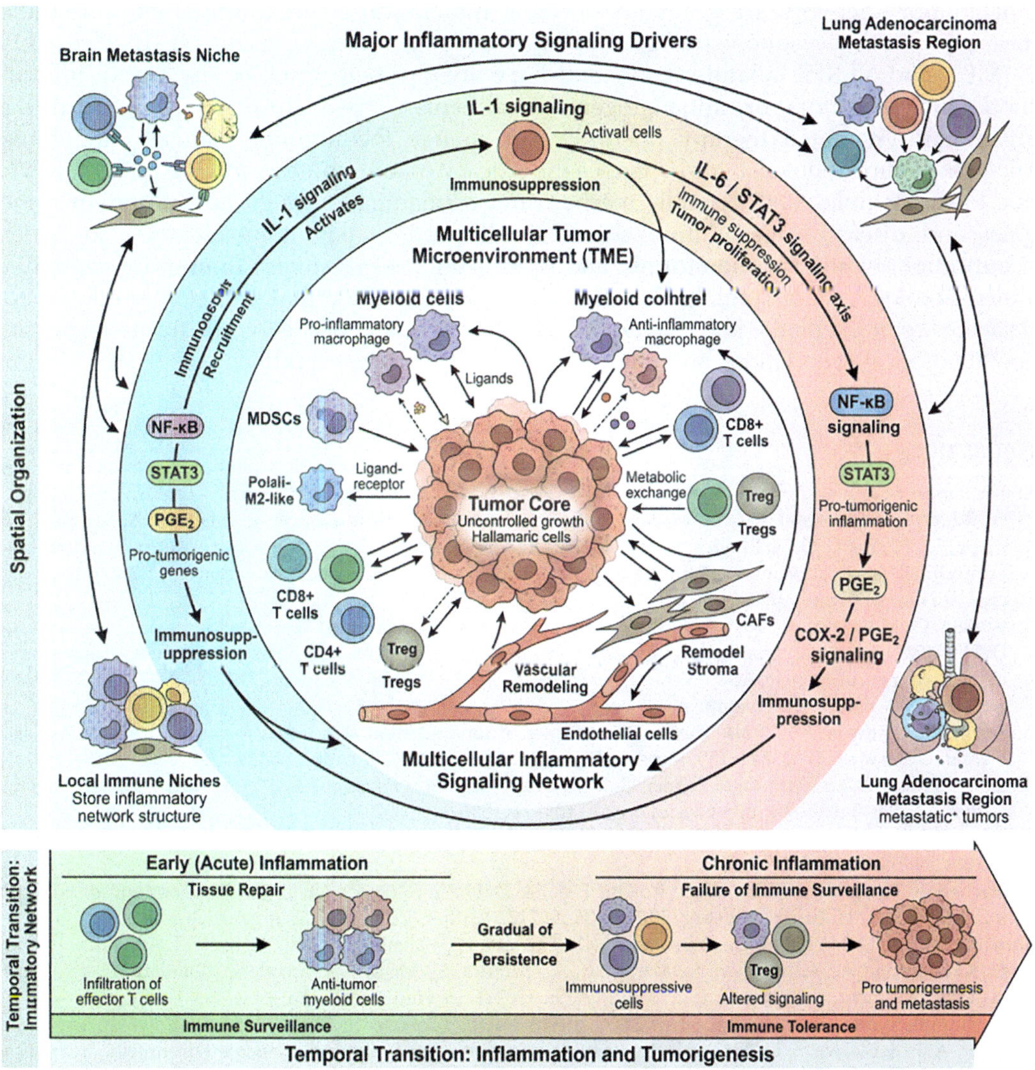

FIGURE 3.3 The inflammatory cancer ecosystem integrates cellular interactions, signaling networks, and therapeutic targeting. Tumor cells interact dynamically with immune cells and stromal cells—including myeloid cells, T cell subsets, fibroblasts, and endothelial cells—forming a multicellular inflammatory ecosystem regulated by signaling pathways such as IL-1, IL-6/STAT3, NF-κB, and COX-2/PGE2. Spatial immune niches, temporal transitions from acute to chronic inflammation, microbiome-derived metabolites, and immunometabolic regulation collectively shape tumor progression and immune suppression. Targeting inflammatory pathways (e.g., IL-1β, IL-6, JAK–STAT3, CCR2, COX-2/PGE2, and NLRP3) offers potential strategies to enhance immunotherapy and improve cancer treatment outcomes. *CAFs*, Cancer-associated fibroblasts.

network is expected to reveal novel regulatory mechanisms between the host, microbiota, and tumor, and provide new ideas for developing treatment strategies based on microbiome or metabolic regulation.

From the perspective of translational medicine, therapeutic strategies targeting the inflammatory network are gradually entering the clinical stage. Multiple clinical studies have explored intervention strategies for inflammatory pathways such as IL-1β, IL-6, COX-2/PGE2, and NLRP3 inflammasome, and have attempted to combine them with immune checkpoint inhibitors or antiangiogenic treatments. These studies have shown that inflammatory-targeted therapy not only can change the immune status in the tumor microenvironment but also may enhance the efficacy of immunotherapy (Fig. 3.3). However, due to the complex and dynamic mechanism of inflammatory signals in different tumor types and disease stages, future clinical trials need to pay more attention to patient stratification, biomarker monitoring, and optimization of treatment timing. By combining systems biology, spatial omics, and clinical data, it is expected that precise immunotherapy strategies centered on the inflammatory network will be established in the future, providing new theoretical foundations and clinical pathways for tumor treatment.

References

Abu-Sultanah, M., Zhou, Z., Jiang, C., Mitchell, D. K., Bessler, W. K., Jiang, L., Li, X., Qian, S., Smith, A. E., Mang, H. E., White, E. E., Ciesielski, M. D., Hickey, B. E., Brewster, K. M., Sandusky, G. E., Masters, A., Angus, S. P., Clapp, D. W., Le, L. Q., & Rhodes, S. D. (2025). TGFβ-dependent signaling drives tumor growth and aberrant extracellular matrix dynamics in NF1-associated plexiform neurofibroma. *Science Advances, 11*(25). https://doi.org/10.1126/sciadv.adu0772.

Anastasaki, C., Mo, J., Chen, J. K., Chatterjee, J., Pan, Y., Scheaffer, S. M., Cobb, O., Monje, M., Le, L. Q., & Gutmann, D. H. (2022). Neuronal hyperexcitability drives central and peripheral nervous system tumor progression in models of neurofibromatosis-1. *Nature Communications, 13*(1). https://doi.org/10.1038/s41467-022-30466-6, https://www.nature.com/ncomms/.

Antonucci, L., & Karin, M. (2024). The past and future of inflammation as a target to cancer prevention. *Cancer Prevention Research, 17*(4), 141–155. https://doi.org/10.1158/1940-6207.capr-23-0423.

Beltran, A., Jiang, X.'er, Shen, Y., & Lehner, B. (2025). Site-saturation mutagenesis of 500 human protein domains. *Nature, 637*(8047), 885–894. https://doi.org/10.1038/s41586-024-08370-4.

Bennour, Haroun, Sicard, Mounien, & Landrier (2022). Vitamin D and obesity/adiposity-a brief overview of recent studies. *Nutrients, 14*(10).

Bhattacharjee, T., Amchin, D. B., Alert, R., Ott, J. A., & Datta, S. S. (2022). Chemotactic smoothing of collective migration. *eLife, 11*. https://doi.org/10.7554/eLife.71226, https://elifesciences.org/articles/71226.

Borrelli, C., Roberts, M., Eletto, D., Hussherr, M.-D., Fazilaty, H., Valenta, T., Lafzi, A., Kretz, J. A., Guido Vinzoni, E., Karakatsani, A., Adivarahan, S., Mannhart, A., Kimura, S., Meijs, A., Baccouche Mhamedi, F., Acar, I. E., Handler, K., Ficht, X., Platt, R. J., ... Moor, A. E. (2024). In vivo interaction screening reveals liver-derived constraints to metastasis. *Nature, 632*(8024), 411–418. https://doi.org/10.1038/s41586-024-07715-3.

Boutilier, A. J., & Elsawa, S. F. (2021). Macrophage polarization states in the tumor microenvironment. *International Journal of Molecular Sciences, 22*(13), 6995. https://doi.org/10.3390/ijms22136995.

Campbell, J. P., & Turner, J. E. (2018). Debunking the myth of exercise-induced immune suppression: Redefining the impact of exercise on immunological health across the lifespan. *Frontiers in Immunology, 9*. https://doi.org/10.3389/fimmu.2018.00648, https://www.frontiersin.org/articles/10.3389/fimmu.2018.00648/full.

Chakraborty, C., Sharma, A. R., Bhattacharya, M., & Lee, S. S. (2022). A detailed overview of immune escape, antibody escape, partial vaccine escape of SARS-CoV-2 and their emerging variants with escape mutations. *Frontiers in Immunology, 13*. https://doi.org/10.3389/fimmu.2022.801522, https://www.frontiersin.org/journals/immunology#.

Chen, H. Y., Almonte-Loya, A., Lay, F. Y., Hsu, M., Johnson, E., González-Avalos, E., Yin, J., Bruno, R. S., Ma, Q., Ghoneim, H. E., Wozniak, D. J., Harrison, F. E., & Lio, C. W. J. (2022). Epigenetic remodeling by vitamin C potentiates plasma cell differentiation. *eLife, 11*. https://doi.org/10.7554/ELIFE.73754, https://elifesciences.org/articles/73754.

Chen, M., Shan, H., Tao, Q., Hu, R., Sun, Q., Zheng, M., Chen, Z., Lin, Q., Yin, M., Zhao, S., Chen, X., & Chen, Z. (2024). Mimicking tumor metastasis using a transwell-integrated organoids-on-A-chip platform. *Small (Weinheim an der Bergstrasse, Germany), 20*(27). https://doi.org/10.1002/smll.202308525.

Chen, S. M., Liu, Y. K., Ma, X. Q., Wei, C. Y., Li, M. Q., & Zhu, X. Y. (2025). Creatine promotes endometriosis progression by inducing M2 polarization of peritoneal macrophages. *Reproduction (Cambridge, England), 169*(3). https://doi.org/10.1530/REP-24-0278, https://rep.bioscientifica.com/view/journals/rep/169/3/rep.169.issue-3.xml.

Chen, X., Ji, Y., Liu, R., Zhu, X., Wang, K., Yang, X., Liu, B., Gao, Z., Huang, Y., Shen, Y., Liu, H., & Sun, H. (2023). Mitochondrial dysfunction. Roles in skeletal muscle atrophy. *Journal of Translational Medicine, 21*(1). https://doi.org/10.1186/s12967-023-04369-z.

Choi, S., Kang, J. G., Tran, Y. T. H., Jeong, S. H., Park, K. Y., Shin, H., Kim, Y. H., Park, M., Nahmgoong, H., Seol, T., Jeon, H., Kim, Y., Park, S., Kim, H. J., Kim, M. S., Li, X., Bou Sleiman, M., Lee, E., Choi, J., ... Suh, J. M. (2024). Hippo–YAP/TAZ signalling coordinates adipose plasticity and energy balance by uncoupling leptin expression from fat mass. *Nature Metabolism, 6*(5), 847–860. https://doi.org/10.1038/s42255-024-01045-4, https://www.nature.com/natmetab/.

Coussens, L. M., & Werb, Z. (2002). Inflammation and cancer. *Nature, 420*(6917), 860–867. https://doi.org/10.1038/nature01322.

Daniel, B., Belk, J. A., Meier, S. L., Chen, A. Y., Sandor, K., Czimmerer, Z., Varga, Z., Bene, K., Buquicchio, F. A., Qi, Y., Kitano, H., Wheeler, J. R., Foster, D. S., Januszyk, M., Longaker, M. T., Chang, H. Y., & Satpathy, A. T. (2023). Macrophage inflammatory and regenerative response periodicity is programmed by cell cycle and chromatin state. *Molecular Cell, 83*(1), 121. https://doi.org/10.1016/j.molcel.2022.11.017, www.molecule.org.

Drougard, A., Ma, E. H., Wegert, V., Sheldon, R., Panzeri, I., Vatsa, N., Apostle, S., Fagnocchi, L., Schaf, J., Gossens, K., Völker, J., Pang, S., Bremser, A., Dror, E., Giacona, F., Sagar, S., Henderson, M. X., Prinz, M., Jones, R. G., & Pospisilik, J. A. (2024). An acute microglial metabolic response controls metabolism and improves memory. *eLife, 12*. https://doi.org/10.7554/elife.87120.

Dunleavy, K. A., Raffals, L. E., & Camilleri, M. (2023). Intestinal barrier dysfunction in inflammatory bowel disease: underpinning pathogenesis and therapeutics. *Digestive Diseases and Sciences, 68*(12), 4306–4320. https://doi.org/10.1007/s10620-023-08122-w, https://www.springer.com/journal/10620.

Fan, Y., Li, Y., Yao, X., Jin, J., Scott, A., Liu, B., Wang, S., Huo, L., Wang, Y., Wang, R., Pool Pizzi, M., Ma, L., Shao, S., Sewastjanow-Silva, M., Waters, R., Chatterjee, D., Liu, B., Shanbhag, N., Peng, G., ... Song, S. (2023). Epithelial SOX9 drives progression and metastases of gastric adenocarcinoma by promoting immunosuppressive tumour microenvironment. *Gut, 72*(4), 624–637. https://doi.org/10.1136/gutjnl-2021-326581.

Feng, K., Zhang, X., Li, J., Han, M., Wang, J., Chen, F., Yi, Z., Di, L., & Wang, R. (2025). Neoantigens combined with in situ cancer vaccination induce personalized immunity and reshape the tumor microenvironment. *Nature Communications, 16*(1). https://doi.org/10.1038/s41467-025-60448-3.

Feng, L., Li, B., Xi, Y., Cai, M., & Tian, Z. (2022). Aerobic exercise and resistance exercise alleviate skeletal muscle atrophy through IGF-1/IGF-1R-PI3K/Akt pathway in mice with myocardial infarction. *American Journal of Physiology-Cell Physiology, 322*(2), C164. https://doi.org/10.1152/ajpcell.00344.2021.

Ferragut Cardoso, A. P., Banerjee, M., Nail, A. N., Lykoudi, A., & States, J. C. (2021). miRNA dysregulation is an emerging modulator of genomic instability. *Seminars in Cancer Biology, 76*, 120–131. https://doi.org/10.1016/j.semcancer.2021.05.004, http://www.elsevier.com/inca/publications/store/6/2/2/9/4/3/index.htt.

Francette, A. M., & Arndt, K. M. (2024). Multiple direct and indirect roles of the Paf1 complex in transcription elongation, splicing, and histone modifications. *Cell Reports, 43*(9), 114730. https://doi.org/10.1016/j.celrep.2024.114730.

Gil-Henn, H., Girault, J. A., & Lev, S. (2024). PYK2, a hub of signaling networks in breast cancer progression. *Trends in Cell Biology, 34*(4), 312–326. https://doi.org/10.1016/j.tcb.2023.07.006, https://www.sciencedirect.com/science/journal/09628924.

Grabowski, M. M., Sankey, E. W., Ryan, K. J., Chongsathidkiet, P., Lorrey, S. J., Wilkinson, D. S., & Fecci, P. E. (2021). Immune suppression in gliomas. *Journal of Neuro-oncology, 151*(1), 3–12. https://doi.org/10.1007/s11060-020-03483-y, www.wkap.nl/journalhome.htm/0167-594X.

Grandi, F. C., Modi, H., Kampman, L., & Corces, M. R. (2022). Chromatin accessibility profiling by ATAC-seq. *Nature Protocols, 17*(6), 1518–1552. https://doi.org/10.1038/s41596-022-00692-9, http://www.natureprotocols.com/.

Greca, F. L., & Magez, S. (2011). Vaccination against trypanosomiasis: Can it be done or is the trypanosome truly the ultimate immune destroyer and escape artist? *Human Vaccines, 7*(11), 1225–1233. https://doi.org/10.4161/hv.7.11.18203, http://www.landesbioscience.com/journals/vaccines/LaGrecaHV7-11.pdf.

Gu, X., Zhu, Y., Su, J., Wang, S., Su, X., Ding, X., Jiang, L., Fei, X., & Zhang, W. (2024). Lactate-induced activation of tumor-associated fibroblasts and IL-8-mediated macrophage recruitment promote lung cancer progression. *Redox Biology, 74*, 103209. https://doi.org/10.1016/j.redox.2024.103209.

He, N., Zhang, J., Liu, M., & Yin, L. (2024). Elucidating the mechanism of plasticizers inducing breast cancer through network toxicology and molecular docking analysis. *Ecotoxicology and Environmental Safety, 284*, 116866. https://doi.org/10.1016/j.ecoenv.2024.116866.

Hou, Y., Yuan, Y., Li, Y., Wang, L., Hu, J., & Liu, X. (2023). The role of histone methylation in renal cell cancer: An update. *Molecular Biology Reports, 50*(3), 2735–2742. https://doi.org/10.1007/s11033-022-08124-3.

Jena, D., Ghosh, A., Jha, A., Prasad, P., & Raghav, S. K. (2024). Impact of vaccination on SARS-CoV-2 evolution and immune escape variants. *Vaccine, 42*(21), 126153. https://doi.org/10.1016/j.vaccine.2024.07.054.

Jeong, H., Koh, J., Kim, S., Yim, J., Song, S. G., Kim, H., Li, Y., Lee, S. H., Chung, Y. K., Kim, H., Lee, C.-H., Kim, H. Y., Keam, B., Lee, S.-H., Chung, D. H., & Jeon, Y. K. (2025). Cell-intrinsic PD-L1 signaling drives immunosuppression by myeloid-derived suppressor cells through IL-6/Jak/Stat3 in PD-L1-high lung cancer. *Journal for ImmunoTherapy of Cancer, 13*(3), e010612. https://doi.org/10.1136/jitc-2024-010612.

Ji, Y., Chen, X., Lin, S., Traw, M. B., Tian, D., Yang, S., Wang, L., & Huang, J. (2023). High level of somatic mutations detected in a diploid banana wild relative *Musa basjoo. Molecular Genetics and Genomics, 298*(1), 67–77. https://doi.org/10.1007/s00438-022-01959-2.

Jing, Y., Zhang, Y., Pan, R., Ding, K., Chen, R., & Meng, Q. (2022). Effect of inhalation anesthetics on tumor metastasis. *Technology in Cancer Research and Treatment, 21*. https://doi.org/10.1177/15330338221121092, https://journals.sagepub.com/home/TCT.

Jones, G. H., Vecera, C. M., Pinjari, O. F., & Machado-Vieira, R. (2021). Inflammatory signaling mechanisms in bipolar disorder. *Journal of Biomedical Science, 28*(1). https://doi.org/10.1186/s12929-021-00742-6, http://www.jbiomedsci.com.

Jovasevic, V., Wood, E. M., Cicvaric, A., Zhang, H., Petrovic, Z., Carboncino, A., Parker, K. K., Bassett, T. E., Moltesen, M., Yamawaki, N., Login, H., Kalucka, J., Sananbenesi, F., Zhang, X., Fischer, A., & Radulovic, J. (2024). Formation of memory assemblies through the DNA-sensing TLR9 pathway. *Nature, 628*(8006), 145–153. https://doi.org/10.1038/s41586-024-07220-7, https://www.nature.com/nature/.

Kaur, B. P., & Secord, E. (2021). Innate immunity. *Immunology and Allergy Clinics of North America, 41*(4), 535–541.

Kennel, K. B., Bozlar, M., De Valk, A. F., & Greten, F. R. (2023). Cancer-associated fibroblasts in inflammation and antitumor immunity. *Clinical Cancer Research, 29*(6), 1009–1016. https://doi.org/10.1158/1078-0432.CCR-22-1031, https://watermark.silverchair.com/1009.pdf.

Kondratyeva, L. G., Rakitina, O. A., Pleshkan, V. V., Kuzmich, A. I., Linge, I. A., Kondratieva, S. A., Snezhkov, E. V., Alekseenko, I. V., & Sverdlov, E. D. (2024). The cellular and transcriptomic early innate immune response to BCG vaccination in mice. *Federation Cells, 13*(24). https://doi.org/10.3390/cells13242043, https://www.mdpi.com/journal/cells.

Li, M., Jiang, Z., Xu, X., Wu, X., Liu, Y., Chen, K., Liao, Y., Li, W., Wang, X., Guo, Y., Zhang, B., Wen, L., Kee, K., & Tang, F. (2025). Chromatin accessibility landscape of mouse early embryos revealed by single-cell NanoATAC-seq2. *Science (New York, N.Y.), 387*(6741). https://doi.org/10.1126/science.adp4319.

Li, Q., Zeng, K., Chen, Q., Han, C., Wang, X., Li, B., Miao, J., Zheng, B., Liu, J., Yuan, X., & Liu, B. (2025). Atractylenolide I inhibits angiogenesis and reverses sunitinib resistance in clear cell renal cell carcinoma through ATP6V0D2-mediated autophagic degradation of EPAS1/HIF2α *Autophagy, 21*(3), 619–638. https://doi.org/10.1080/15548627.2024.2421699.

Li, Y., Chen, Y., Zhou, L., You, S., Deng, H., Chen, Y., Alseekh, S., Yuan, Y., Fu, R., Zhang, Z., Su, D., Fernie, A. R., Bouzayen, M., Ma, T., Liu, M., & Zhang, Y. (2020). MicroTom metabolic network: rewiring tomato metabolic regulatory network throughout the growth cycle. *Molecular Plant, 13*(8), 1203–1218. https://doi.org/10.1016/j.molp.2020.06.005.

Lin, A., Brittan, M., Baker, A. H., Dimmeler, S., Fisher, E. A., Sluimer, J. C., & Misra, A. (2024). Clonal expansion in cardiovascular pathology. *JACC: Basic to Translational Science, 9*(1), 120–144. https://doi.org/10.1016/j.jacbts.2023.04.008, https://www.sciencedirect.com/science/journal/2452302X.

Lin, J., Rao, D., Zhang, M., & Gao, Q. (2024). Metabolic reprogramming in the tumor microenvironment of liver cancer. *Journal of Hematology & Oncology, 17*(1). https://doi.org/10.1186/s13045-024-01527-8.

Liu, C., Zhai, W. W., & Lu, X. M. (2025). Evolutionary ecology in tumor evolution: Concept, application and innovation. *Yi chuan = Hereditas, 47*(2), 228–236. https://doi.org/10.16288/j.yczz.24-264.

Mao, G., Zeng, R., Peng, J., Zuo, K., Pang, Z., & Liu, J. (2022). Reconstructing gene regulatory networks of biological function using differential equations of multilayer perceptrons. *BMC Bioinformatics, 23*(1). https://doi.org/10.1186/s12859-022-05055-5.

Medina Ferrer, F., & Nayak, D. D. (2025). An archaeal transcription factor bridges prokaryotic and eukaryotic regulatory paradigms. *Cell, 188*(26), 7366. https://doi.org/10.1016/j.cell.2025.10.036, https://www.sciencedirect.com/science/journal/00928674.

Mikami, Y., & Kanai, T. (2023). Network approaches to uncover pathogenesis and therapeutic targets of inflammatory bowel diseases. *The Keio Journal of Medicine, 72*(2), 29–43. https://doi.org/10.2302/kjm.2022-0015-ir.

Mily, A., Kalsum, S., Loreti, M. G., Rekha, R. S., Muvva, J. R., Lourda, M., & Brighenti, S. (2020). Polarization of m1 and m2 human monocyte-derived cells and analysis with flow cytometry upon mycobacterium tuberculosis infection. *Journal of Visualized Experiments, Sweden Journal of Visualized Experiments, 2020*(163), 1–20. https://doi.org/10.3791/61807, https://www.jove.com/pdf/61807.

Mo, J., Anastasaki, C., Chen, Z., Shipman, T., Papke, J., Yin, K., Gutmann, D. H., & Le, L. Q. (2021). Humanized neurofibroma model from induced pluripotent stem cells delineates tumor pathogenesis and developmental origins. *Journal of Clinical Investigation, 131*(1). https://doi.org/10.1172/jci139807.

Neurath, M. F. (2024). Strategies for targeting cytokines in inflammatory bowel disease. *Nature Reviews. Immunology, 24*(8), 559–576. https://doi.org/10.1038/s41577-024-01008-6, https://www.nature.com/nri/.

Palatianou, M. E., Karamanolis, G., Tsentidis, C., Gourgiotis, D., Papaconstantinou, I., & Vezakis, A. (2023). M. Tzouvala, Signaling pathways associated with bone loss in inflammatory bowel disease. *Annals of Gastroenterology, 36*(2), 132–140. https://doi.org/10.20524/aog.2023.0785, http://www.annalsgastro.gr/index.php/annalsgastro/article/download/6903/5512.

Pang, L., Dunterman, M., Guo, S., Khan, F., Liu, Y., Taefi, E., Bahrami, A., Geula, C., Hsu, W.-H., Horbinski, C., James, C. D., & Chen, P. (2023). Kunitz-type protease inhibitor TFPI2 remodels stemness and immunosuppressive tumor microenvironment in glioblastoma. *Nature Immunology, 24*(10), 1654–1670. https://doi.org/10.1038/s41590-023-01605-y.

Patritti Cram, J., Wu, J., Coover, R. A., Rizvi, T. A., Chaney, K. E., Ravindran, R., Cancelas, J. A., Spinner, R. J., & Ratner, N. (2022). P2RY14 cAMP signaling regulates Schwann cell precursor self-renewal, proliferation, and nerve tumor initiation in a mouse model of neurofibromatosis. *eLife, 11*. https://doi.org/10.7554/elife.73511.

Pea, A., Bevere, M., Gkountakos, A., Pasini, D., Fiorini, D., Mafficini, A., Golovco, S., Simbolo, M., Pedron, S., Sciammarella, C., Mattiolo, P., Mombello, A., Villanova, M., Franzina, C., Masetto, F., Ciulla, C., Sperandio, N., Fujikura, K., Ahadi, M. S., ... Luchini, C. (2025). Mucinous cystic neoplasms and simple mucinous cysts are two distinct precursors of pancreatic cancer: Clinicopathological, genomic, and transcriptomic characterization. *The Journal of Pathology, 266*(4-5), 421–434. https://doi.org/10.1002/path.6437.

Picard, M., & Shirihai, O. S. (2022). Mitochondrial signal transduction. *Cell Metabolism, 34*(11), 1620–1653. https://doi.org/10.1016/j.cmet.2022.10.008, http://www.cellmetabolism.org/.

Powers, J., Zhang, X., Reyes, A. V., Zavaliev, R., Ochakovski, R., Xu, S.-L., & Dong, X. (2024). Next-generation mapping of the salicylic acid signaling hub and transcriptional cascade. *Molecular Plant, 17*(10), 1558–1572. https://doi.org/10.1016/j.molp.2024.08.008.

Qin, X., Zhang, J., Wang, M., Feng, Y., Zhao, Y., Zhang, H., & Guo, W. (2023). The effect of thalidomide on the invasive ability of gastric cancer cells by regulating miR-524-5p/FSTL1. *Cellular and Molecular Biology, 69*(14), 137–142. https://doi.org/10.14715/cmb/2023.69.14.22, https://www.cellmolbiol.org/index.php/CMB/article/view/5128/2880.

Qing, X., Zhang, G., & Wang, Z. Q. (2023). DNA damage response in neurodevelopment and neuromaintenance. *FEBS Journal, 290*(13), 3300–3310. https://doi.org/10.1111/febs.16535, http://onlinelibrary.wiley.com/journal/10.1111/(ISSN)1742-4658.

Ravari, A., Ghoreishi, S. F., & Imani, M. (2023). Optimal recursive expert-enabled inference in regulatory networks. *IEEE Control Systems Letters, 7*, 1027–1032. https://doi.org/10.1109/LCSYS.2022.3229054, http://ieeexplore.ieee.org/xpl/aboutJournal.jsp?punumber=7782633.

Richardson, T. E., Walker, J. M., Abdullah, K. G., McBrayer, S. K., Viapiano, M. S., Mussa, Z. M., Tsankova, N. M., Snuderl, M., & Hatanpaa, K. J. (2022). Chromosomal instability in adult-type diffuse gliomas. *Acta Neuropathologica Communications, 10*(1). https://doi.org/10.1186/s40478-022-01420-w, https://actaneurocomms.biomedcentral.com/.

Robinson, P. Z., Frank, D. N., & Ramakrishnan, V. R. (2023). Inflammation resolution and specialized pro-resolving lipid mediators in chronic rhinosinusitis. *Expert Review of Clinical Immunology, 19*(8), 969–979. https://doi.org/10.1080/1744666X.2023.2232554, http://www.tandfonline.com/loi/ierm20.

Roeck, B. F., Lotfipour Nasudivar, S., Vorndran, M. R. H., Schueller, L., Yapici, F. I., Rübsam, M., von Karstedt, S., Niessen, C. M., & Garcia-Saez, A. J. (2025). Ferroptosis spreads to neighboring cells via plasma membrane contacts. *Nature Communications, 16*(1). https://doi.org/10.1038/s41467-025-58175-w, https://www.nature.com/ncomms/.

Roerden, M., & Spranger, S. (2025). Cancer immune evasion, immunoediting and intratumour heterogeneity. *Nature Reviews. Immunology, 25*(5), 353–369. https://doi.org/10.1038/s41577-024-01111-8.

Rzeszotarska, E., Sowinska, A., Stypinska, B., Lutkowska, A., Felis-Giemza, A., Olesinska, M., Puszczewicz, M., Majewski, D., Jagodzinski, P. P., Haładyj, E., & Paradowska-Gorycka, A. (2022). IL-1β, IL-10 and TNF-α polymorphisms may affect systemic lupus erythematosus risk and phenotype. *Clinical and Experimental Rheumatology, 40*(9), 1708–1717. https://doi.org/10.55563/clinexprheumatol/qdgq0v, https://www.clinexprheumatol.org/a.asp?IDArchivio=265.

Singh, N., Baby, D., Rajguru, J., Patil, P., Thakkannavar, S., & Pujari, V. (2019). Inflammation and cancer. *Annals of African Medicine, 18*(3), 121–126. https://doi.org/10.4103/aam.aam_56_18, http://www.annalsafrmed.org/backissues.asp.

Sloan, E. K., & Chang, A. (2025). Wired to spread: Neural regulation of metastasis. *Neuron, 113*(17), 2726–2728. https://doi.org/10.1016/j.neuron.2025.07.009, https://www.sciencedirect.com/science/journal/08966273.

Sribnick, E. A., Popovich, P. G., & Hall, M. W. (2022). Central nervous system injury-induced immune suppression. *Neurosurgical Focus, 52*(2). https://doi.org/10.3171/2021.11.FOCUS21586, http://thejns.org/action/showCoverGallery?journalCode=foc.

Sun, Y., Gao, L., Han, Y., Feng, C., Liu, Z., Li, C., Dong, Y., Yin, S., Liu, L., Yang, M., Niu, Q., Kong, D., Liu, L., Zhang, J., Tian, W., Luan, S., Li, L., & Hou, C. (2025). Activation of the CNGC2–CNGC4 channel complex by P2K1-mediated phosphorylation links extracellular ATP perception to calcium signaling in plant immunity. *Molecular Plant, 18*(7), 1130–1142. https://doi.org/10.1016/j.molp.2025.06.001.

Tanwar, V. S., Reddy, M. A., Dey, S., Malek, V., Lanting, L., Chen, Z., Ganguly, R., & Natarajan, R. (2025). Palmitic acid alters enhancers/super-enhancers near inflammatory and efferocytosis-associated genes in human monocytes. *Journal of Lipid Research, 66*(4), 100774. https://doi.org/10.1016/j.jlr.2025.100774.

Theis, A., & Harrison, M. M. (2023). Reprogramming of three-dimensional chromatin organization in the early embryo. *Current Opinion in Structural Biology, 81*, 102613. https://doi.org/10.1016/j.sbi.2023.102613.

Tian, D., Sun, Y., Zhou, J., & Ye, Q. (2021). The global epidemic of the SARS-CoV-2 delta variant, key spike mutations and immune escape. *Frontiers in Immunology, 12*. https://doi.org/10.3389/fimmu.2021.751778.

Tian, S., Liu, M., Han, S., Wu, H., Qin, R., Ma, K., Liu, L., Zhao, H., & Li, Y. (2025). Novel first-trimester serum biomarkers for early prediction of gestational diabetes mellitus. *Nutrition and Diabetes, 15*(1). https://doi.org/10.1038/s41387-025-00372-z, https://www.nature.com/nutd/.

Tisch, N., & Ruiz de Almodóvar, C. (2021). Contribution of cell death signaling to blood vessel formation. *Cellular and Molecular Life Sciences, 78*(7), 3247–3264. https://doi.org/10.1007/s00018-020-03738-x.

Valentini, E., D'Aguanno, S., Di Martile, M., Montesano, C., Ferraresi, V., Patsilinakos, A., Sabatino, M., Antonini, L., Chiacchiarini, M., Valente, S., Mai, A., Colotti, G., Ragno, R., Trisciuoglio, D., & Bufalo, D. D. (2022). Targeting the anti-apoptotic Bcl-2 family proteins: Machine learning virtual screening and biological evaluation of new small molecules. *Theranostics, 12*(5), 2427–2444. https://doi.org/10.7150/thno.64233.

Wang, M., Sunkel, B. D., Ray, W. C., & Stanton, B. Z. (2022). Chromatin structure in cancer. *BMC Molecular and Cell Biology, 23*(1). https://doi.org/10.1186/s12860-022-00433-6, https://bmcmolcellbiol.biomedcentral.com.

Wang, Y., Zhang, C., Yan, M., Ma, X., Song, L., Wang, B., Li, P., & Liu, P. (2024). PD-L1 regulates tumor proliferation and T-cell function in NF2-associated meningiomas. *CNS Neuroscience and Therapeutics, 30*(6). https://doi.org/10.1111/cns.14784, http://onlinelibrary.wiley.com/journal/10.1111/(ISSN)1755-5949.

Wang, Z., Li, Z., Han, C., Cheng, Y., & Wang, K. (2022). TRIM47 promotes glioma angiogenesis by suppressing Smad4. *In Vitro Cellular & Developmental Biology - Animal, 58*(9), 771–779. https://doi.org/10.1007/s11626-022-00722-6.

Wu, M. Y., Ge, Y. J., Wang, E. J., Liao, Q. W., Ren, Z. Y., Yu, Y., Zhu, G., Liu, C. P., Zhang, M. N., Su, H., Shen, H. M., Chen, Y., Wang, L., Wang, Y. T., Li, M., Bian, Z., Chai, J., Ye, R. D., & Lu, J. H. (2023). Enhancement of efferocytosis through biased FPR2 signaling attenuates intestinal inflammation. *EMBO Molecular Medicine, 15*(12). https://doi.org/10.15252/emmm.202317815, http://embomolmed.embopress.org/.

Xu, J., Jia, C., Qiu, Q., Qin, Y., Wang, Y., Wu, S., Li, W., Ren, S., & Wang, Y. (2025). NLRP3 proteins translocation into nuclei mediates SV40 T-antigen-induced corneal epithelial cell immortalization. *Experimental Eye Research, 258*, 110455. https://doi.org/10.1016/j.exer.2025.110455.

Yang, B., & Moss, J. (2023). Cell survival pathways targeted in rare lung disease affecting women. *Science Advances, 9*(19). https://doi.org/10.1126/sciadv.adi1215.

Yu, X., Mukwaya, V., Mann, S., & Dou, H. (2023). Signal transduction in artificial cells. *Small Methods, 7*(12). https://doi.org/10.1002/smtd.202300231.

Zhang, G., Ma, L., Bai, L., Li, M., Guo, T., Tian, B., He, Z., & Fu, Q. (2021). Inflammatory microenvironment-targeted nanotherapies. *Journal of Controlled Release, 334*, 114–126. https://doi.org/10.1016/j.jconrel.2021.04.018.

Zhang, L., Zhou, J., & Kong, W. (2025). Extracellular matrix in vascular homeostasis and disease. *Nature Reviews Cardiology, 22*(5), 333–353. https://doi.org/10.1038/s41569-024-01103-0.

Zhang, X., Zhang, L., Li, T., Zhang, Z., Shang, X., Bai, H., Liu, Y., Zong, X., Shang, C., Song, D., Zhang, X., Fan, L., & Liu, Z. (2024). Investigating bacteria-induced inflammatory responses using novel endometrial epithelial gland organoid models. *Frontiers in Reproductive Health, 6*. https://doi.org/10.3389/frph.2024.1490520.

Zhang, X., Li, B., Lan, T., Chiari, C., Ye, X., Wang, K., & Chen, J. (2025). The role of interleukin-17 in inflammation-related cancers. *Frontiers in Immunology, 15*. https://doi.org/10.3389/fimmu.2024.1479505.

Zhou, C., Wang, M., Zhang, C., & Zhang, Y. (2025). The transcription factor GABPA is a master regulator of naive pluripotency. *Nature Cell Biology, 27*(1), 48–58. https://doi.org/10.1038/s41556-024-01554-0.

CHAPTER

4

Micro/nano-modulation of inflammatory signaling pathways in cancer

Xilong Wu[1,2], *Yundi Wu*[1,2], *Cong Wang*[1], *Huanran Qu*[1,2], *and Ruocan Liu*[1,2]

[1]School of Biomedical Engineering, School of Pharmaceutical Sciences, Key Laboratory of Tropical Biological Resources of Ministry of Education, Hainan University, Haikou, P.R. China
[2]State Key Laboratory of Digital Medical Engineering, Hainan Engineering Research Center for Drug Screening and Evaluation, Collaborative Innovation Center of One Health, Hainan University, Haikou, P.R. China

4.1 Core mechanisms and biological implications of inflammatory signaling pathways in cancer

In 1863 German pathologist Rudolf Virchow first observed the infiltration of chronic inflammatory cells (including macrophages and lymphocytes) in tumor tissues, and based on this, proposed the classic hypothesis that chronic inflammation is the soil for cancer development (Balkwill & Mantovani, 2001). Based on systematic histopathological analysis, he established the disease progression framework of "inflammation-cell proliferation-carcinogenesis," laying the foundation for subsequent tumor inflammation theory. Limited by the level of development of microscopy in the 19th century, Virchow failed to reveal the molecular mechanisms behind the process, especially the regulatory roles of key inflammatory factors and their signaling pathways. It was not until the late 20th and early 21st centuries, driven by the rapid development of molecular biology and immunology techniques, that the theory was widely validated at the level of experimental evidence after more than a hundred years of silence (Balkwill et al., 2005; Coussens & Werb, 2002; Mantovani et al., 2008). Recently, a large number of basic studies and clinical data have consistently shown that inflammatory mediators and related signaling pathways serve as central drivers of the occurrence, growth, and treatment response of various tumors. According to statistics from the World Health Organization (WHO), about 15%–20% of

Inflammation in Tumorigenesis and Cancer Treatment
DOI: https://doi.org/10.1016/B978-0-443-36649-9.00007-4

human cancers are closely related to chronic inflammation, including liver cancer (hepatitis B/C-related), stomach cancer (*Helicobacter pylori* infection), and colorectal cancer (inflammatory bowel disease) (Akkız et al., 2025; Eden et al., 2016; Njunge et al., 2020; Wu, Xiao, et al., 2025). More importantly, persistent and unresolving dysregulated inflammation has been shown to significantly increase an individual's risk of cancer and accelerate the invasion and metastasis of tumors. In this context, immune cells, stromal cells, and tumor cells in the TME interact through a complex network of cytokines to form a self-sustaining procancer inflammatory state.

Chronic inflammation, a "booster" for tumor progression. In the chronic inflammatory microenvironment, nontumor cells such as tumor-associated macrophages (TAMs) and cancer-associated fibroblasts (CAFs) continuously release proinflammatory cytokines such as tumor necrosis factor-α (TNF-α) and interleukin-6 (IL-6). These factors significantly enhance the proliferation ability and antiapoptotic potential of tumor cells by activating key signaling pathways, including NF-κB and STAT3 (Li et al., 2022; Liu, Yang, et al., 2025; Tolomeo & Cascio, 2021; Yamaguchi et al., 2023). Moreover, chronic inflammation promotes tumor neovascularization through upregulation of vascular endothelial growth factor (VEGF), providing it with adequate nutrition and oxygen support, thereby promoting local infiltration and distant metastasis of the tumor. It is notable that the impact of inflammation on tumors is a typical "double-edged sword," and its biological effects are highly dependent on the duration, intensity, and microenvironmental background of the inflammation. Acute inflammation is the "first line of defense" of antitumor immunity. From a positive regulatory perspective, acute inflammation, as the body's natural defense mechanism against injury and infection, is critical for immune surveillance. When cells undergo genetic mutations or abnormal proliferation, damp-associated molecular patterns (DAMPs) are released, such as high mobility group protein B1 (HMGB1), ATP, and DNA fragments. These molecules can be recognized by pattern recognition receptors (PRRs) on the surface of innate immune cells (macrophages and neutrophils), triggering an inflammatory cascade. And recruit dendritic cells (DCs) to take up and present tumor antigens, thus activating tumor-specific adaptive immunity (Huang et al., 2022; Li & Kroemer, 2023; Ren et al., 2024). In addition, the moderate levels of reactive oxygen species (ROS) and reactive nitrogen species (RNS) released during inflammation not only participate in pathogen clearance but also enhance the phagocytic and cytotoxic activity of immune cells, further strengthening the antitumor immune response (Checa & Aran, 2020; Lin, 2019). This mechanism provides an important theoretical basis for tumor prevention strategies based on immune activation. The "double-edged sword" nature of inflammatory signaling pathways in clinical practice presents both prevention and treatment opportunities and severe challenges. On the one hand, interventions targeting chronic inflammation have been shown to be effective in reducing the incidence of certain cancers. For example, long-term use of nonsteroidal antiinflammatory drugscan significantly reduce the risk of colorectal cancer and gastric cancer by inhibiting cyclooxygenase-2 (COX-2) activity and reducing the synthesis of prostaglandin E_2 (PGE_2) (Cheng et al., 2024; Feng et al., 2021; Li et al., 2020) (Tacconel). On the other hand, exogenous-induced acute inflammation can enhance antitumor immunity by promoting DC maturation and effector T cell activation, providing the possibility of synergistic immunotherapy (Fu et al., 2025; Xu, Yu, et al., 2025). In summary, the study of tumor-inflammatory signaling pathways is not only a key entry point for understanding the intrinsic mechanisms of tumorigenesis and development but also provides a solid theoretical support for the development of novel targeted therapies and combined immunotherapies.

In the complex network of tumor inflammatory signaling pathways, there are multiple key signaling pathways, each playing a unique and important role. These pathways, by transmitting inflammatory signals, regulate immune cell infiltration, cell proliferation and apoptosis, angiogenesis, and other processes, ultimately affecting the malignant phenotype of tumors. The inflammatory signaling pathway simplicated in the regulation of the TME can be classified into the following four categories: (1) PRR pathways: Represented by the cyclic guanylate–adenylate synthase [cGAS]–STING pathway, which initiates an inflammatory cascade by sensing danger signals (DAMPs/pathogen-associated molecular patterns [PAMPs]) in the tumor microenvironment (TME). Specifically, cGAS acts as a cytoplasmic DNA sensor that recognizes free DNA fragments resulting from DNA leakage caused by tumor cell necrosis, radiotherapy, or chemotherapy, thereby catalyzing the generation of the second messenger cGAMP. The latter binds and activates the interferon gene-stimulating protein (STING), induces the expression of type I interferons (IFN-α/β) and proinflammatory cytokines, promotes DC activation and $CD8^+$ T cell infiltration, and plays a key role in antitumor immunity (Huang, Liang, et al., 2024; Wang, Zhang, et al., 2023). (2) Transcription factor-mediated pathways: The NF-κB signaling pathway, as the core hub of "inflammation-tumor" transformation, is continuously activated in a variety of solid tumors. On one hand, it maintains the chronic inflammatory microenvironment by upregulating proinflammatory factors (IL-6 and TNF-α); On the other hand, it directly regulates the expression of functional genes such as cyclin D1 (promoting cell cycle progression) and MMP9 (enhancing invasive ability), promoting malignant transformation of tumors (Cao et al., 2024; Lemieszek et al., 2019). Abnormal activation of NF-κB is also closely associated with chemotherapy resistance in digestive system tumors such as liver cancer and gastric cancer (Kumar et al., 2021; Li et al., 2024). In addition to the NF-κB signaling pathway, the mitogen-activated protein kinase (MAPK) pathway is a core pathway that receives upstream inflammatory signals and activates downstream transcription factors, including three subbranches: ERK, JNK, and p38. Although MAPK itself does not directly recognize DAMPs or cytokines, it can phosphorylate transcription factors such as c-Fos and c-Jun by responding to signaling molecules such as TNF-α and IL-1β released after activation by the TLR/NLR or cGAS–STING pathway through upstream kinase cascades such as MEK/MKK, regulating inflammation and oncogene expression (Wang, Wang, et al., 2025; Wu et al., 2024). The core function of the MAPK pathway is to promote the expression of inflammatory genes and oncogenes by phosphorylating downstream transcription factors. (3) Cytokine-mediated pathways: The JAK–STAT pathway is a classic executor of cytokine signaling, and its activation is strictly dependent on the binding of soluble factors such as IL-6 and IFN-γ to their transmembrane receptors. Receptor dimerization recruits and activates Janus kinase (JAK), which then phosphorylates the signal transducer and activator of transcription (STAT) protein. Phosphorylated STAT forms dimers that enter the nucleus, regulating the expression of a range of target genes involved in cell proliferation (c-Myc), antiapoptosis (Bcl-2), angiogenesis (VEGF), and immune escape (PD-L1, Treg amplification), and has become an important target for tumor treatment (Sim et al., 2024; Xue et al., 2023). (4) Metabolism-related inflammatory signaling pathways: The PI3K/AKT/mTOR pathway not only regulates cell growth and metabolism but is also deeply involved in inflammatory regulation. At the metabolic level, the pathway promotes aerobic glycolysis (Warburg effect) and protein synthesis in tumor cells by activating mTORC1 to meet the energy requirements for their rapid proliferation (Hoxhaj & Manning, 2019). At the inflammatory level, AKT can indirectly activate NF-κB by phosphorylating IκB kinase (IKK), promoting IL-6 and TNF-α secretion; Meanwhile, mTORC1 regulates the polarization direction of macrophages, tends to induce M2-type antiinflammatory/procancer phenotypes, and enhances the translation efficiency of inflammatory factors, thereby maintaining the immunosuppressive state of the TME (Sun et al., 2024; Xu et al., 2024). It is notable that the aforementioned pathways are tightly interconnected and collectively constitute a dynamic, malleable regulatory network through multilevel cross-dialogue that jointly drives tumorigenesis, immune escape, and treatment resistance.

4.2 Material design strategies for micro/nanotechnology to regulate inflammatory pathways in cancer

With the rapid development of micro/nanobiotechnology, functionalized micro/nanomaterials have become a frontier tool for precise intervention in tumor inflammatory signaling pathways due to their excellent designability, targeting, and biocompatibility. The current design strategies mainly revolve around the "direct intervention-indirect delivery-precise response" trinity framework, forming a complementary and synergistic regulatory system (Fig. 4.1).

4.2.1 Intrinsic micro/nanomaterials: direct regulation based on their own properties

Functional micro/nanomaterials do not load traditional drugs but directly target and regulate key nodes in the inflammatory pathway by their inherent physical properties (size, charge, etc.), chemical properties (catalytic activity, photosensitivity, acoustic sensitivity, etc.), or biological characteristics (biomimetic structure) to achieve "drug-free" antitumor effects.

Studies have shown that the size and morphology of nanomaterials significantly affect their cellular uptake pathways and subcellular localization, thereby influencing the localization, interaction, or biological effects of proteins related to inflammatory pathways (Gu et al., 2022; Zeng et al., 2025). Zhu et al. (2024) found that 30 nm diameter gold nanoparticles (Au NPs) could significantly inhibit the activation of NLRP3 inflammasomes by suppressing ROS generation and blocking NLRP3–NEK7 interactions, thereby reducing the release of IL-1β in bone marrow-derived suppressor cells (MDSCs). Further, the researchers designed an H6 peptide-modified Au-H6 NPs that specifically targeted MDSCs and showed significant tumor suppressor effects in colon cancer, lung cancer, and melanoma models, accompanied by increased infiltration of antitumor immune cells in the TME to reshape the TME. Liu's team systematically investigated the effect of iron oxide NP (IONPs) morphology on inflammasome activation. The study found that octapod-

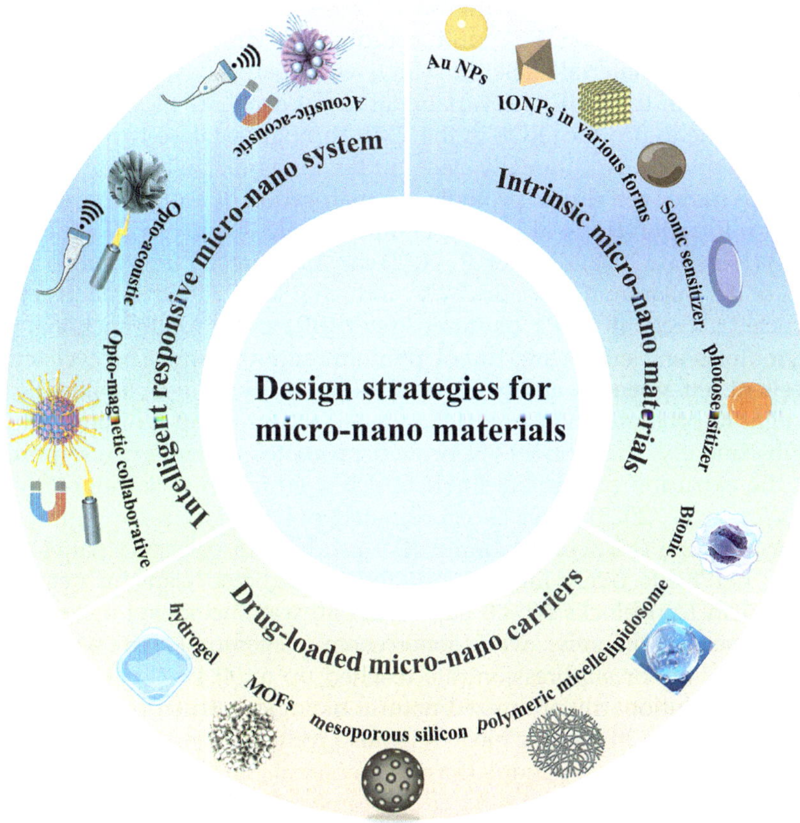

FIGURE 4.1 Design strategies for micro/nanomaterials. The current design strategies mainly revolve around the "direct intervention-indirect delivery-precise response" trinity framework, forming a complementary and synergistic regulatory system.

shaped and plate-shaped IONPs showed a stronger NLRP3 activation ability compared to cubic and spherical IONPs, and the mechanism was associated with higher ROS generation, lysosomal damage, and the degree of potassium efflux, suggesting that material morphology can be an important parameter for regulating immune response (Liu et al., 2018). Besides, the inherent chemical properties of functional micro/nanomaterials, such as enzyme-like activity, photosensitivity, and sonosensitivity, are critical in regulating tumor-associated inflammatory signaling pathways (Li et al., 2024; Xu et al., 2020; Xue et al., 2024). Nanomaterials with enzyme-like activity can intervene in inflammatory pathways by regulating REDOX balance, such as oxidase, peroxidase, catalase, superoxide dismutase, and glutathione peroxidase, by catalyzing the consumption/production of key ROS, RNS, or small-molecule signaling substances, direct regulation of REDOX balance or key molecules in inflammatory pathways. For example, materials based on variational metals such as Fe^{3+} (Sun, Ou, et al., 2019), Cu^{2+} (Ma et al., 2018), and Mn^{2+}(Ruan et al., 2021) can induce ferroptosis in tumor cells by generating ROS or consuming glutathione (GSH) through peroxidase-like or catalase-like activity. Li's team used porous metal-organic frameworks (MOFs) based on Fe^{3+} and coordinated with organic ligands containing disulfide bonds as the material skeleton. MnO_2 was coated on Fe-MOF and then loaded with procybrin (PB). In the TME, the variational metal elements Fe and Mn in the material consume glutathione to produce ROS in the TME through catalase-like activity and induce ferroptosis in tumor cells. Additionally, Mn^{2+} in the material can activate the cGAS–STING pathway, induce tumor cell death, promote the maturation of antigen-presenting cells, and increase T cell infiltration (Li et al., 2025). Photodynamic therapy (PDT) and sonodynamic therapy (SDT) (Hu et al., 2022; Zhou et al., 2022) can also directly intervene in key molecules or organelles of the inflammatory pathway by inducing ROS with exogenous energy. Wen's team constructed a cyclic BODIPY photosensitizer (BR) and a multifunctional platform for inducing pyroptosis and enhancing tumor photoimmunotherapy. The cyclization strategy gave BR excellent self-assembly ability (forming BR NPs, BRNs) and stability. BRNs produce ROS under light to promote mitochondrial damage, activate caspase-1 and induce GSDMD cleavage. Subsequently, the GSDMD-N protein promotes cell membrane pore formation, resulting in the extrusion of cytokines and DAMPs, which in turn induces immunogenic pyroptosis (Wen et al., 2025). Li et al. coordinated polymers of poly (γ-glutamic acid) (γ-PGA) grafted histidine (H) with platinum (IV) prodrug to construct nanosonosensitizers (PHPt). While PHPt effectively inhibits glutathione-mediated cisplatin detoxification, the addition of aspirin (As) blocks NF-κB signaling pathway, achieving a double reversal of cisplatin resistance. Ultimately, with sonodynamic chemotherapy without additional sonosensitizers, the tumor suppression rate reached up to 99.4% (Li et al., 2025). Drawing inspiration from evolutionarily optimized natural biological structures, the development of nanostructures derived with unique bioactivity also provides new impetus for the design of personalized antitumor micro/nanoplatforms (Liao et al., 2025; Zhang, Wang, et al., 2024). For example, several bacterial species-based antitumor strategies have entered clinical trials for antitumor treatment so far, yet achieving the best balance between antitumor efficacy and systemic safety remains an ongoing challenge. Wu's team coated an attenuated strain of *Salmonella typhimurium* expressing bacterial luciferase (*S.t. ΔppGpp/Lux*, denoted as *S.t.*) with a zirconium-based nano-MOF (UiO-66-NH_2) loaded with indocyanine green and the flavonoid luteolin through electrostatic interaction. A biological/abiotic hybrid nanoplatform was developed (Wu, Xiao, et al., 2025). The system enhances tumor targeting and penetration while using mild hyperthermia and autophagy to trigger ICD. Second, the system induces excessive autophagy, resulting in DAMPs release and promoting strong immunity. In addition, the ability of *S. typhimurium* to self-replicate and lyse tumor cells enhances cell-mediated immunity by promoting $CD8^+$ T cell infiltration.

4.2.2 Drug-loaded micro/nanocarriers: indirect regulation based on drug delivery

Drug-loaded micro/nanocarriers are one of the core strategies for regulating tumor inflammatory signaling pathways. Their primary strength resides in overcoming the drawbacks of conventional drug molecules such as low bioavailability, poor targeting, and high toxicity and side effects, and in achieving precise intervention on specific cells, subcellular organelles, and key nodes of specific inflammatory pathways. These vectors encapsulate small-molecule inhibitors, agonizts, nucleic acid drugs (siRNA, miRNA, mRNA, and DNA plasmids), gene editing tools (CRISPR–Cas9), and protein drugs, and combine active/passive targeting design, environmental response release, and other strategies. Significantly, increase the accumulation concentration and action efficiency of the drug at the tumor site, thereby achieving effective regulation of the inflammatory pathway.

Liposomes, as a classic nanodelivery system, have good biocompatibility and modifiability. The concept of liposomes was first proposed by Bangham in 1965 (Bangham et al., 1965). Liposomes are nanoscale, spherical vesicles composed of lipid bilayers that resemble biological membranes, typically ranging in size from 25 to 1000 nm. Liposomes self-assemble into a unique structure with a lipid membrane and a hydrophilic core, similar to the structure of cell membranes, which can be used to deliver hydrophobic and hydrophilic molecules and are biocompatible and biodegradable. Liposomes have properties such as enhanced solubility of encapsulated substances, reduced adverse reactions and toxicity of free drugs, flexible charge and size control, and the ability to be surface-modified (Han et al., 2025; Wang, Wang, et al., 2025; Zhao, Wu, et al., 2025). Yang, Wang, et al. (2025) designed a size-tunable micro/nanoliposome system PCAL@TM for targeted delivery of paclitaxel and oxygen to lung tumors. By interacting biotin–avidin with a matrix metalloproteinase-9 (MMP-9) cleavable linker, PtX-loaded coroxoic acid (CA) nanoliposomes (PCAL, 100 nm) were anchored to the surface of oxygen-containing perfluorotributylamine (TBA) loaded polyvesicular liposomes (TM, 10 μm). After intravenous administration to lung tumor-bearing mice, PCAL@TM exhibited markedly greater accumulation in the lungs compared to the liver and spleen. TM can rupture into smaller vesicles under vascular pressure and release oxygen, resulting in downregulation of HIF-1α and TGF-β. At the same time, PCAL can penetrate deep into tumors through the tumor-targeted penetrating CA liposomes, promoting a reduction in inflammation levels and enhancing PtX-induced immunogenic cell death.

Polymer micelles are also among the most watched nanocarriers in cancer theranostics. The polymer micelle structure is formed in aqueous solution by self-assembling amphiphilic block copolymers with spherical structures of hydrophobic nuclei and hydrophilic crowns. Hydrophobic drugs can be loaded at the center of the micelles. Polymer micelles as drug delivery carriers enhance drug solubility as well as improve drug stability and offer in vivo pharmacokinetic advantages over free drugs (Peng et al., 2025; Wang, Wang, et al., 2025; Wang, Zhang, et al., 2023). Li et al. (2020) developed a biomimetic polymer magnetic polymer micelle carrier that selectively targets and polarizes TAMs to enhance the immunotherapy effect of breast cancer. The polymer micelles are based on a highly biocompatible and fully biodegradable polylactic acolate-glycolate (PLGA) matrix and are loaded with Fe_3O_4 and Toll-like receptor 7 (TLR7) agonist imiquimod (R837) to form magnetic polymer NPs in the PLGA polymer micelles. After intracellular uptake, the polymer NPs, in synergy with Fe_3O_4 NPs and R837, can greatly polarize TAMs from the M2 phenotype to the antitumor M1 phenotype. Unlike previous reports, this polarization is attributed to Fe_3O_4 NPs activating the interferon regulatory factor 5 (IRF5) signaling pathway mainly through iron ions, rather than the reactive oxygen-induced NF-κB signaling pathway.

The drug-type micro/nanocarriers have also become important tools for tumor treatment, owing to their unique rigid structure, large specific surface area, tunable pore size, and excellent stimulus–response (Liu, Zhen, et al., 2019; Narayan et al., 2021; Ramos-Valle et al., 2025; Shanmugam & Jayaraman, 2025). They significantly enhance drug bioavailability by efficiently loading chemotherapeutic drugs, nucleic acids, or immunomodulators, combined with targeted modifications (such as folic acid [FA] and peptide ligands) and intelligent response designs (pH/light/magnetic trigger release), overcome the TME barrier, and regulate tumor-associated inflammatory pathways through drugs. Wang's team designed mesoporous silica nanocapsules (MSNCs) for codelivery of T-type Ca^{2+} channel siRNA and doxorubicin (DOX) to conquer drug-resistant breast cancer. MSNCs, with mesoporous/hollow structures and abundant primary amino groups, can efficiently load drugs and siRNA, and have pH-sensitive release properties (Wang et al., 2018). Through treatment experiments, the well-designed MSNCs achieved synergistic therapeutic effects on drug-resistant MCF-7/ADR cells by delivering a combination of siRNA and DOX, which was attributed to decreased expression of T-type Ca^{2+} channels and intracellular calcium ion concentration, cell cycle arrest at G0/G1, and increased intracellular drug accumulation. In addition, Qian et al. also developed a drug-hybrid silica framework based on a drug-skeleton hybridization strategy, and by integrating DOX into the framework, the researchers achieved superior interface performance compared to traditional structures. The hybrid system enabled drug delivery during the operation and demonstrated excellent tumor attachment ability, hemostatic performance, and immune activation effects mediated by TLR4 (Qian et al., 2025).

MOFs are a special class of organic-inorganic hybrid materials composed of metal ions and organic ligands. Due to their diverse structure, large pore size, and specific surface area, high loading capacity, and inherent biodegradability, MOFs have shown unique advantages in the field of tumor diagnosis and treatment (Fang et al., 2023; Rajeev et al., 2025; Yan, Hu, et al., 2025). Yu's team designed an acid-responsive iron/manganese bimetallic organic framework nanosystem loaded with metal ions and the immune adjuvant R848 (FeMn@R@H) and used it in combination with pyroptosis and enhanced immunotherapy. In an acidic TME, FeMn@R@H is triggered to decompose to release Fe^{3+} and Mn^{2+} ions, thereby initiating a Fenton-like reaction for ROS-mediated pyroptosis. Pyroptosia-induced cell rupture induces tumor cells to release proinflammatory cytokines and immunogenic components, further leading to immunogenic cell death, promoting the antitumor immune response. Meanwhile, the codelivery of R848 reverses the inhibitory tumor immune microenvironment by activating the TLR7/8 pathway and induces an inflammatory response (Feng et al., 2023).

Organic micro/nano drug delivery systems are also an important part of the field of drug delivery carriers, among which hydrogel-based drug delivery systems have become one of the most representative carrier types in this class due to their unique physicochemical properties and biocompatibility (Xiao et al., 2025; Yu et al., 2023). Lin's team (Yıldırım et al., 2025) developed an injectable hydrogel designed to boost antitumor effects and suppress postoperative recurrence and metastasis. The PSBMA polymer was synthesized via free radical polymerization and, driven by electrostatic forces, self-assembled in saline into a hydrogel exhibiting resistance to protein adsorption. This platform was coloaded with tumor-targeting NPs (M/CuO/DOX) and the STING agonist 2′,3′-cGAMP to construct the final system (Gel@M/CuO2/DOX/STING). The interaction between DOX and CDT markedly induces tumor cell apoptosis and restores recognition of tumor antigens. The released agonist, along with DOX-triggered DNA damage, activates the STING signaling pathway, leading to increased production of type I interferons. These immune mediators facilitate DC maturation, enhance infiltration of tumor-specific T cells, and support prolonged modulation of the TIME.

4.2.3 Intelligent responsive micro/nanosystems: precise regulation based on external physical fields

With the continuous evolution of tumor immunotherapy and targeted intervention strategies, how to achieve precise spatiotemporal control of inflammatory signaling pathways has become one of the core challenges in current research. While traditional drug delivery or static nanoplatforms can improve pharmacokinetics and targeting to some extent, they often struggle to achieve on-demand release, site-specific activation, and multimodal synergistic regulation in the face of highly heterogeneous and dynamically evolving TMEs. For this reason, intelligent responsive micro/nanosystems have emerged. The core design concept is to introduce external physical stimuli as "switches" to perceive and transform external energy input, thereby triggering internal structural changes or functional responses of nanomaterials, ultimately achieving precise, controllable, and reversible intervention in inflammatory signaling pathways. These systems not only break through the limitations of traditional passive targeting, but also endow the treatment process with unprecedented dynamic regulation capabilities, marking an important transition from static to dynamic in precision oncology. At present, the external physical fields applied to intelligent responsive micro/nanosystems mainly include three categories: light (Han et al., 2025; Liu, Zhen, et al., 2019; Song, Guan, et al., 2024; Wang, Wang, et al., 2025), acoustic (Wu et al., 2023; Yang, Wang, et al., 2025; Zhou et al., 2021), and magnetism (Liu, Yang, et al., 2025; Wang et al., 2024; Xiong et al., 2025), as well as multiple stimulus–response (Liu, Yang, et al., 2025; Qu et al., 2025; Silva et al., 2023; Yang et al., 2023), each with its unique advantages and applicable tumor model treatment. Intelligent responsive micro/nanosystems achieve spatiotemporal dynamic intervention of tumor inflammatory pathways by integrating the energy of external physical fields such as light, magnetism, and sound, as well as multiple stimuli. These systems utilize the local energy conversion (such as thermal/mechanical force) generated by functionalized materials under external field stimulation to trigger signal molecule regulation and precisely control key inflammatory pathways. Intelligent responsive micro/nanosystems, starting from the intrinsic properties of materials, drug delivery efficiency, and external controllability, provide multiple technical approaches to address issues such as insufficient specificity, significant side effects, and poor controllability in the regulation of cancer-related inflammation, and jointly promote the clinical transformation of micro/nanomaterials in antiinflammatory treatment of cancer.

Light-magnetic synergy platform: Integrating light–stimulus–responsive materials with magnetic NPs in the same carrier, it can achieve targeted enrichment through magnetic fields and photothermal or photodynamic effects through near-infrared (NIR) illumination. The combination of the two can not only significantly reduce the shortcomings of a single mode, but also achieve dynamic regulation of tumor-inflammatory pathways. Liu, Yang, et al. (2025) developed a dual-magnetically driven ultrasmall nanozyme $Mo_{0.2}Fe_{2.8}O_4@CeO_x$/FA (MFCF), which exhibited multiple enzyme-like activities and dual responsiveness to AMF and static magnetic fields, in synergy with FA-mediated molecular targeting. Enhanced blood–brain barrier penetration and achieved high-precision glioblastoma localization. Under simultaneous exposure to AMF and NIR laser irradiation, the nanozyme amplifies ROS production, depletes glutathione, alleviates hypoxia, and achieves dynamic regulation of the hypoxia pathway and ferroptosis pathway by synergistic magnetothermal effects, PDT, and its inherent multienzyme catalytic activity. In addition, macrophage polarization can be reprogrammed to a proinflammatory M1 phenotype based on the nanozyme. Further activating systemic immunity, quantifying serum cytokines by ELISA, MFCF showed the highest secretion of proinflammatory cytokines (IL-6 and IL-12) under dual stimulation of laser and magnetic field, significantly reduced levels of antiinflammatory cytokine IL-10, and elevated levels of antitumor cytokines TNF-α and IFN-γ. This indicates that the intelligent responsive nanosystem, under the precise regulation of the external physical field, can effectively reverse the immunosuppressive TME, release inflammatory factors, and activate systemic antitumor immunity.

Photoacoustic coupling platform: utilizing the cascade of ultrasound-responsive and photoresponsive materials to construct a "acousto-photo-dynamic" cascade reaction chain. This strategy ingeniously circumvented the problem of insufficient light penetration depth, enabling photothermal therapy (PTT)/PDT to be applied to deep tumors. For example, Lv et al. developed a Schottky heterojunction model composed of Ti_3C_2 (TC) and $BaTiO_3$ TC@BTO, and the Schottky interface enables the integration of the two tumor ablation modalities, SDT and PTT, in a dynamic state. After successive ultrasound and NIR irradiation, the Schottky heterojunction enhanced TC@BTO promoted the accumulation of Fe^{2+}, ROS, and lipid ROS in osteosarcoma cells, ultimately inducing cell ferroptosis and eradicating osteosarcoma. In addition, in the static state, the Schottky heterojunction promotes superior carrier mobility, thereby enhancing the efficacy of bone regeneration by activating the Wnt signaling pathway (Lv et al., 2023).

Magneto-acoustic platform: Under the combined effect of an alternating magnetic field and NIR laser, the magneto-acoustic platform not only achieves the superposition of thermal effect and ROS effect but also enhances the activity of magneto-acoustic platform-like enzymes through magneto-thermal and ultrasound, further increasing ROS production and regulating the corresponding inflammatory pathway. The Jiang team developed a biodegradable $ZnFe_2O_4$@Pt@PEG-GOx NP (ZFPG NPs) with five types of enzyme activity, good sonosensitivity, and significant magnetic targeting properties, which is beneficial for sonoelectrometal-immunotherapy of prostate cancer in male mice. The magnetic targeting ability effectively improved their accumulation in tumors while still showing enrichment in the liver and kidneys. The multienzyme cascade catalysis and photosensitivity of these NPs effectively consumed glutathione and glucose and enhanced H_2O_2 production, thereby inducing multiple ROS bursts. In addition, these combined effects upregulate HMOX1 to promote Fe^{2+} and lipid peroxide accumulation, thereby inducing immunogenic ferroptosis. Exploring the potential mechanisms of multiphysical field synergistic therapy at the genetic level through animal RNA sequencing, it was found that after ZFPG+US treatment, significant changes occurred in genes associated with multiple inflammatory and metabolic pathways such as MAPK signaling pathway, PI3K–AKT signaling pathway, oxidative phosphorylation (OXPHOS), cell homeostasis, ferroptosis, p53 signaling pathway, glutathione metabolism, etc. (Wang, Wang, et al., 2025).

To sum up, intelligent responsive micro/nanosystems represent the direction of the next generation of precision anticancer platforms. The advantages lie in: (1) achieving spatio-temporal controllability of the treatment process; (2) support for multimodal synergistic treatment to enhance the therapeutic effect; (3) it can induce persistent antitumor immune memory and prevent recurrence and metastasis. However, the field still faces many challenges, such as insufficient long-term biosafety assessment, complex large-scale preparation processes, and unclear clinical translational pathways. Future studies should prioritize the design of highly biocompatible stimuli–responsive materials, establishing standardized stimulation parameter systems, and promoting the development of intelligent closed-loop control systems (such as combining wearable devices to monitor physiological indicators in real time and automatically adjust stimulation intensity) to truly realize the ideal vision of "treatment on demand."

4.3 Micro/nanotechnology for the regulation of key inflammatory signaling pathways

Inflammatory signaling networks in the TME form the "information superhighway" that drives malignant progression of tumors. Understanding and precisely intervening in these pathways is at the core of developing a new generation of antitumor therapies. Micro/nanotechnologies, with their programmable material properties and precise delivery capabilities, offer an unprecedented toolkit for targeting and regulating these complex pathways. The following will delve into the molecular mechanisms of the five core pathways and the corresponding micro/nano intervention strategies.

4.3.1 NF-κB pathway

This is the core hub of the connection between inflammation and cancer. Nuclear factor kappa B (NF-κB) is a transcription factor dimer composed of the Rel protein family (such as p65/RelA, p50, and RelB). The NF-κB pathway plays a typical "double-edged sword" role in tumors, and its tumor suppressive effect is mainly achieved by regulating the cell cycle, apoptosis, immune microenvironment, and characteristics of tumor stem cells (Catz & Johnson, 2001; Guldenpfennig et al., 2023; Haselager et al., 2021; Khan et al., 2024; Sun et al., 2013). The NF-κB pathway is composed of classical and nonclassical pathways (Iacobazzi et al., 2023; Liu et al., 2017; Mao et al., 2025; Shih et al., 2012), as shown in Fig. 4.2. Typical NF-κB signaling is activated by a variety of immune receptors, including B-cell receptor, T-cell receptor, TLR, interleukin-1 receptor (IL-1R), and tumor necrosis factor receptor (TNFR). These receptors initiate signal cascade reactions (e.g., CARMA1/BCL10/MALT1 or TAK1/TAB complexes) that converge on the IKK complex (IKKα/IKKβ/NEMO). IKKβ's phosphorylation of IκBα triggers its ubiquitination and proteasome degradation, releasing the p50/RelA dimer for nuclear translocation. The pathway drives the expression of genes for survival, inflammation, and immune response. Nonclassical NF-κB signaling is mainly

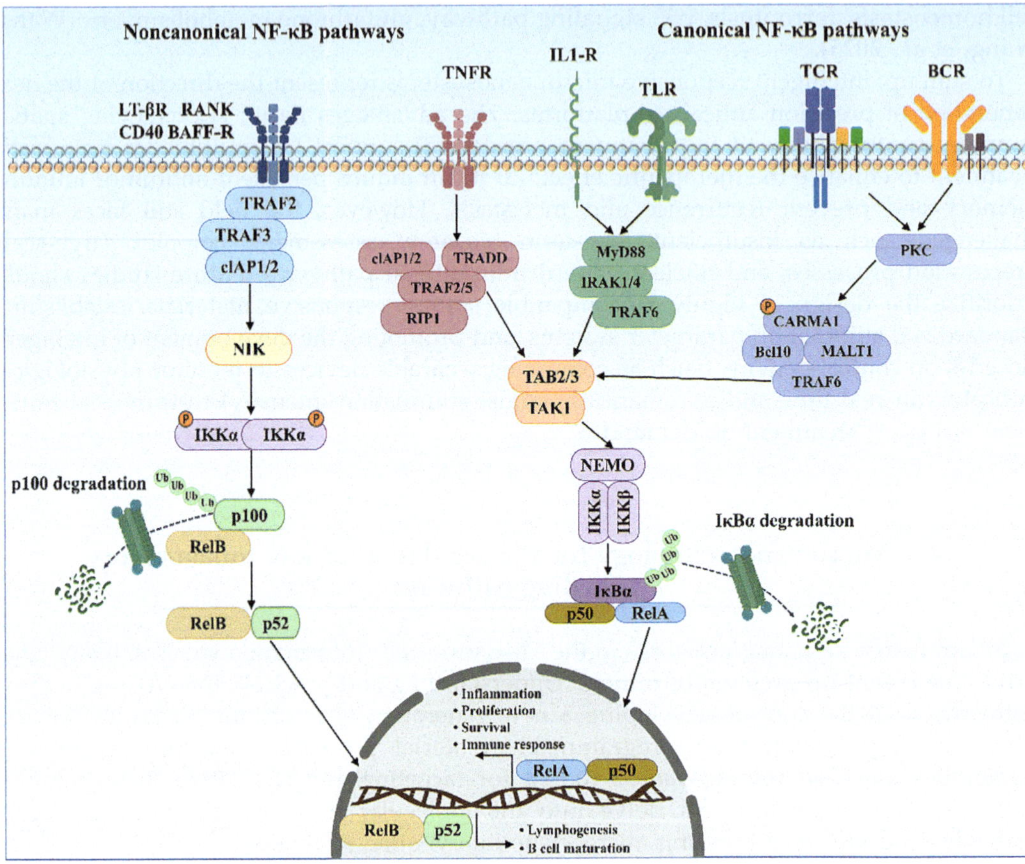

FIGURE 4.2 Schematic diagram of the activation mechanisms and biological functions of classical and nonclassical NF-κB signaling pathways. The NF-κB pathway is composed of classical and nonclassical pathways. *BCR*, B-cell receptor; *TCR*, T-cell receptor; *TLR*, toll-like receptor; *TNFR*, tumor necrosis factor receptor.

triggered by ligand binding of TNFR superfamily members such as CD40, RANK, LT-βR, and BAFF-R, which stabilize NF-κ B-induced kinase (NIK) by disrupting the c-IAP/TRAF2/3 E3 ubiquitin ligase complex. NIK activates IKKα, phosphorylates NF-κB2 precursor p100 and triggers its conversion to p52 through proteasome processing. The p52/RelB dimer translocates to the nucleus, where it regulates genes that are crucial for lymphoid organogenesis, B lymphocyte survival, and maturation. Micro/nanotechnologies targeting the NF-κB pathway mainly focus on the "blocking activation—inhibiting transcription-reshaping the microenvironment" trinity strategy. Wang's team, considering that ion inflows and outflows are strictly regulated by ion channels on the cell membrane, used a strategy of chelating L-phenylalanine (L-Phe) nanostructures with metal ions to modulate the electrophysiological behavior of DCs for enhancing the immune checkpoint blockade (ICB) immunotherapy effect (Tan et al., 2024). L-Phe chelated metal ions ($Mg^{2+}/Fe^{2+}/Zn^{2+}$)

to build three different pH-responsive nanostructures (Ph-Mg nanospheres /Ph-Fe nanoneedles /Ph-Zn nanosheets). After disintegrating in the lysosomal acidic environment, it induces Ca^{2+} influx through K^+ efflux, activates the calmodulin-dependent NF-κB pathway, and synergizes with cathepsin B-triggered inflammatome activation to promote DC maturation and proinflammatory factor secretion, enhancing the ICB effect. Hou's team developed a TME-responsive core-shell structured polymer nanomodulator n(Cat)-Smac-PEG. The catalase (Cat) core decomposes H_2O_2 in the tumor acidic microenvironment to relieve hypoxia, downregulates HIF-1α, and then upregulates the endogenous apoptotic initiation $protein_2$ Sm_2ac. The exogenous Smac peptide on the NP surface synergizes with the endogenous Smac to antagonize the inhibitor of apoptosis proteins. Blocking caspase inhibition and weakening NF-κB-mediated prosurvival signaling ultimately breaks the "hypoxia-apoptosis escape" positive feedback loop and significantly enhances radiosensitivity, offering a novel approach to overcoming resistance to radiotherapy (Hou et al., 2025). A cationic antitumor and anticancer NP (denoted as mt-NP) developed by Tang et al. can specifically anchor and disrupt $cell^{Bodipy}$ membrane stability under NIR light irradiation of PDT, photoimmunotherapy, and NIR-II fluorescence bioimaging. This unique design ensures that quaternary ammonium cations can interact directly with cell membranes, causing cell membrane instability. In addition, $mt\text{-}NP^{Bodipy}$ generates a large amount of ROS under continuous light exposure, leading to lipid peroxidation and further instability of the cell membrane, and fighting tumors by activating a strong immune response. RNA sequencing analysis showed that CT26 cells treated with $mt\text{-}NP^{Bodipy}$ plus laser irradiation significantly affected cell cycle, DNA replication, homologous recombination, and a range of immune and inflammation-related NF-κB signaling pathways, etc. (Tan et al., 2024). The Wang's team constructed a codelivery system of aggregation-induced emission luminescent source AIEgen (TPE-Py) and mitochondrial-targeted naphthalenhydroquinone dimer Rubioncolin C (RC). RC improves tumor hypoxia by inhibiting OXPHOS, enhancing PDT efficiency of TPE-Py. Simultaneously, RC can inhibit the NF-κB signaling pathway and act synergistically with the burst of ROS to trigger tumor cell apoptosis, offering a promising therapeutic approach for triple-negative breast cancer (Wang et al., 2022).

4.3.2 Janus kinase–signal transducer and activator of transcription pathway

The JAK–STAT signaling pathway is an important cellular signal transduction mechanism, mainly involving the transmission of external signals such as cytokines, hormones, and growth factors (Boengler et al., 2008; O'shea et al., 2015; Stark & Darnell, 2012; Valle-Mendiola et al., 2023; Xin et al., 2020; Yu et al., 2009). The main components of this pathway are JAK (Janus kinase) and STAT (signal transducer and activator of transcription) proteins. The activation and negative regulation of the JAK–STAT signaling pathway are shown in Fig. 4.3. Activation of the JAK/STAT signaling pathway: It is currently known that nearly 60 cytokines, including interleukins (ILs), colony-stimulating factors, hormone-like cytokines, and growth factors, initiate transcription through the JAK–STAT pathway as their primary and essential mode of transcription (Brooks et al., 2014; Hu, Zhang, et al., 2021; Kramer et al., 2006; Krause et al., 2006). First, cytokines and growth factors bind to their respective receptors, leading to the recruitment of receptor dimers and associated JAKs. Second, JAK activation leads to tyrosine phosphorylation of the receptor and the formation of

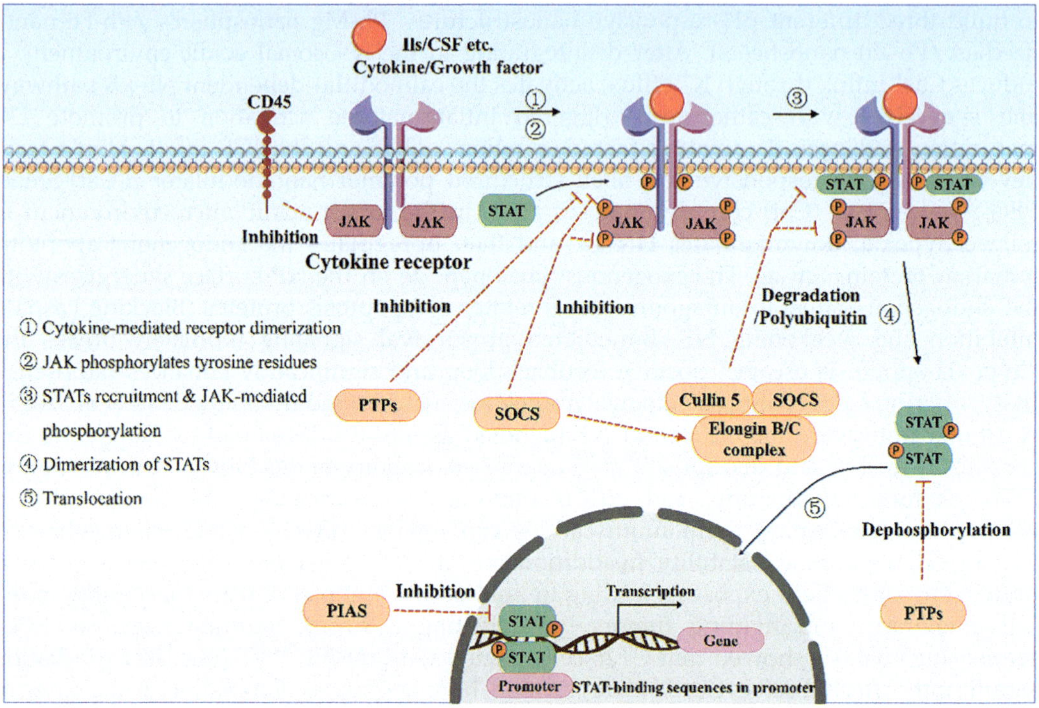

FIGURE 4.3 Schematic diagram of the activation process of the JAK–STAT signaling pathway and its multiple negative regulatory mechanisms. The activation and negative regulation of the JAK–STAT signaling pathway are shown in Figure 3.3. *CSF*, Colony-stimulating factor.

STAT docking sites; again, STAT is phosphorylated by tyrosine. Further, STAT dissociates from the receptor to form homodimers or heterodimers. Finally, the STAT dimer enters the nucleus, binds to DNA, and regulates transcription. The negative regulation involved in the AK-STAT signaling pathway mainly includes PIAS (activated STAT protein suppressor), CIS/SOCS (cytokine signal suppressor family), and PTPs (protein tyrosine phosphatases) (Frankson et al., 2017; Kershaw et al., 2013; Liang, Li, et al., 2024; Seif et al., 2017). PIAS mainly interacts with STAT dimers to inhibit STAT binding to DNA, thereby blocking JAK–STAT signal transduction. The most typical example is SHP-1. The CIS/SOCS family negatively regulates the JAK/STAT pathway in three ways: (1) binding to tyrosine kinase receptors to prevent STAT recruitment; (2) binding directly to JAK and inhibiting its kinase activity; and (3) forming the elongin B/C-cullin5 complex to degrade JAK or STAT bound to SOCS proteins through polyubiquitination and proteasome degradation. PTPs inhibit the JAK/STAT pathway by interacting with JAK, STAT, or receptors: (1) dephosphorylating the STAT dimer; (2) interacting with the receptor to dephosphorylate the associated JAK; and (3) CD45 (a transmembrane PTP) inhibits the phosphorylation of JAK. The JAK–STAT pathway is a vital signal transduction pathway within cells. It acts like a bridge connecting the external environment of the cell to the internal gene expression, providing a continuous power for the cell's life activities. The JAK–STAT signaling pathway is a chain of interactions between intracellular proteins that are involved in processes such as immunity, cell division, cell death, and tumor formation. This pathway transmits extracellular chemical signals to the nucleus, activating genes through transcriptional processes. Zhao's team designed a Cu_2O/V_2C/Cur heterojunction system that synergistically activates antitumor immunity through a sonodynamic-enhanced copper death mechanism, significantly enhancing the therapeutic effect on breast cancer. The study innovatively utilized the interface electric field of the heterojunction to enhance the piezoelectric catalytic effect, thereby strengthening the sonodynamic performance. Simultaneously, by down-regulating the expression of copper death-related genes and activating the JAK–STAT pathway, mitochondrial Cu^{2+} super-accumulation was induced to amplify the copper death effect. Further confirmed that the system can reshape the TME and achieve a triple synergy of sonodynamic–copper death–immunotherapy, providing a new strategy for overcoming the insufficiency of tumor immunogenicity (Zhao, Wu, et al., 2025). Zheng's team constructed a surface-exposed IFN-γ gene modified bacterial bionic vesicle (BBV) and used a nanoassembled membrane pore structure. Engineered IFN-γ BBVS have nanoscale protein and lipid vesicle structures with abundant PAMPs and costimulations of introduced IFN-γ molecules. In vitro, IFN-γ BBV may reprogram M2 macrophages to M1 through NF-κB and JAK–STAT signaling pathways, release NO and inflammatory cytokines IL-1β, IL-6, and TNF-α, and increase the expression of IL-12 and iNOS. In tumor-bearing mice, IFN-γ BBV showed targeted enrichment in tumors and successfully reprogrammed TAMs to the M1 phenotype (Zheng, He, et al., 2024). IFN-γ-modified BBV, which has strong tumor-targeting ability and the ability to modulate cold tumors to heat through reprogramming TAMs, provides an effective approach for tumor immunotherapy. Xu et al. designed a biodegradable organic molecule ferroelectric nanoplatform (C60-TCNQ, CT) to promote effective ferroelectrocatalysis, thereby enhancing tumor immunotherapy through apoptosis and ferroptosis. CT-mediated ultrasound-triggered ferroelectrocatalysis promotes ferroelectric polarization and significantly increases ROS production, leading to massive apoptosis of tumor cells. The polycyano groups of CT NPs selectively react with cysteine under mild conditions, leading to redox imbalance and accumulation of lipid peroxides, which helps induce ferroptosis in tumor cells. Furthermore, CT-induced apoptosis and ferroptosis stimulate the progression of immunogenic cell death, triggering a strong immune response. RNA sequencing analysis indicated that CT treatment led to downregulation of genetic profiles associated with the immune-related JAK–STAT signaling pathway (Xu, Yu, et al., 2025). The study opens up a new path for the development of organic molecule ferroelectric nanomedicines for tumor immunotherapy. Yan et al. designed and prepared NP interferon-γ (nano-IFN-γ) using a bisphosphonate mineralization strategy. In the final stage of radiofrequency ablation surgery, the mineralized nano-IFN-γ was dispersed in alginate gels and injected into peripheral tumors. IFN-γ promotes the transdifferentiation of TAMs from M2 to M1 through the IFNγ receptor-mediated JAK/STAT1 signaling pathway. Due to the persistence of NPs and gels, IFN-γ can remain in the residual tumor site for a long time and exert its immunomodulatory effect, while avoiding its systemic toxicity and adverse reactions in normal peripheral tissues (Yan, Hu, et al., 2025). The JAK–STAT signaling pathway has become an important target for cancer drug development. In cancer treatment, targeting the JAK–STAT pathway can inhibit tumor growth, metastasis, angiogenesis, and, in autoimmune diseases, it can reduce inflammation and abnormal activation of immune cells.

4.3.3 Cyclic guanylate–adenylate synthase–interferon gene-stimulating protein pathway

The cGAS–STING signaling pathway is a signaling pathway that plays a key role in the innate immune system and is the core regulatory network for cytoplasmic DNA triggering immune responses (Briard et al., 2020; Han et al., 2025; Harding et al., 2017; Shen et al., 2015; Yu et al., 2022; Zheng et al., 2020). The activation mechanism is shown in Fig. 4.4: (1) Sensing and initiation: Cytoplasmic DNA sensor cGAS recognizes abnormal double-stranded DNA (dsDNA). These dsDNAs may originate from pathogen infection, genomic instability, or treatment-induced cell damage (such as nuclear DNA or mitochondrial DNA [mtDNA] leakage caused by radiotherapy/chemotherapy). After dsDNA is identified, the cGAS undergoes conformational changes and is activated. (2) Second messenger synthesis: After cGAS activation, the cyclic dinucleotide second messenger 2′,3′-cGAMP is catalyzed using ATP and GTP as substrates. (3) STING activation and translocation: cGAMP binds and activates the interferon gene-stimulating factor (STING) located on the endoplasmic reticulum (ER) membrane. Binding induces conformational changes in STING, driving its

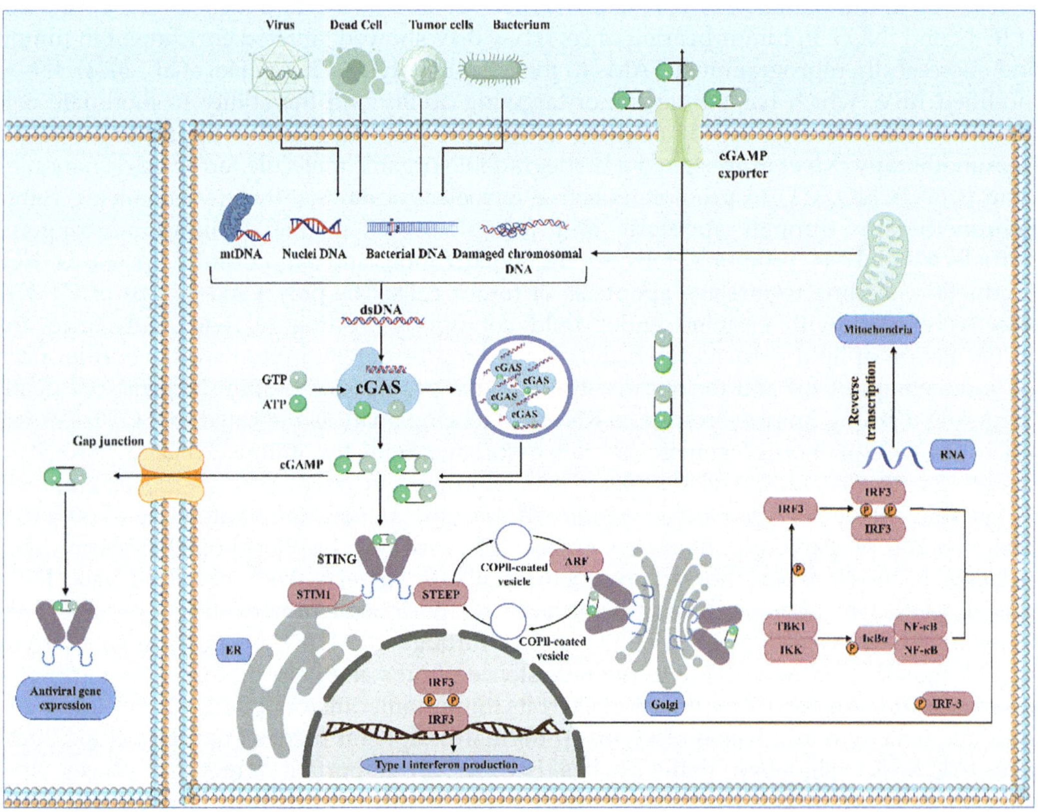

FIGURE 4.4 Schematic diagram of the cyclic guanylate–adenylate synthase (cGAS)–STING signaling pathway. The activation mechanism is shown in Figure 3.4. *dsDNA*, Double-stranded DNA; *mtDNA*, mitochondrial DNA.

transport from the ER to the Golgi apparatus. In the Golgi, STING undergoes palmitoylation modification. (4) Signal cascade amplification and effects: STING recruits and activates Tank-binding kinase 1 (TBK1). TBK1 phosphorylates the C-terminal domain of STING and simultaneously phosphorylates interferon regulatory factor 3 (IRF3). Phosphorylated IRF3 forms a dimer, translocates into the nucleus, and initiates the transcription of type I interferon (IFN-I) genes. In addition, the STING-TBK1 signaling axis also activates NF-κB, coinducing the expression of IFN-I and a variety of proinflammatory cytokines. (5) Immune response and remodeling: Secreted IFN-I collaborates to activate a wide range of immune effects through its downstream JAK–STAT signaling pathway, including antigen-presenting cell maturation, T cell activation, enhanced killing activity of NK cells, and antibody production. By bridging innate and adaptive immunity, the activation of the cGAS–STING pathway can remodel the immunosuppressive TME into an immune-activated state, making it a highly promising target for cancer immunotherapy (Zhang et al., 2020). Wang et al. designed a functional nanosheet (Ti_3C_2@Au-PEG-DMXAA) based on Ti_3C_2 MXene, with gold NPs attached to the surface, modified with polyethylene glycol and loaded with STING agonizts (DMXAA). Improving the tumor immune microenvironment by activating the cGAS–STING signaling pathway in immune cells and mild PTT (mPTT) before cryoablation (CRA). The synergistic effects of mPTT and STING pathway activation promote immunogenic death of tumor cells, activation of DCs, repolarization of TAMs, and enrichment of cytotoxic T cells in the TME. Subsequently, sequential CRA eradicates the local "hot" tumor by gradually releasing tumor-associated antigens in situ, initiates the "cancer vaccine" effect, enhances systemic antitumor immunity, and effectively generates long-term immune memory, thereby suppressing tumor recurrence and distant metastasis (Wang, Wang, et al., 2025). An increasing number of studies have shown that activating the cGAS–STING pathway with the help of nanomaterials can effectively stimulate tumor immune responses and exert effective antitumor effects (He et al., 2021; Li, Jiang, et al., 2022; Li, Ren, et al., 2022; Zhang et al., 2023). Tian et al. developed a nanoadjuvant formed by metal coordination self-assembly of Mn ions and pH-sensitive phenolic polymers (PEG-b-Pho), which also included acoustic-sensitive polymers (PEG-b-IR) and glutathione inhibitors. The SDT-mediated ICD effect binding to the Mn ion promotes the activation of the cGAS–STING pathway and significantly enhances DC maturation. In particular, the nanoadjuvant enhanced the sensitivity of tumors to ICI treatment, thereby effectively inhibiting distant tumor progression and metastasis (Tian et al., 2022). In addition, Chen's team also used manganese-based nanomaterials as STING agonizts to effectively regulate the cGAS–STING pathway, thereby triggering the activation of the host immune system. In the study, the manganese ferrite nanohybrid $MnFe_5O_8$@(M1M-DOX) was used to activate cGAS–STING and NF-κB crosstalk in DCs and TAMs. $MnFe_5O_8$ acts as a source of Fe^{2+}/Fe^{3+} and Mn^{2+}, and the release of these ions has an intrinsic dual immunomodulatory effect on the activation of DCs and the reprogramming of TAMs from M2 phenotype to M1 phenotype. Fe^{2+}/Fe^{3+} activates the NF-κB signaling pathway, triggering the activation of the STING signaling pathway. Meanwhile, Mn^{2+} further enhances STING activation in a cascading manner and stimulates NF-κB. Therefore the mutually enhanced dual activation of cGAS–STING and NF-κB crosstalk promotes the vigorous maturation of DCs and TAMs, synergistically promoting T cell infiltration, thereby inhibiting primary tumor growth and local recurrence (Chen, Fei, et al., 2025). Chen's group developed pegylated manganese-doped calcium sulfide NPs (MCSP) that, through gas-amplified metal immunotherapy, dual-activate pyroptosis and STING pathways, effectively enhancing the antitumor immune response in cervical cancer (Li et al., 2024). Bioactive MCSP can rapidly release Ca^{2+}, Mn^{2+}, and H_2S in response to the TME. H_2S disrupts the calcium buffering system of cancer cells by interfering with the OXPHOS pathway, leading to pyroptosis caused by calcium overload. On the other hand, H_2S-mediated mitochondrial dysfunction further promotes the release of mtDNA and enhances the activation of Mn^{2+} on the cGAS–STING signaling axis, thereby activating immunosuppressed DCs. The released H_2S acts as an important synergist between Mn^{2+} and Ca^{2+}, bridging innate and adaptive immune responses by modulating dual signaling mechanisms. The study reveals potential synergies between H_2S gas therapy and metal immunotherapy and provides ideas for designing nanoimmunomodulators to improve the tumor immunosuppressive microenvironment. The cGAS–STING pathway has emerged as a highly promising target for therapeutic interventions and has gained significant momentum in tumor biology and anticancer treatment, and the integration of nanomaterials holds great potential for advancing the development of STING agonizts and expanding their future applications.

4.3.4 Mitogen-activated protein kinase pathway

The MAPK signaling pathway plays a crucial role in biological processes such as cell response to external stimuli, regulation of cell proliferation, differentiation, survival, and stress response. The three classic subfamilies of the MAPK signaling pathway include ERK (extracellular signal-regulated kinases), JNK (amino-terminal kinases), and p38 MAPK, each of which plays a significant role in different biological functions and pathological processes (Cheng et al., 2020; Duan et al., 2017; Sui et al., 2023; Wang, Zhang, et al., 2023; Xie et al., 2018). Persistent activation of MAPK signaling has been found in many malignancies. The RAS–RAF–MEK–ERK signaling pathway is the most important of the MAPK signaling pathways (transmitting extracellular stimulatory signals into the cell to regulate a variety of physiological functions of the cell, including proliferation, differentiation, survival, apoptosis, and migration). It plays a key role in a variety of physiological and pathological processes such as proliferation, differentiation, survival, migration, and apoptosis of cells (Guo et al., 2020; Moon & Ro, 2021; Shi et al., 2024; Soleimani et al., 2019; Zheng, He, et al., 2024).

The activation mechanism of the RAS–RAF–MEK–ERK signaling pathway (Fig. 4.5): extracellular growth factors (such as epidermal growth factor EGF and platelet-derived growth factor PDGF) bind to receptor tyrosine kinases (RTKs) on the cell membrane, causing dimerization and self-phosphorylation of RTKs. Phosphorylated RTKs provide binding sites for proteins containing the SH2 domain, such as GEFs. When GEFs bind to RTKs, it promotes the binding of RAS proteins to GTP and activates them. The activated RAS protein recruits and activates RAF protein, and the activated RAF protein phosphorylates MEK protein to activate it. The activated MEK protein further phosphorylates the ERK protein, and the activated ERK protein enters the nucleus and phosphorylates a variety of transcription factors (such as Elk-1 and c-Myc), which, when activated, can regulate the expression of genes related to cell proliferation, differentiation, etc.

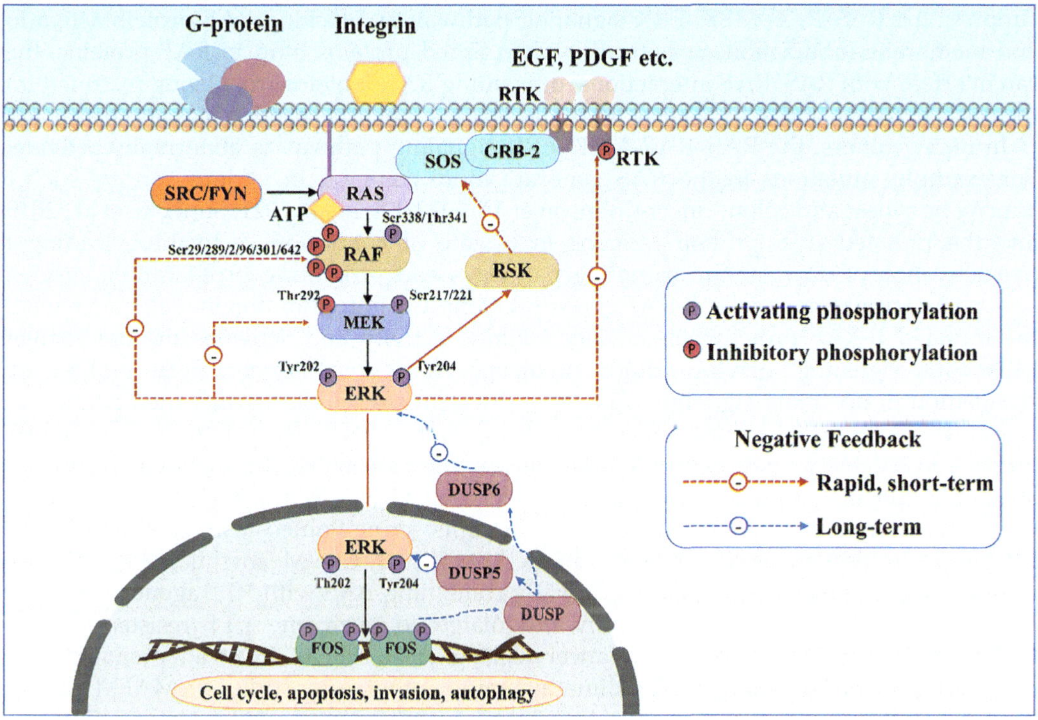

FIGURE 4.5 Schematic diagram of the activation, regulation, and downstream biological effect mechanisms of the mitogen-activated protein kinase signaling pathway. The activation mechanism of the RAS–RAF–MEK–ERK signaling pathway.

The inhibition mechanism of the RAS–RAF–MEK–ERK signaling pathway: (1) Feedback regulation mediated by ERK: Activated ERK can phosphorylate upstream RAF proteins. When activated, ERK can phosphorylate multiple sites of the C-RAF protein. This phosphorylation can inhibit the activity of RAF protein, thereby creating a negative feedback regulation of the RAS–RAF–MEK–ERK signaling pathway. This is because RAF protein is the key kinase in the signaling pathway, and the inhibition of its activity weakens the signaling of the entire signaling pathway. Additionally, ERK can also regulate the activity of RAS proteins. Activated ERK can phosphorylate and activate RAS–GAP (GTP-activating protein), which promotes the hydrolysis of GTP by RAS protein, transforming it from the activated GTP-bound state to the nonactivated GDP-bound state, thereby reducing the activation of RAS protein and inhibiting the conduction of signaling pathways. (2) Endogenous protein inhibitor: Sprouty proteins (such as Sprouty1 and Sprouty2) are important endogenous inhibitors. They are mainly located near the cell membrane and can bind directly to growth factor receptors. When growth factors activate RTKs, Sprouty proteins can inhibit RTK-mediated RAS activation. For example, Sprouty proteins can compete with GEFs (guanine nucleotide exchange factors) for binding sites and prevent GEFs from activating RAS proteins, thereby suppressing the initiation stage of the signaling pathway. Spred proteins (such as Spred1 and Spred2) can bind to RAF proteins. They suppress the RAS–RAF–MEK–ERK signaling pathway by blocking RAF protein activation and membrane localization. Specifically, when Spred proteins bind to RAF proteins, they can interfere with RAS–RAF interactions, preventing RAF proteins from being recruited into the cell membrane and activated by RAS proteins, thereby interrupting signal transduction.

In many tumors, the RAS–RAF–MEK–ERK signaling pathway is abnormally activated. For example, mutations in the RAS gene are more common in various cancers such as pancreatic cancer and colon cancer (Johnson et al., 2022; Lin et al., 2021; Sun, Ou, et al., 2019), and the mutated RAS protein remains in a state of continuous activation, leading to overactivation of downstream signaling pathways and promoting proliferation, survival, and metastasis of tumor cells. B-RAF gene mutations are more common in melanoma, where the mutated B-RAF protein has sustained kinase activity and activates the downstream MEK–ERK signaling, driving tumor occurrence and development, even without the stimulation of upstream signaling. Zheng's team delivered photothermal therapeutics and artesunate (ARS) to CAFs and cancer cells using aminoethylanisamide-modified nanobiomimetic low-density lipoprotein (A-aLDL) in combination with PTT, achieving significant antitumor effects in multiple models. Serine metabolism was found to play a major role in CAF resistance through spatial omics. ARS disrupts serine homeostasis, thereby reducing the cascade activity of small G proteins in the MAPK pathway. Meanwhile, MAP2K7 is the most promising target for sensitizing PTT. By combining ARS with PTT agents, the serine-MAPK axis in CAFs was successfully modulated to overcome PTT resistance in the treatment of triple-negative breast cancer (Zheng et al., 2025). Li et al. prepared PEG-modified polymethacrylate 2-(*N*,*N*-dimethylamino) ethyl ester (PEG-PDMAEMA)-based NPs (NP-PTPN6) loaded with protein tyrosine phosphatase nonreceptor type 6 (PTPN6). It was subsequently conjugated with atezolizumab (aPD-L1), a monoclonal antibody against programmed death ligand 1 (PD-L1) (aPD-L1NP-PTPN6). The antitumor effect assessment showed that aPD-L1NP-PTPN6 had a stronger ability to inhibit the growth, invasion, and migration of colorectal cancer cells compared with other treatments and ultimately prolonged the survival time of tumor-bearing mice. Further mechanistic studies showed that treatment of colorectal cancer cells with aPD-L1NP-PTPN6 significantly inhibited the MAPK–ERK signaling pathway (Li et al., 2020). Abnormal activation of specific proteins in the MAPK signaling pathway is a significant cause of various cancers. Therefore therapeutic intervention in this signaling pathway is an effective tumor treatment strategy.

4.3.5 PI3K–AKT–mTOR pathway

The phosphatidylinositol 3-kinase (PI3K)–AKT–mTOR pathway is one of the most common activation pathways in human cancers (Jian et al., 2018; Pierobon et al., 2017; Qian et al., 2025). Under physiological conditions, the pathway is activated by insulin, growth factors, and cytokines, and regulates key metabolic processes, including glucose metabolism, macromolecular biosynthesis, and maintaining REDOX balance to support systemic metabolic dynamic balance and growth and metabolism of individual cells (Fig. 4.6). Oncogenic activation of the PI3K–AKT–mTOR pathway in cancer cells reprograms cellular metabolism by enhancing the activity of nutrient transporters and metabolic enzymes, thereby supporting the anabolic requirements of abnormally growing cells (Hu, Zhang, et al., 2021; Janku et al., 2018; King et al., 2015). As shown in Fig. 4.7, in the inactive

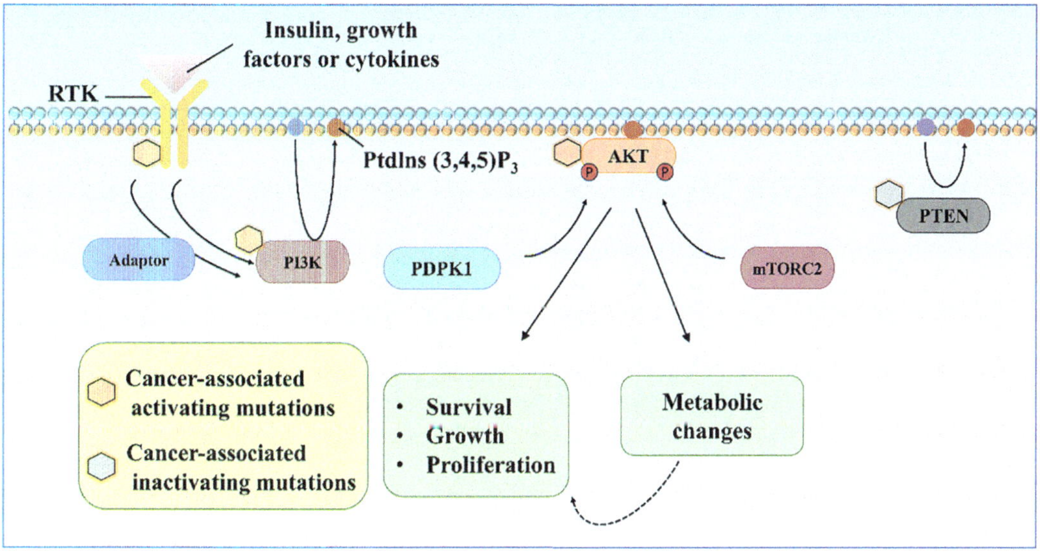

FIGURE 4.6 Diagram of the activation of the PI3K–AKT–mTOR signaling pathway. Under physiological conditions, the pathway is activated by insulin, growth factors, and cytokines and regulates key metabolic processes, including glucose metabolism, macromolecular biosynthesis, and maintaining REDOX balance to support systemic metabolic dynamic balance and growth and metabolism of individual cells.

state of the PI3K–AKT–mTOR pathway, the catalytic subunit p110 of PI3K forms a heterodimer with the regulatory subunit p85, thereby inhibiting the activation of PI3K. Under physiological conditions, the SH2 domain in the p85 regulatory subunit of PI3K is "occupied" to prevent it from binding to the catalytic subunit p110, thus transforming PI3K from an inactive state to an activated one, influenced by stimulators such as upstream growth factors and cytokines (such as insulin automatically released by elevated blood glucose in the human body). This will further catalyze PIP2 downstream to produce PIP3, which then transmits signals down to activate AKT and mTOR components downstream, opening up pathways for cell growth and survival. Due to the importance of the PI3K–AKT–mTOR pathway, abnormal activation of the pathway directly promotes tumor cell growth and reduces tumor cell senescence. The abnormal activation of the pathway is usually mediated by the amplification of component gene mutations within the pathway, the loss or inactivation of the tumor suppressor PTEN (homologous phosphatase-tensin), and the activation of PI3K upstream proto-oncogenes such as RAS in the ERK/MAPK pathway (Totan et al., 2020). Yao's group previously discovered that abnormal expression of the PI3K subunit p85β protein could activate the PI3K–AKT–mTOR pathway to induce tamoxifen resistance, and based on this, they jointly constructed two-dimensional copper-palladium (2D-CuPd) nanozymes with oxygenase-like activity and peroxidase-like activity. 2D-CuPd degrades the PI3K subunit p85β protein by generating ROS and inhibits the activity of the PI3K/AKT/mTOR signaling pathway, thereby reversing tamoxifen resistance. To verify its ability to reverse tamoxifen resistance in both tamoxifen-resistant breast cancer cell line animal models and human tumor xenograft models (Jiang et al., 2023).

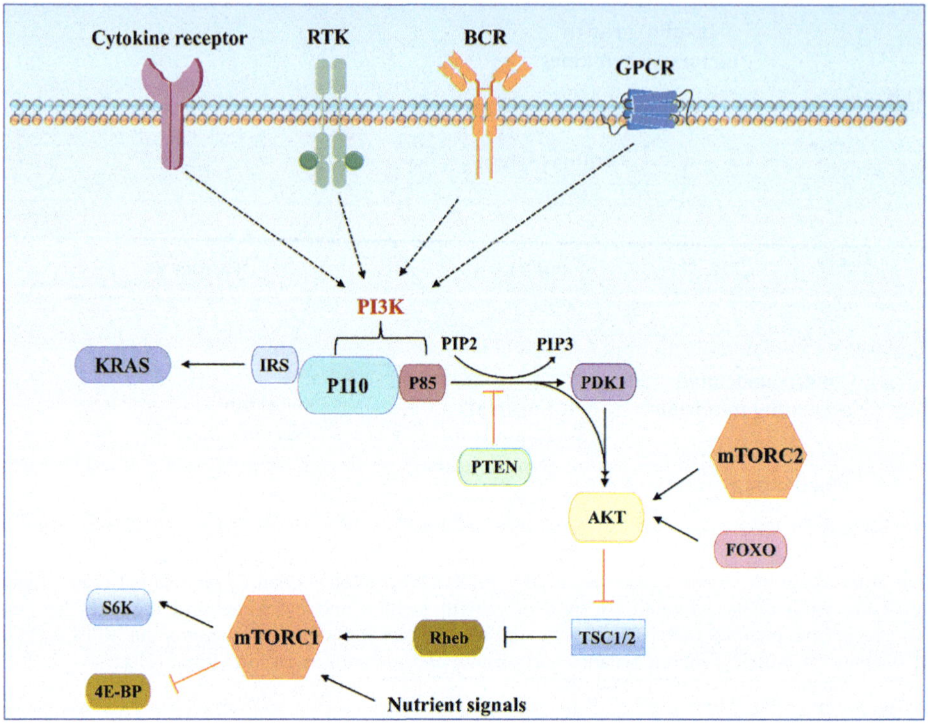

FIGURE 4.7 Schematic diagram of the multireceptor activation and downstream regulatory mechanisms of the PI3K–AKT–mTOR signaling pathway. In the inactive state of the PI3K–AKT–mTOR pathway, the catalytic subunit p110 of PI3K forms a heterodimer with the regulatory subunit p85, thereby inhibiting the activation of PI3K. *BCR*, B-cell receptor.

Likewise, Cui's team designed a microenvironment responsive NP that uses the decomposition products of the ZR-metal-organic skeleton (Zr-MOF) to suppress cisplatin resistance, thereby suppressing the PI3K–AKT–mTOR pathway in tumor cells and overcoming cisplatin resistance in A549R cells (Song, Guan, et al., 2024). Li et al. developed a novel 450 nm laser-mediated sodium porphyrin (DVDMS)-based PDT therapy that induces significant growth inhibition and apoptosis induction in vitro by generating excessive ROS, and the laser-mediated PDT (BL-PDT) also induces autophagic flux in GC cells. Through transcriptomic analysis and functional studies, it was determined that the ROS–PI3-K–AKT–mTOR pathway was involved in regulating BL-PDT-induced autophagy (Li et al., 2022). The Wang team designed a photosensitive lipid NP (LNP) formulation for the combined delivery of FSP1 siRNA with the photosensitizer verteporfin to achieve a synergistic effect in immunotherapy for colon cancer. Photosensitive LNPs (FSP1/LNPs) initiate synergistic ferroptosis effects in colon cancer cells by silencing the FSP1 gene and generating ROS. This mechanism further induces ICD and tumor antigen release, thereby promoting DC maturation and CTL activation. RNA sequencing analysis showed that signaling pathways such as cholesterol metabolism, IL-17, apoptosis, and PI3K–AKT were significantly affected after FSP1/LNPs treatment. These pathways are involved in lipid peroxidation, cellular REDOX balance, and cell proliferation in colon cancer cells. The study confirmed that FSP1 gene silencing and PDT have significant synergistic effects in colon cancer cells, opening up new avenues for the clinical translation of photosensitive lipid NPs in cancer treatment (Liu, Yang, et al., 2025). The PI3K–AKT pathway acts like the "metabolic commander" of cancer cells—it not only commands to "grow fast" but also personally arranges food, fuel, and building materials to allow cancer cells to multiply infinitely. Cutting off its chain of command or cutting off its food supply is the new battlefield for us to fight cancer.

4.4 Summary and outlook

This chapter systematically reviews the research progress of micro/nanotechnology in regulating cancer-related inflammatory signaling pathways, forming a complete research framework from mechanism analysis, material design to pathway intervention. At the mechanism level, the pivotal roles of five core pathways NF-κB, JAK–STAT, cGAS–STING, MAPK, and PI3K–AKT–mTOR in the "inflammation-canceration" transformation of tumors are clarified, revealing their "double-edged sword" characteristics—providing signal support for acute antitumor immunity It can also drive tumor proliferation, immune escape, and therapeutic resistance in the chronic inflammatory microenvironment, providing a theoretical anchor for targeted intervention. In terms of pathway intervention mechanisms, micro/nanotechnology can do so by directly targeting key molecules (such as inhibiting NF-κB nuclear translocation and activating the cGAS–STING pathway), reshaping the TME (such as polarization of M2-type macrophages to M1-type and promoting $CD8^+$ T cell infiltration), and coordinating multiple therapeutic modalities. Multidimensional regulation of the inflammatory signaling network is achieved, providing new pathways to overcome tumor heterogeneity and treatment resistance. However, the field still faces key challenges: first, the long-term biosafety assessment is insufficient, and the in vivo metabolic mechanisms and potential immunogenicity of some nanomaterials remain unclear; second, clinical translation bottlenecks. Existing studies are mostly based on ideal models, and the penetration efficiency of complex physiological barriers (such as the blood–brain barrier) and large-scale preparation processes still need to be optimized; third, it is difficult to precisely regulate the cross-dialogue of pathways. A single pathway intervention is prone to trigger compensatory activation, and a multipathway coordinated regulation strategy needs to be strengthened.

Future research could focus on three directions: first, develop biodegradable/metabolizable intelligent response materials and build a "monitoring-regulation" closed-loop system in combination with wearable devices to achieve "treatment on demand"; second, deepen the application of single-cell sequencing and spatial omics technology to analyze the dynamic evolution of inflammatory pathways in the tumor-heterogeneous microenvironment and guide the design of personalized nanomedicines; third, promote interdisciplinary integration, explore the synergistic mechanisms of micro/nanotechnology with gene editing and microbiological therapy, and provide a new paradigm for the clinical translation of cancer inflammation-targeted therapy.

References

Akkız, H., Şimşek, H., Balcı, D., Ülger, Y., Onan, E., Akçaer, N., & Delik, A. (2025). Inflammation and cancer: Molecular mechanisms and clinical consequences. *Frontiers in Oncology, 15*. https://doi.org/10.3389/fonc.2025.1564572.

Boengler, K., Hilfikerkleiner, D., Drexler, H., Heusch, G., & Schulz, R. (2008). The myocardial JAK/STAT pathway: From protection to failure. *Pharmacology & Therapeutics, 120*(2), 172–185. https://doi.org/10.1016/j.pharmthera.2008.08.002.

Balkwill, F., Charles, K. A., & Mantovani, A. (2005). Smoldering and polarized inflammation in the initiation and promotion of malignant disease. *Cancer Cell, 7*(3), 211–217. https://doi.org/10.1016/j.ccr.2005.02.013.

Balkwill, F., & Mantovani, A. (2001). Inflammation and cancer: Back to virchow? *Lancet, 357*(9255), 539–545. https://doi.org/10.1016/s0140-6736(00)04046-0.

Bangham, A. D., S, M. M., & Watkins, J. C. (1965). Diffusion of univalent ions across the lamellae of swollen phospholipids. *Journal of Molecular Biology, 3*, 238–252. https://doi.org/10.1016/s0022-2836(65)80093-6.

Briard, B., Place, D. E., & Kanneganti, T.-D. (2020). DNA sensing in the innate immune response. *Physiology, 35*(2), 112–124. https://doi.org/10.1152/physiol.00022.2019.

Brooks, A. J., Dai, W., O'Mara, M. L., Abankwa, D., Chhabra, Y., Pelekanos, R. A., Gardon, O., Tunny, K. A., Blucher, K. M., Morton, C. J., Parker, M. W., Sierecki, E., Gambin, Y., Gomez, G. A., Alexandrov, K., Wilson, I. A., Doxastakis, M., Mark, A. E., & Waters, M. J. (2014). Mechanism of activation of protein kinase JAK2 by the growth hormone receptor. *Science (New York, N.Y.), 344*(6185). https://doi.org/10.1126/science.1249783, http://www.sciencemag.org/content/344/6185/1249783.full.pdf.

Cao, Y., Yi, Y., Han, C., & Shi, B. (2024). NF-κB signaling pathway in tumor microenvironment. *Frontiers in Immunology, 15*. https://doi.org/10.3389/fimmu.2024.1476030.

Catz, S. D., & Johnson, J. L. (2001). Transcriptional regulation of bcl-2 by nuclear factor κB and its significance in prostate cancer. *Oncogene, 20*(50), 7342–7351. https://doi.org/10.1038/sj.onc.1204926.

Checa, J., & Aran, J. M. (2020). Reactive oxygen species: Drivers of physiological and pathological processes. Journal of Inflammation Research, *13*, 1057–1073. https://doi.org/10.2147/jir.S275595.

Chen, H., Wang, D., Liu, J., Chen, J., Hu, Y., & Ni, Y. (2025). Augmenting antitumor immune effects through the coactivation of cGAS-STING and NF-κB crosstalk in dendritic cells and macrophages by engineered manganese ferrite nanohybrids. ACS Applied Materials and Interfaces, *17*(9), 13375–13390. https://doi.org/10.1021/acsami.4c18570.

Chen, J., Fei, S., Cao, Z., Liu, X., Ji, W., Chen, H., Niu, Y., & Yang, Z. (2025). Tumor microenvironment metabolism-modulating nanomedicines for enhancing anti-tumor immunity. *Small (Weinheim an der Bergstrasse, Germany)* e09685. https://doi.org/10.1002/smll.202509685.

Chen, M., Winston, D. D., Wang, M., Niu, W., Cheng, W., Guo, Y., Wang, Y., Luo, M., Xie, C., Leng, T., Qu, X., & Lei, B. (2022). Hierarchically multifunctional bioactive nanoglass for integrated tumor/infection therapy and impaired wound repair. Materials Today, *53*, 27–40. https://doi.org/10.1016/j.mattod.2022.01.019.

Cheng, L., Hu, Z., Gu, J., Li, Q., Liu, J., Liu, M., Li, J., & Bi, X. (2024). Exploring COX-independent pathways: A novel approach for meloxicam and other NSAIDs in cancer and cardiovascular disease treatment. *Pharmaceuticals, 17*(11), 1488. https://doi.org/10.3390/ph17111488.

Cheng, M., & Dou, H. (2022). Nano-assemblies based on biomacromolecules to overcome cancer drug resistance. Polymer International, *71*(4), 371–378. https://doi.org/10.1002/pi.6310.

Cheng, Y., Sun, F., Wang, L., Gao, M., Xie, Y., Sun, Y., Liu, H., Yuan, Y., Yi, W., Huang, Z., Yan, H., Peng, K., Wu, Y., & Cao, Z. (2020). Virus-induced p38 MAPK activation facilitates viral infection. *Theranostics, 10*(26), 12223–12240. https://doi.org/10.7150/thno.50992.

Coussens, L. M., & Werb, Z. (2002). Inflammation and cancer. *Nature, 420*(6917), 860–867. https://doi.org/10.1038/nature01322.

D'ambrosio, A., Bressan, D., Ferracci, E., Carbone, F., Mulè, P., Rossi, F., Barbieri, C., Sorrenti, E., Fiaccadori, G., Detone, T., Vezzoli, E., Bianchi, S., Sartori, C., Corso, S., Fukuda, A., Bertalot, G., Falqui, A., Barbareschi, M., Romanel, A., ... Chiacchiera, F. (2024). Increased genomic instability and reshaping of tissue microenvironment underlie oncogenic properties of Arid1a mutations. *Science Advances, 10*(11). https://doi.org/10.1126/sciadv.adh4435 eadh4435.

Dong, X., Xia, S., Du, S., Zhu, M., Lai, X., Yao, S. Q., Chen, H., & Fang, C. (2023). Tumor metabolism-rewriting nanomedicines for cancer immunotherapy. ACS Central Science, *9*(10), 1864–1893. https://doi.org/10.1021/acscentsci.3c00702.

Du, F., Zhao, H., Song, Y., Feng, Z., Liu, K., Wang, Z., Guo, R., Qiu, L., Chen, Q., & Zhou, L. (2024). Apoptosis-sensitizing tumor nanomedicine by regulating pyroptosis-associated inflammatory cell death. Advanced Functional Materials, *34*(44), 2406150. https://doi.org/10.1002/adfm.202406150.

Duan, B., Niu, H., Zhang, W., Ma, Y., Yuan, Y., & Liu, C. (2017). Microporous density-mediated response of MSCs on 3D trimodal macro/micro/nano-porous scaffolds via fibronectin/integrin and FAK/MAPK signaling pathways. *Journal of Materials Chemistry B, 5*(19), 3586–3599. https://doi.org/10.1039/c7tb00041c, http://pubs.rsc.org/en/journals/journalissues/tb.

Eden, C. O., Edwards, D. K., Eide, C. A., Traer, E., Tyner, J. W., McWeeney, S. K., & Agarwal, A. (2016). Cytokine-mediated inflammatory pathways promote clonal evolution and disease progression in acute myeloid leukemia. *Blood, 128*(22), 1688. https://doi.org/10.1182/blood.v128.22.1688.1688 1688.

Fang, Y., Huang, S., Hu, Q., Zhang, J., King, J. A., Wang, Y., Wei, Z., Lu, J., He, Z., Kong, X., Yang, X., Ji, J., Li, J., Zhai, G., & Ye, L. (2023). Injectable zwitterionic physical hydrogel with enhanced chemodynamic therapy and tumor microenvironment remodeling properties for synergistic anticancer therapy. *ACS Nano, 17*(24), 24883–24900. https://doi.org/10.1021/acsnano.3c05898, http://pubs.acs.org/journal/ancac3.

Feng, Y., Tao, L., Wang, G., Li, Z., Yang, M., He, W., Zhong, X., Zhang, Y., Yang, J., Cheung, S., McDonald, F., & Chen, L. (2021). Aspirin inhibits prostaglandins to prevents colon tumor formation via down-regulating Wnt production. *European Journal of Pharmacology, 906*, 174173. https://doi.org/10.1016/j.ejphar.2021.174173.

Feng, Z., Chen, G., Zhong, M., Lin, L., Mai, Z., Tang, Y., Chen, G., Ma, W., Li, G., Yang, Y., Yu, Z., & Yu, M. (2023). An acid-responsive MOF nanomedicine for augmented anti-tumor immunotherapy via a metal ion interference-mediated pyroptotic pathway. *Biomaterials, 302*, 122333. https://doi.org/10.1016/j.biomaterials.2023.122333.

Frankson, R., Yu, Z.-H., Bai, Y., Li, Q., Zhang, R.-Y., & Zhang, Z.-Y. (2017). Therapeutic targeting of oncogenic tyrosine phosphatases. *Cancer Research, 77*(21), 5701–5705. https://doi.org/10.1158/0008-5472.can-17-1510.

Fu, Y., Duan, B., Zheng, P., Chu, H., Li, W., Yang, Y., Yang, Z., He, J., Wang, M., Li, S., Ding, Y., Ruan, B., Bai, J., Luo, Y., Hu, Y., Liu, Q., Long, Q., & Ma, Y. (2025). Genetically modified bacterial vesicles with interferon-γ and tumor antigen remodel anti-tumor cellular immunity by modulating dendritic cells. *Biomaterials, 324*, 123524. https://doi.org/10.1016/j.biomaterials.2025.123524.

Graván, P., Marchal, J. A., & Galisteo-González, F. (2025). Improving tumor treatment: Cell membrane-coated nanoparticles for targeted therapies. Materials Today *Bio, 32*, 101716. https://doi.org/10.1016/j.mtbio.2025.101716.

Gu, D., Qiao, Y., Fu, H., Zhao, H., Yue, X., Wang, S., Yin, Y., Xi, R., Fu, X., Zhao, X., & Meng, M. (2022). Size-controllable DNA origami-stacked gold nanoparticles for deep tumor-penetrating therapy. *ACS Applied Materials and Interfaces, 14*(33), 38048–38055. https://doi.org/10.1021/acsami.2c05750, http://pubs.acs.org/journal/aamick.

Gu, Z., Liu, T., Liu, C., Yang, Y., Tang, J., Song, H., Wang, Y., Yang, Y., & Yu, C. (2021). Ferroptosis-strengthened metabolic and inflammatory regulation of tumor-associated macrophages provokes potent tumoricidal activities. *Nano Letters, 21*(15), 6471–6479. https://doi.org/10.1021/acs.nanolett.1c01401.

Guldenpfennig, C., Teixeiro, E., & Daniels, M. (2023). NF-κB's contribution to B cell fate decisions. *Frontiers in Immunology, 14*, 1214095. https://doi.org/10.3389/fimmu.2023.1214095.

Guo, Pan, Liu, Shen, Xu, & Hu (2020). ERK/MAPK signalling pathway and tumourigenesis. *Experimental and Therapeutic Medicine, 19*, 1997–2007. https://doi.org/10.3892/etm.2020.8454.

Han, X., Cheng, Y., Wan, D., Alu, A., Zhang, Z., Bi, Z., Wang, M., Tang, Y., Hong, W., Chen, S., Chen, L., & Wei, Y. (2025). Enhancing antitumor immunity through the combination of cholesterolized TLR7 agonist liposomes and radiotherapy: A role for IL-1β and the inflammasome pathway. *Cancer Communications, 45*(7), 794–812. https://doi.org/10.1002/cac2.70024.

Harding, S. M., Benci, J. L., Irianto, J., Discher, D. E., Minn, A. J., & Greenberg, R. A. (2017). Mitotic progression following DNA damage enables pattern recognition within micronuclei. *Nature, 548*(7668), 466–470. https://doi.org/10.1038/nature23470, http://www.nature.com/nature/index.html.

Haselager, M., Thijssen, R., West, C., Young, L., Van Kampen, R., Willmore, E., Mackay, S., Kater, A., & Eldering, E. (2021). Regulation of Bcl-XL by non-canonical NF-κB in the context of CD40-induced drug resistance in CLL. *Cell Death & Differentiation, 28*(5), 1658–1668. https://doi.org/10.1038/s41418-020-00692-w.

He, G., Mei, C., Chen, C., Liu, X., Wu, J., Deng, Y., & Liao, Y. (2024). Application and progress of nanozymes in antitumor therapy. *International Journal of Biological Macromolecules, 265*, 130960. https://doi.org/10.1016/j.ijbiomac.2024.130960.

He, T., Jiang, C., He, J., Zhang, Y., He, G., Wu, J., Lin, J., Zhou, X., & Huang, P. (2021). Manganese-dioxide-coating-instructed plasmonic modulation of gold nanorods for activatable duplex-imaging-guided NIR-II photothermal-chemodynamic therapy. *Advanced Materials, 33*(13). https://doi.org/10.1002/adma.202008540.

He, Y., Zha, J., Wang, Y., Liu, W., Yang, X., & Yu, P. (2013). Tissue damage–associated "danger signals" influence t-cell responses that promote the progression of preneoplasia to cancer. *Cancer Research, 73*(2), 629–639. https://doi.org/10.1158/0008-5472.Can-12-2704.

Hou, X., Wang, C., Zhao, Y., Wang, Q., Wang, D., Zhao, J., Liu, Y., Huang, F., & Liu, J. (2025). Tumor-specific activated polymeric nanotuners disrupt positive feedback cycle of hypoxia and apoptosis evasion for potent cancer radiotherapy. *Biomaterials, 322*, 123361. https://doi.org/10.1016/j.biomaterials.2025.123361.

Hoxhaj, G., & Manning, B. D. (2019). The PI3K–AKT network at the interface of oncogenic signalling and cancer metabolism. *Nature Reviews Cancer, 20*(2), 74–88. https://doi.org/10.1038/s41568-019-0216-7.

Hu, Y., Zhang, Y., Ding, M., & Xu, R. (2021). Long noncoding RNA TMPO-AS1/miR-126-5p/BRCC3 axis accelerates gastric cancer progression and angiogenesis by activating PI3K/AKT/mTOR pathway. Journal of Gastroenterology and Hepatology, *36*(7), 1877–1888. https://doi.org/10.1111/jgh.15362.

Hu, Z., Song, X., Ding, L., Cai, Y., Yu, L., Zhang, L., Zhou, Y., & Chen, Y. (2022). Engineering Fe/Mn-doped zinc oxide nanosonosensitizers for ultrasound-activated and multiple ferroptosis-augmented nanodynamic tumor suppression. *Materials Today Bio, 16*, 100452. https://doi.org/10.1016/j.mtbio.2022.100452.

Huang, H., Li, N., Zeng, L., Zeng, Q., Yang, Z., Shen, J., Wei, X., Yang, H., Wang, D., Liu, Y., & Wu, C. (2025). Smart biomimetic "nano-med-fireman" blocking inflammation and lactate metabolism crosstalk for normalized spatiotemporal photo-immunotherapy. Bioactive Materials, *51*, 431–449. https://doi.org/10.1016/j.bioactmat.2025.05.012.

Huang, L., Rong, Y., Tang, X., Yi, K., Qi, P., Hou, J., Liu, W., He, Y., Gao, X., Yuan, C., & Wang, F. (2022). Engineered exosomes as an in situ DC-primed vaccine to boost antitumor immunity in breast cancer. *Molecular Cancer, 21*(1). https://doi.org/10.1186/s12943-022-01515-x.

Huang, R., Lin, C., Jiang, G., Zhang, M., Gao, W., Aihemaiti, K., Liu, Q., Shi, J., Shi, W., & Huang, R. (2024). BBB-penetrating magnetoelectric nanoparticles with sustainable Gel formulation for enhanced chemotherapy and reduced postoperative glioma recurrence. Chemical Engineering Journal, *496*, 154208. https://doi.org/10.1016/j.cej.2024.154208.

Huang, X., Liang, N., Zhang, F., Lin, W., & Ma, W. (2024). Lovastatin-induced mitochondrial oxidative stress leads to the release of mtdna to promote apoptosis by activating cGAS-STING pathway in human colorectal cancer cells. *Antioxidants, 13*(6), 679. https://doi.org/10.3390/antiox13060679.

Iacobazzi, D., Convertini, P., Todisco, S., Santarsiero, A., Iacobazzi, V., & Infantino, V. (2023). New Insights into NF-κB Signaling in Innate Immunity: Focus on Immunometabolic Crosstalks. *Biology, 12*(6), 776. https://doi.org/10.3390/biology12060776.

Janku, F., Yap, T. A., & Meric-Bernstam, F. (2018). Targeting the PI3K pathway in cancer: Are we making headway? *Nature Reviews Clinical Oncology, 15*(5), 273–291. https://doi.org/10.1038/nrclinonc.2018.28.

Jian, M., Yunjia, Z., Zhiying, D., Yanduo, J., & Guocheng, J. (2018). Interleukin-7 receptor activates PI3K/AKT/mTOR signalling pathway via downregulation of Beclin-1 in lung cancer. Molecular Carcinogenesis, *58*(3), 358–365. https://doi.org/10.1002/mc.22933.

Jiang, W., Zhong, S., Chen, Z., Qian, J., Huang, X., Zhang, H., Wen, L., Zhang, Y., & Yao, G. (2023). 2D-CuPd nanozyme overcome tamoxifen resistance in breast cancer by regulating the PI3K/AKT/mTOR pathway. *Biomaterials, 294*, 121986. https://doi.org/10.1016/j.biomaterials.2022.121986.

Jin, Y., Huang, Y., Ren, H., Huang, H., Lai, C., Wang, W., Tong, Z., Zhang, H., Wu, W., Liu, C., Bao, X., Fang, W., Li, H., Zhao, P., & Dai, X. (2024). Nano-enhanced immunotherapy: Targeting the immunosuppressive tumor microenvironment. *Biomaterials, 305*, 122463. https://doi.org/10.1016/j.biomaterials.2023.122463.

Jing, G., Fan, J., Zhang, X., Zeng, X., Song, Z., Ding, W., & Ju, D. (2025). Improved biodistribution and antitumor effects of a Nectin4 and Trop2 bispecific fatty acid-modified nanobody conjugate. *Journal of Controlled Release: Official Journal of the Controlled Release Society, 388*, 114325. https://doi.org/10.1016/j.jconrel.2025.114325.

Johnson, R. M., Qu, X., Lin, C. F., Huw, L. Y., Venkatanarayan, A., Sokol, E., Ou, F. S., Ihuegbu, N., Zill, O. A., Kabbarah, O., Wang, L., Bourgon, R., de Sousa e Melo, F., Bolen, C., Daemen, A., Venook, A. P., Innocenti, F.,

Lenz, H. J., & Bais, C. (2022). ARID1A mutations confer intrinsic and acquired resistance to cetuximab treatment in colorectal cancer. *Nature Communications, 13*(1). https://doi.org/10.1038/s41467-022-33172-5, https://www.nature.com/ncomms/.

Kershaw, N. J., Murphy, J. M., Liau, N. P. D., Varghese, L. N., Laktyushin, A., Whitlock, E. L., Lucet, I. S., Nicola, N. A., & Babon, J. J. (2013). SOCS3 binds specific receptor-JAK complexes to control cytokine signaling by direct kinase inhibition. *Nature Structural and Molecular Biology, 20*(4), 469–476. https://doi.org/10.1038/nsmb.2519.

Khan, A., Zhang, Y., Ma, N., Shi, J., & Hou, Y. (2024). NF-κB role on tumor proliferation, migration, invasion and immune escape. *Cancer Gene Therapy, 31*(11), 1599–1610. https://doi.org/10.1038/s41417-024-00811-6.

King, D., Yeomanson, D., & Bryant, H. E. (2015). PI3King the lock: Targeting the PI3K/AKT/mTOR pathway as a novel therapeutic strategy in neuroblastoma. *Journal of Pediatric Hematology/Oncology, 37*(4), 245–251. https://doi.org/10.2174/156800909789271521.

Kramer, J. M., Yi, L., Shen, F., Maitra, A., Jiao, X., Jin, T., & Gaffen, S. L. (2006). Cutting edge: Evidence for ligand-independent multimerization of the IL-17 receptor. *Journal of Immunology, 176*(2), 711–715. https://doi.org/10.4049/jimmunol.176.2.711, http://www.jimmunol.org/.

Krause, C. D., Mei, E., Mirochnitchenko, O., Lavnikova, N., Xie, J., Jia, Y., Hochstrasser, R. M., & Pestka, S. (2006). Interactions among the components of the interleukin-10 receptor complex. *Biochemical and Biophysical Research Communications, 340*(2), 377–385. https://doi.org/10.1016/j.bbrc.2005.11.182.

Kumar, S., Nandi, A., Singh, S., Regulapati, R., Li, N., Tobias, J. W., Siebel, C. W., Blanco, M. A., Klein-Szanto, A. J., Lengner, C., Welm, A. L., Kang, Y., & Chakrabarti, R. (2021). Dll1+ quiescent tumor stem cells drive chemoresistance in breast cancer through NF-κB survival pathway. *Nature Communications, 12*(1). https://doi.org/10.1038/s41467-020-20664-5, http://www.nature.com/ncomms/index.html.

Lemieszek, M. K., Nunes, F. M., Marques, G., & Rzeski, W. (2019). Cantharellus cibarius branched mannans inhibits colon cancer cells growth by interfering with signals transduction in NF-κB pathway. *International Journal of Biological Macromolecules, 134*, 770–780. https://doi.org/10.1016/j.ijbiomac.2019.05.072, www.elsevier.com/locate/ijbiomac.

Li, J., Ren, H., Qiu, Q., Yang, X., Zhang, J., Zhang, C., Sun, B., Lovell, J. F., & Zhang, Y. (2022). Manganese coordination micelles that activate stimulator of interferon genes and capture in situ tumor antigens for cancer metalloimmunotherapy. *ACS Nano, 16*(10), 16909–16923. https://doi.org/10.1021/acsnano.2c06926, http://pubs.acs.org/journal/ancac3.

Li, M., Jiang, H., Chen, S., & Ma, Y. (2022). GATA binding protein 1 recruits histone deacetylase 2 to the promoter region of nuclear receptor binding protein 2 to affect the tumor microenvironment and malignancy of thyroid carcinoma. *Bioengineered, 13*(4), 11336–11357. https://doi.org/10.1080/21655979.2022.2068921.

Li, T., & Kroemer, G. (2023). Mechanisms of programmed cell death. *Immunological Reviews, 321*(1), 5–6. https://doi.org/10.1111/imr.13303.

Li, W., Xu, M., Li, Y., Huang, Z., Zhou, J., Zhao, Q., Le, K., Dong, F., Wan, C., & Yi, P. (2020). Comprehensive analysis of the association between tumor glycolysis and immune/inflammation function in breast cancer. *Journal of Translational Medicine, 18*(1). https://doi.org/10.1186/s12967-020-02267-2.

Li, X., Cheng, G., Chen, N., Ding, Z., Dai, Z., Wang, W., Li, L., Li, C., Liu, C., & Zheng, X. (2025). MnO_2-mediated cGAS-STING signaling and photothermal effect amplify chemodynamic therapy induced by Fe-Based nanoparticle in tumor therapy. ACS Applied Nano Materials, *8*(6), 2986–2996. https://doi.org/10.1021/acsanm.4c06622.

Li, X.-P., Hou, D.-Y., Wu, J.-C., Zhang, P., Wang, Y.-Z., Lv, M.-Y., Yi, Y., & Xu, W. (2024). Stimuli-responsive nanomaterials for tumor immunotherapy. *ACS Biomaterials Science & Engineering, 10*(9), 5474–5495. https://doi.org/10.1021/acsbiomaterials.4c00388.

Li, Y., Qi, M., Ding, F., Lv, Y., Ma, J., & Zhu, Y. (2020). Tumour-targetable and microenvironment-responsive nanoparticles simultaneously disrupt the PD-1/PD-L1 and MAPK/ERK/JNK pathways for efficient treatment of colorectal cancer. *Journal of Drug Targeting, 29*(4), 454–465. https://doi.org/10.1080/1061186x.2020.1853750.

Li, Z., Chu, Z., Yang, J., Qian, H., Xu, J., Chen, B., Tian, T., Chen, H., Xu, Y., & Wang, F. (2022). Immunogenic cell death augmented by manganese zinc sulfide nanoparticles for metastatic melanoma immunotherapy. *ACS Nano, 16*(9), 15471–15483. https://doi.org/10.1021/acsnano.2c08013.

Liang, D., Wang, Q., Zhang, W., Tang, H., Song, C., Yan, Z., Liang, Y., & Wang, H. (2024). JAK/STAT in leukemia: A clinical update. *Molecular Cancer, 23*(1), 25. https://doi.org/10.1186/s12943-023-01929-1.

Liang, X., Li, Y., Guo, B., Zeng, Z., Deng, K., Zou, D., Xie, Y., Xu, Y., Shen, C., & Xu, X. (2024). Inherent tumor microenvironment-reversing hydrogels: Potentiating molecular therapy efficacy against drug-resistant tumors. Advanced Functional Materials, *34*(21), 2314772. https://doi.org/10.1002/adfm.202314772.

Liao, Z., Liao, H., Luo, Y., Chen, S., Chen, M., He, J., Xu, Y., Wang, L., & Niu, C. (2025). Red blood cell membrane-camouflaged nanoparticles for synergistic sonodynamic therapy and TGF-β inhibition to reprogram immunosuppressive tumor microenvironment. *ACS Applied Materials & Interfaces, 17*(29), 41680–41695. https://doi.org/10.1021/acsami.5c07008.

Lin, R., Bao, X., Wang, H., Zhu, S., Liu, Z., Chen, Q., Ai, K., & Shi, B. (2021). TRPM2 promotes pancreatic cancer by PKC/MAPK pathway. *Cell Death and Disease, 12*(6). https://doi.org/10.1038/s41419-021-03856-9, https://www.nature.com/cddis/.

Lin, Y.-H. (2019). MicroRNA networks modulate oxidative stress in cancer. *International Journal of Molecular Sciences, 20*(18), 4497. https://doi.org/10.3390/ijms20184497.

Liu, H., Yang, X., Liang, X., & Xia, Y. (2025). Dual-magnetically driven nanozymes for glioblastoma immunotherapy via magnetothermal and nir-amplified ferroptosis and apoptosis. Materials Today *Bio, 35*, 102363. https://doi.org/10.1016/j.mtbio.2025.102363.

Liu, L., Sha, R., Yang, L., Zhao, X., Zhu, Y., Gao, J., Zhang, Y., & Wen, L. P. (2018). Impact of morphology on iron oxide nanoparticles-induced inflammasome activation in macrophages. *ACS Applied Materials and Interfaces, 10*(48), 41197–41206. https://doi.org/10.1021/acsami.8b17474, http://pubs.acs.org/journal/aamick.

Liu, T., Zhang, L., Joo, D., & Sun, S.-C. (2017). NF-κB signaling in inflammation. *Signal Transduction and Targeted Therapy, 2*(1). https://doi.org/10.1038/sigtrans.2017.23.

Liu, Y., Zhen, W., Wang, Y., Liu, J., Jin, L., Zhang, T., Zhang, S., Zhao, Y., Song, S., Li, C., Zhu, J., Yang, Y., & Zhang, H. (2019). One-dimensional fe_2p acts as a fenton agent in response to NIR II light and ultrasound for deep tumor synergetic theranostics. Angewandte Chemie International Edition, *58*(8), 2407–2412. https://doi.org/10.1002/anie.201813702.

Lv, Z., Wu, Y., Lin, J., Li, W., Weisbecker, H., Wang, P., Song, X., Sun, W., Sun, Z., Xie, Y., Meng, J., Dong, J., An, X., Chen, J., Yang, S., Yuan, T., Jiang, H., Sun, C., Yang, X., ... Bao, N. (2023). Schottky heterojunction facilitates osteosarcoma ferroptosis and enhances bone formation in a switchable mode. Advanced Functional Materials, *34*(10), 2312032. https://doi.org/10.1002/adfm.202312032.

Ma, B., Wang, S., Liu, F., Zhang, S., Duan, J., Li, Z., Kong, Y., Sang, Y., Liu, H., Bu, W., & Li, L. (2018). Self-assembled copper–amino acid nanoparticles for in situ glutathione "AND" H_2O_2 sequentially triggered chemodynamic therapy. *Journal of the American Chemical Society, 141*(2), 849–857. https://doi.org/10.1021/jacs.8b08714.

Mantovani, A., Allavena, P., Sica, A., & Balkwill, F. (2008). Cancer-related inflammation. *Nature, 454*(7203), 436–444. https://doi.org/10.1038/nature07205.

Mao, H., Zhao, X., & Sun, S. (2025). NF-κB in inflammation and cancer. *Cellular & Molecular Immunology, 22*(8), 811–839. https://doi.org/10.1038/s41423-025-01310-w.

Moon, H., & Ro, S. W. (2021). MAPK/ERK signaling pathway in hepatocellular carcinoma. *Cancers, 13*(12), 3026. https://doi.org/10.3390/cancers13123026.

Narayan, R., Gadag, S., Cheruku, S. P., Raichur, A. M., Day, C. M., Garg, S., Manandhar, S., Pai, K. S. R., Suresh, A., Mehta, C. H., Nayak, Y., Kumar, N., & Nayak, U. Y. (2021). Chitosan-glucuronic acid conjugate coated mesoporous silica nanoparticles: A smart pH-responsive and receptor-targeted system for colorectal cancer therapy. *Carbohydrate Polymers, 261*. https://doi.org/10.1016/j.carbpol.2021.117893, http://www.elsevier.com/wps/find/journaldescription.cws_home/405871/description#description.

Njunge, L. W., Estania, A. P., Guo, Y., Liu, W., & Yang, L. (2020). Tumor progression locus 2 (TPL2) in tumor-promoting inflammation, tumorigenesis and tumor immunity. *Theranostics, 10*(18), 8343–8364. https://doi.org/10.7150/thno.45848, http://www.thno.org/.

Oliver Metzig, M., Tang, Y., Mitchell, S., Taylor, B., Foreman, R., Wollman, R., & Hoffmann, A. (2020). An incoherent feedforward loop interprets NFκB/RelA dynamics to determine TNF-induced necroptosis decisions. Molecular Systems Biology, *16*(12), e9677. https://doi.org/10.15252/msb.20209677.

O'shea, J. J., Schwartz, D. M., Villarino, A. V., Gadina, M., Mcinnes, I. B., & Laurence, A. (2015). The JAK-STAT pathway: Impact on human disease and therapeutic intervention. *Annual Review of Medicine, 66*(1), 311–328. https://doi.org/10.1146/annurev-med-051113-024537.

Peng, S., Hou, X., Liu, J., & Huang, F. (2025). Advances in polymer nanomaterials targeting cGAS-STING pathway for enhanced cancer immunotherapy. *Journal of Controlled Release, 381*, 113560. https://doi.org/10.1016/j.jconrel.2025.02.056.

Pierobon, M., Ramos, C., Wong, S., Hodge, K. A., Aldrich, J., Byron, S., Anthony, S. P., Robert, N. J., Northfelt, D. W., Jahanzeb, M., Vocila, L., Wulfkuhle, J., Gambara, G., Gallagher, R. I., Dunetz, B., Hoke, N., Dong, T., Craig, D. W., Cristofanilli, M., ... Petricoin, E. F. (2017). Enrichment of PI3K-AKT–mTOR pathway activation in hepatic metastases from breast cancer. *Clinical Cancer Research, 23*(16), 4919–4928. https://doi.org/10.1158/1078-0432.CCR-16-2656, http://clincancerres.aacrjournals.org/content/23/16/4919.full-text.pdf.

Qian, M., Jiang, G., Zhao, S., Guo, W., Wang, Y., Xu, Y., Lv, W., Li, W., Nie, H., Lin, C., Qin, Y., Aihemaiti, K., Zhang, M., Yang, L., Gao, W., Li, H., Tao, W., & Huang, R. (2025). Modulating nano-bio interface via drug-framework hybridization to activate chemoimmunotherapy against glioma postoperative recurrence. *Cell Biomaterials, 1*(3), 100025. https://doi.org/10.1016/j.celbio.2025.100025.

Qu, H., Zhang, Y., Chen, M., Shao, S., Chen, J., Wu, Y., & Wu, X. (2025). NIR-II photo- and sono-responsive hyaluronic acid-capped nanozymes for glioblastoma-targeting theranostics. *International Journal of Biological Macromolecules, 306*(Pt 3), 141737. https://doi.org/10.1016/j.ijbiomac.2025.141737.

Rajeev, S., Hasoon K T, N., & Panicker, U. G. (2025). Sodium alginate/polyvinylpyrrolidone/lapatinib-loaded Zr–Metal organic framework: Biocompatibility evaluation and pH-responsive in vitro drug release for oral delivery applications. Journal of Materials Chemistry B, *13*(38), 12205–12223. https://doi.org/10.1039/d5tb01449b.

Ramos-Valle, A., Domínguez, A., Navarro, N., Márquez-López, A., Aviñó, A., Eritja, R., Fàbrega, C., García-Hevia, L., & Fanarraga, M. L. (2025). Targeted tumor microenvironment delivery of floxuridine prodrug via soluble silica nanoparticles in malignant melanoma as a model for aggressive cancer treatment. *Small (Weinheim an der Bergstrasse, Germany), 21*(20), 2407752. https://doi.org/10.1002/smll.202407752.

Ren, X., Xue, R., Luo, Y., Wang, S., Ge, X., Yao, X., Li, L., Min, J., Li, M., Luo, Z., & Wang, F. (2024). Programmable melanoma-targeted radio-immunotherapy via fusogenic liposomes functionalized with multivariate-gated aptamer assemblies. *Nature Communications, 15*(1). https://doi.org/10.1038/s41467-024-49482-9.

Ruan, J., Liu, H., Chen, B., Wang, F., Wang, W., Zha, Z., Qian, H., Miao, Z., Sun, J., Tian, T., He, Y., & Wang, H. (2021). Interfacially engineered ZnxMn1- xS@polydopamine hollow nanospheres for glutathione depleting photothermally enhanced chemodynamic therapy. *ACS Nano, 15*(7), 11428–11440. https://doi.org/10.1021/acsnano.1c01077, http://pubs.acs.org/journal/ancac3.

Rucker, A. J., Park, C. S., Li, Q. J., Moseman, E. A., & Chan, F. K.-M. (2024). Necroptosis stimulates interferon-mediated protective anti-tumor immunity. *Cell Death Disease, 15*(6), 403. https://doi.org/10.1038/s41419-024-06801-8.

Sangaletti, S., Tripodo, C., Ratti, C., Piconese, S., Porcasi, R., Salcedo, R., Trinchieri, G., Colombo, M. P., & Chiodoni, C. (2010). Oncogene-driven intrinsic inflammation induces leukocyte production of tumor necrosis factor that critically contributes to mammary carcinogenesis. *Cancer Research, 70*(20), 7764–7775. https://doi.org/10.1158/0008-5472.Can-10-0471.

Seif, F., Khoshmirsafa, M., Aazami, H., Mohsenzadegan, M., Sedighi, G., & Bahar, M. (2017). The role of JAK-STAT signaling pathway and its regulators in the fate of T helper cells. *Cell Communication and Signaling, 15*(1). https://doi.org/10.1186/s12964-017-0177-y, http://www.biosignaling.com/.

Shanmugam, L., & Jayaraman, M. (2025). Hyaluronan-decorated-phloroglucinol-loaded mesoporous silica nanoparticles downregulate GLI1 and SMO genes of hedgehog signaling pathway in gastrointestinal cancer stem-like cells. *International Journal of Biological Macromolecules, 315*, 144372. https://doi.org/10.1016/j.ijbiomac.2025.144372.

Shen, Y. J., Le Bert, N., Chitre, A. A., Koo, C. X.'E., Nga, X. H., Ho, S. S. W., Khatoo, M., Tan, N. Y., Ishii, K. J., & Gasser, S. (2015). Genome-derived cytosolic DNA mediates type I interferon-dependent rejection of B cell lymphoma cells. *Cell Reports, 11*(3), 460–473. https://doi.org/10.1016/j.celrep.2015.03.041.

Shi, A., Liu, L., Li, S., & Qi, B. (2024). Natural products targeting the MAPK-signaling pathway in cancer: Overview. *Journal of Cancer Research and Clinical Oncology, 150*(1). https://doi.org/10.1007/s00432-023-05572-7.

Shih, V. F. S., Davis-Turak, J., MacAl, M., Huang, J. Q., Ponomarenko, J., Kearns, J. D., Yu, T., Fagerlund, R., Asagiri, M., Zuniga, E. I., & Hoffmann, A. (2012). Control of RelB during dendritic cell activation integrates canonical and noncanonical NF-κB pathways. *Nature Immunology, 13*(12), 1162–1170. https://doi.org/10.1038/ni.2446.

Silva, F.a L. S., Chang, H. P., Incorvia, J.a C., Oliveira, M. J., Sarmento, B., Santos, S. G., Magalhães, F. D., & Pinto, A. M. (2023). 2D nanomaterials and their drug conjugates for phototherapy and magnetic hyperthermia therapy of cancer and infections. *Small (Weinheim an der Bergstrasse, Germany), 20*(13), 2306137. https://doi.org/10.1002/smll.202306137.

Sim, D. Y., Lee, H.-J., Ahn, C.-H., Park, J. E., Park, S.-Y., Kil, B.-J., Shim, B.-S., Kim, B., & Kim, S.-H. (2024). Negative regulation of CPSF6 suppresses the warburg effect and angiogenesis leading to tumor progression via c-Myc signaling network: Potential therapeutic target for liver cancer therapy. *International Journal of Biological Sciences, 20*(9), 3442–3460. https://doi.org/10.7150/ijbs.93462.

Soleimani, A., Rahmani, F., Saeedi, N., Ghaffarian, R., Khazaei, M., Ferns, G. A., Avan, A., & Hassanian, S. M. (2019). The potential role of regulatory microRNAs of RAS/MAPK signaling pathway in the pathogenesis of colorectal cancer. *Journal of Cellular Biochemistry, 120*(12), 19245–19253. https://doi.org/10.1002/jcb.29268, http://onlinelibrary.wiley.com/journal/10.1002/(ISSN)1097-4644.

Song, C., Guan, X., Xie, C., Jiang, S., Hong, Z., Wu, Q., Qu, G., Ma, T., & Cui, Y. (2024). Inhibiting PI3K/AKT/mTOR signaling by metal-organic frameworks for overcoming multiple drug resistance in chemoradiotherapy. *Science China Materials, 67*(5), 1631–1645. https://doi.org/10.1007/s40843-023-2774-8, https://www.springer.com/journal/40843.

Stark, G.r, & Darnell, J.e (2012). The JAK-STAT pathway at twenty. *Immunity, 36*(4), 503–514. https://doi.org/10.1016/j.immuni.2012.03.013.

Su, X., Su, M., Guo, E., Zhou, Y., Yang, X., Li, S., & Ye, Y. (2025). Tissue-resident macrophage membrane-coated nanomedicine for targeted tumor therapy. *ACS Nano, 19*(29), 26296–26319. https://doi.org/10.1021/acsnano.5c04463.

Sui, A., Yao, C., Chen, Y., Li, Y., Yu, S., Qu, J., Wei, H., Tang, J., & Chen, G. (2023). Polystyrene nanoplastics inhibit StAR expression by activating HIF-1α via ERK1/2 MAPK and AKT pathways in TM3 Leydig cells and testicular tissues of mice. *Food and Chemical Toxicology, 173*, 113634. https://doi.org/10.1016/j.fct.2023.113634.

Sun, H., Ou, B., Zhao, S., Liu, X., Song, L., Liu, X., Wang, R., & Peng, Z. (2019). USP11 promotes growth and metastasis of colorectal cancer via PPP1CA-mediated activation of ERK/MAPK signaling pathway. *EBioMedicine, 48*, 236–247. https://doi.org/10.1016/j.ebiom.2019.08.061.

Sun, S., Chang, J., & Jin, J. (2013). Regulation of nuclear factor-κB in autoimmunity. *Trends in Immunology, 34*(6), 282–289. https://doi.org/10.1016/j.it.2013.01.004.

Sun, Y., Zhou, P., Qian, J., Zeng, Q., Wei, G., Li, Y., Liu, Y., Lai, Y., Zhan, Y., Wu, D., & Fang, Y. (2024). Spermine synthase engages in macrophages M2 polarization to sabotage antitumor immunity in hepatocellular carcinoma. *Cell Death and Differentiation, 32*(3), 573–586. https://doi.org/10.1038/s41418-024-01409-z.

Tan, M., Cao, G., Wang, R., Cheng, L., Huang, W., Yin, Y., Ma, H., Ho, S.-H., Wang, Z., Zhu, M., Ran, H., Nie, G., & Wang, H. (2024). Metal-ion-chelating phenylalanine nanostructures reverse immune dysfunction and sensitize breast tumour to immune checkpoint blockade. *Nature Nanotechnology, 19*(12), 1903–1913. https://doi.org/10.1038/s41565-024-01758-3.

Tian, H., Wang, G., Sang, W., Xie, L., Zhang, Z., Li, W., Yan, J., Tian, Y., Li, J., Li, B., & Dai, Y. (2022). Manganese-phenolic nanoadjuvant combines sonodynamic therapy with cGAS-STING activation for enhanced cancer immunotherapy. *Nano Today, 43*, 101405. https://doi.org/10.1016/j.nantod.2022.101405.

Tilg, H., Ianiro, G., Gasbarrini, A., & Adolph, T. E. (2025). Adipokines: Masterminds of metabolic inflammation. *Nature Reviews. Immunology, 25*(4), 250–265. https://doi.org/10.1038/s41577-024-01103-8.

Tolomeo, M., & Cascio, A. (2021). The multifaced role of STAT3 in cancer and its implication for anticancer therapy. *International Journal of Biological Sciences, 22*(2), 603. https://doi.org/10.3390/ijms22020603.

Totan, D. M. A., Stanescu Spinu, I.-I., S, C. B., S, C., & G, M. (2020). PI3K/AKT/mTOR signalling pathway in breast cancer: From molecular landscape to clinical aspects. *International Journal of Biological Sciences, 22*(1), 173. https://doi.org/10.3390/ijms.

Valle-Mendiola, A., Gutiérrez-Hoya, A., & Soto-Cruz, I. (2023). JAK/STAT signaling and cervical cancer: From the cell surface to the nucleus. *Genes, 14*(6). https://doi.org/10.3390/genes14061141.

Van Elsland, D., & Neefjes, J. (2018). Bacterial infections and cancer. *EMBO Reports, 19*(11), e46632. https://doi.org/10.15252/embr.201846632.

Wang, J., Wu, H., Zhao, Q., Zou, Y., Ding, D., Yin, H., & Xu, H. (2022). Aggregation-induced emission photosensitizer synergizes photodynamic therapy and the inhibition of the NF-κB signaling pathway to overcome hypoxia in breast cancer. *ACS Applied Materials & Interfaces, 14*(26), 29613–29625. https://doi.org/10.1021/acsami.2c06063.

Wang, M., Yi, H., Zhan, Z., Feng, Z., Yang, G., Zheng, Y., & Zhang, D. (2024). A self-assembled nanomedicine for glucose supply interruption-amplified low-temperature photothermal therapy and anti-prometastatic inflammatory processes of triple-negative breast cancer. *Aggregate, 5*(6), e622. https://doi.org/10.1002/agt2.622.

Wang, R., Wang, Z., Zhang, M., Zhong, D., & Zhou, M. (2025). Application of photosensitive microalgae in targeted tumor therapy. *Advanced Drug Delivery Reviews, 219*, 115519. https://doi.org/10.1016/j.addr.2025.115519.

Wang, S., Liu, X., Chen, S., Liu, Z., Zhang, X., Liang, X., & Li, L. (2018). Regulation of Ca^{2+} signaling for drug-resistant breast cancer therapy with mesoporous silica nanocapsule encapsulated doxorubicin/siRNA cocktail. *ACS Nano, 13*(1), 274–283. https://doi.org/10.1021/acsnano.8b05639.

Wang, S., Liu, X., Wei, D., Zhou, H., Zhu, J., Yu, Q., Luo, L., Dai, X., Jiang, Y., Yu, L., Yang, Y., & Tan, W. (2024). Polyvalent aptamer nanodrug conjugates enable efficient tumor cuproptosis therapy through copper overload and glutathione depletion. *Journal of the American Chemical Society, 146*(44), 30033–30045. https://doi.org/10.1021/jacs.4c06338.

Wang, X., Zhang, M., Li, Y., Cong, H., Yu, B., & Shen, Y. (2023). Research status of dendrimer micelles in tumor therapy for drug delivery. *Small (Weinheim an der Bergstrasse, Germany), 19*(50), 2304006. https://doi.org/10.1002/smll.202304006

Wang, Y., Li, H., Lin, J., Li, Y., Zhang, K., Li, H., Fu, Q., & Jiang, Y. (2025). Engineering nanozyme immunomodulator with magnetic targeting effect for cascade-enzyodynamic and ultrasound-reinforced metallo-immunotherapy in prostate carcinoma. Nature Communications, *16*(1), 1876. https://doi.org/10.1038/s41467-025-57190-1.

Wei, D., Sun, Y., Zhu, H., & Fu, Q. (2023). Stimuli-responsive polymer-based nanosystems for cancer theranostics. *ACS Nano, 17*(23), 23223–23261. https://doi.org/10.1021/acsnano.3c06019.

Wen, H., Xiang, X., Li, Z., Sun, T., & Xie, Z. (2025). A cyclic photosensitizer nanoplatform for effective pyroptosis and enhanced photoimmunotherapy. *ACS Nano, 19*(39), 35181–35192. https://doi.org/10.1021/acsnano.5c13927.

Werfel, T. A., Elion, D. L., Rahman, B., Hicks, D. J., Sanchez, V., Gonzales-Ericsson, P. I., Nixon, M. J., James, J. L., Balko, J. M., Scherle, P. A., Koblish, H. K., & Cook, R. S. (2019). Treatment-induced tumor cell apoptosis and secondary necrosis drive tumor progression in the residual tumor microenvironment through mertk and ido1. *Cancer Research, 79*(1), 171–182. https://doi.org/10.1158/0008-5472.Can-18-1106.

Wu, W., Xu, M., Qiao, B., Huang, T., Guo, H., Zhang, N., Zhou, L., Li, M., Tan, Y., Zhang, M., Xie, X., Shuai, X., & Zhang, C. (2023). Nanodroplet-enhanced sonodynamic therapy potentiates immune checkpoint blockade for systemic suppression of triple-negative breast cancer. *Acta Biomaterialia, 158*, 547–559. https://doi.org/10.1016/j.actbio.2022.12.023.

Wu, Z., Xiao, H., Kloeber, J. A., Ouyang, Y., Yin, P., Huang, J., Chen, B., Zhu, S., Lu, J., Han, Y., Tu, X., Dragojevic, S., Luo, K., Ting, A. T., Welliver, M., & Lou, Z. (2025). Parkin deficiency promotes colorectal tumorigenesis and progression through RIPK3-dependent necroptotic inflammation. *Cancer Communications, 45*(4), 406–410. https://doi.org/10.1002/cac2.12648, https://onlinelibrary.wiley.com/journal/25233548.

Wu, Z., Zhang, W., Wang, L., Leng, J., Li, Y., Fan, Z., Zhan, M., Cao, L., Jiang, Y., Jiang, Y., Sun, B., Fu, J., Li, J., Shi, W., & Jin, H. (2024). Multi-omics integration reveals the oncogenic role of eccDNAs in diffuse large B-cell lymphoma through STING signalling. *Clinical and Translational Medicine, 14*(8). https://doi.org/10.1002/ctm2.1815.

Xiao, L., Hou, J., Liu, H., & Lu, Q. (2025). Targeting drug cocktail hydrogel platform for inhibiting tumor growth and metastasis. *Materials Today Bio, 32*, 101798. https://doi.org/10.1016/j.mtbio.2025.101798.

Xie, S.-J., Li, J.-H., Chen, H.-F., Tan, Y.-Y., Liu, S.-R., Zhang, Y., Xu, H., Yang, J.-H., Liu, S., Zheng, L.-L., Huang, M.-B., Guo, Y.-H., Zhang, Q., Zhou, H., & Qu, L.-H. (2018). Inhibition of the JNK/MAPK signaling pathway by myogenesis-associated miRNAs is required for skeletal muscle development. *Cell Death & Differentiation, 25*(9), 1581–1597. https://doi.org/10.1038/s41418-018-0063-1.

Xie, Y., Liu, F., Wu, Y., Zhu, Y., Jiang, Y., Wu, Q., Dong, Z., & Liu, K. (2025). Inflammation in cancer: Therapeutic opportunities from new insights. *Molecular Cancer, 24*(1), 51. https://doi.org/10.1186/s12943-025-02243-8.

Xin, P., Xu, X., Deng, C., Liu, S., Wang, Y., Zhou, X., Ma, H., Wei, D., & Sun, S. (2020). The role of JAK/STAT signaling pathway and its inhibitors in diseases. *International Immunopharmacology, 80*. https://doi.org/10.1016/j.intimp.2020.106210, www.elsevier.com/locate/intimp.

Xiong, L., Liang, B., & Yu, K. (2025). Magnetic hyperthermia in oncology: Nanomaterials-driven combinatorial strategies for synergistic therapeutic gains. Materials Today *Bio, 33*, 102070. https://doi.org/10.1016/j.mtbio.2025.102070.

Xu, B., Cui, Y., Wang, W., Li, S., Lyu, C., Wang, S., Bao, W., Wang, H., Qin, M., Liu, Z., Wei, W., & Liu, H. (2020). Immunomodulation-enhanced nanozyme-based tumor catalytic therapy. *Advanced Materials, 32*(33). https://doi.org/10.1002/adma.202003563, http://onlinelibrary.wiley.com/journal/10.1002/(ISSN)1521-4095.

Xu, B., Li, S., Han, A., Zhou, Y., Sun, M., Yang, H., Zheng, L., Shi, R., & Liu, H. (2024). Engineering atomically dispersed Cu–N1S2 sites via chemical vapor deposition to boost enzyme-like activity for efficient tumor therapy. *Advanced Materials, 36*(13). https://doi.org/10.1002/adma.202312024, http://onlinelibrary.wiley.com/journal/10.1002/(ISSN)1521-4095.

Xu, Z., Yu, J., Zhang, Y., Wang, Y., Li, W., Zhang, B., Cui, W., Li, Y., Wang, Y., Yang, Z., Liu, Y., Li, X., Wang, Y., He, Z., & Liu, H. (2025). In situ oxidation-responsive nanovaccine coordinates photosensitizer and STING agonist for cancer photo-immunotherapy. *Nano Today, 62*, 102726. https://doi.org/10.1016/j.nantod.2025.102726.

Xue, C., Yao, Q., Gu, X., Shi, Q., Yuan, X., Chu, Q., Bao, Z., Lu, J., & Li, L. (2023). Evolving cognition of the JAK-STAT signaling pathway: Autoimmune disorders and cancer. *Signal Transduction and Targeted Therapy, 8*(1). https://doi.org/10.1038/s41392-023-01468-7.

Xue, Z., Liu, J., Xing, W., Mu, F., Wu, Y., Zhao, J., Liu, X., Wang, D., Wang, J., Li, X., Wang, J., & Huang, B. (2024). Hypoxic glioma-derived exosomal miR-25-3p promotes macrophage M2 polarization by activating the PI3K-AKT-mTOR signaling pathway. Journal of Nanobiotechnology, *22*(1), 628. https://doi.org/10.1186/s12951-024-02888-5.

Yadav, P., Mandal, S. K., Tang, B., & Sheth, R. A. (2025). Liposomal nanoparticle mediated gene modulation for the treatment of melanoma in murine models. *Cancer Research, 85*, 4473. https://doi.org/10.1158/1538-7445.Am2025-4473 4473.

Yamaguchi, M., Hashimoto, K., Jijiwa, M., & Murata, T. (2023). The inflammatory macrophages repress the growth of bone metastatic human prostate cancer cells via TNF-α and IL-6 signaling: Involvement of cell signaling regulator regucalcin. *Cellular Signalling, 107*, 110663. https://doi.org/10.1016/j.cellsig.2023.110663.

Yan, Y., Hu, J., Han, N., Li, H., Yang, X., Li, L., Xu, Z., Xia, F., Li, J., Li, T., & Chen, R. (2025). Sorafenib-loaded metal-organic framework nanoparticles for anti-hepatocellular carcinoma effects through synergistically potentiating ferroptosis and remodeling tumor immune microenvironment. Materials Today *Bio, 32*, 101848. https://doi.org/10.1016/j.mtbio.2025.101848.

Yang, G., Su, Q., Lv, J., Zheng, Y., Song, T., Zhang, H., Li, M., Zhou, W., Li, T., Qin, X., Li, S., Wu, C., Liao, X., Liu, Y., & Yang, H. (2023). Bio-inspired oxidative stress amplifier for suppressing cancer metastasis and imaging-guided combination therapy. *ACS Applied Materials & Interfaces, 15*(5), 6572–6583. https://doi.org/10.1021/acsami.2c22558.

Yang, J., Wang, H., Liu, J., Ding, M., Xie, X., Yang, X., Peng, Y., Zhou, S., Ouyang, R., & Miao, Y. (2021). Recent advances in nanosized metal organic frameworks for drug delivery and tumor therapy. *RSC Advances, 11*(6), 3241–3263. https://doi.org/10.1039/D0RA09878G.

Yang, Y., Wang, N., Wang, Z., Yan, F., Shi, Z., & Feng, S. (2025). Glutathione-responsive metal–organic-framework-derived MnxOy/(A/R)TiO_2 nanoparticles for enhanced synergistic sonodynamic/chemodynamic/immunotherapy. *ACS Nano, 19*(1), 885–899. https://doi.org/10.1021/acsnano.4c12304.

Yao, W., Lin, Y., Weng, Y., Wu, Y., Zheng, L., Zheng, D., Xi, Q., & Zhao, J. (2025). Lipid-based nanoparticles in cancer therapy: Advances in targeted drug delivery and therapeutic potential for renal cell carcinoma. *Advancement of Science, 12*(36), e07666. https://doi.org/10.1002/advs.202507666.

Yıldırım, E., Şengelen, A., Yücel, O., Aksüt, Y., Öğütcü, İ., Bayrakçı, A., Gencel-Güler, C., Güneş, U., İldeş, C., Pekmez, M., & Emik, S. (2025). Methotrexate-loaded Sr-BDC metal-organic frameworks attenuate glioblastoma and cervical-carcinoma cells and spheroids' growth and motility by reducing the inflammation-EMT axis and inducing apoptosis. *Journal of Drug Delivery Science and Technology, 111*. https://doi.org/10.1016/j.jddst.2025.107160, https://www.sciencedirect.com/science/journal/17732247.

Yu, H., Gao, R., Liu, Y., Fu, L., Zhou, J., & Li, L. (2023). Stimulus-responsive hydrogels as drug delivery systems for inflammation targeted therapy. *Advancement of Science, 11*(1), 2306152. https://doi.org/10.1002/advs.202306152.

Yu, H., Pardoll, D., & Jove, R. (2009). STATs in cancer inflammation and immunity: A leading role for STAT3. *Nature Reviews Cancer, 9*(11), 798–809. https://doi.org/10.1038/nrc2734.

Yu, Y., Liu, J., Liu, C., Liu, R., Liu, L., Yu, Z., Zhuang, J., & Sun, C. (2022). Post-translational modifications of cGAS-STING: A critical switch for immune regulation. *Cells, 11*(19), 3043. https://doi.org/10.3390/cells11193043.

Zeng, X., Tang, L., Zhang, W., Hong, X., & Xiao, Y. (2025). Shape and size effects of gold nanoparticles for tumor photoacoustic imaging and photothermal therapy within the NIR-I and NIR-II biowindows. *Small (Weinheim an der Bergstrasse, Germany), 21*(21). https://doi.org/10.1002/smll.202412296.

Zhang, J. A., Feng, K., Shen, W. T., Gao, W., & Zhang, L. (2024). Research advances of cellular nanoparticles as multiplex countermeasures. *ACS Nano, 18*(44), 30211–30223. https://doi.org/10.1021/acsnano.4c09830, http://pubs.acs.org/journal/ancac3.

Zhang, M., Wang, Y., Han, L., Liu, X., Xie, Y., Xu, Z., & Sun, Z. (2024). Biomaterials elicit pyroptosis enhancing cancer immunotherapy. Advanced Functional Materials, *34*(7), 2311362. https://doi.org/10.1002/adfm.202311362.

Zhang, S., Zeng, Y., Wang, K., Song, G., Yu, Y., Meng, T., Yuan, H., & Hu, F. (2023). Chitosan-based nano-micelles for potential anti-tumor immunotherapy: Synergistic effect of cGAS-STING signaling pathway activation and tumor antigen absorption. *Carbohydrate Polymers, 321*, 121346. https://doi.org/10.1016/j.carbpol.2023.121346.

Zhang, X., Bai, X.-C., & Chen, Z. J. (2020). Structures and mechanisms in the cGAS-STING innate immunity pathway. *Immunity, 53*(1), 43–53. https://doi.org/10.1016/j.immuni.2020.05.013.

Zhang, X., Chen, Y., He, X., Zhang, Y., Zhou, M., Peng, C., He, Z., Gui, S., & Li, Z. (2021). Smart nanogatekeepers for tumor theranostics. *Small (Weinheim an der Bergstrasse, Germany), 17*(47), 2103712. https://doi.org/10.1002/smll.202103712.

Zhao, X., Wu, K., Zhang, Y., Zhang, H., Zhang, X., Ni, Q., Wang, Z., & Xia, Y. (2025). Targeted biomimetic fusogenic liposome enhances tumor accumulation, penetration, and therapeutic efficacy of sirna therapeutics. Materials Today *Bio, 35*, 102414. https://doi.org/10.1016/j.mtbio.2025.102414.

Zheng, D., Yan, J., Liu, X., Zhang, Z., Jin, A., Zhao, Y., Bai, L., Quan, M., Qi, X., Fu, B., Wu, Z., Zhou, J., Han, H., Wang, Z., Wang, S., Deng, C., Sun, W., Chang, C., Zhou, S., & Zhang, H. (2025). Artesunate nanoplatform targets the serine–MAPK axis in cancer-associated fibroblasts to reverse photothermal resistance in triple-negative breast cancer. *Advanced Materials, 37*(35). https://doi.org/10.1002/adma.202502617, http://onlinelibrary.wiley.com/journal/10.1002/(ISSN)1521-4095.

Zheng, J., Mo, J., Zhu, T., Zhuo, W., Yi, Y., Hu, S., Yin, J., Zhang, W., Zhou, H., & Liu, Z. (2020). Comprehensive elaboration of the cGAS-STING signaling axis in cancer development and immunotherapy. *Molecular Cancer, 19*(1). https://doi.org/10.1186/s12943-020-01250-1, http://www.molecular-cancer.com/start.asp.

Zheng, P., He, J., Fu, Y., Yang, Y., Li, S., Duan, B., Yang, Y., Hu, Y., Yang, Z., Wang, M., Liu, Q., Zheng, X., Hua, L., Li, W., Li, D., Ding, Y., Yang, X., Bai, H., Long, Q., ... Ma, Y. (2024). Engineered bacterial biomimetic vesicles reprogram tumor-associated macrophages and remodel tumor microenvironment to promote innate and adaptive antitumor immune responses. *ACS Nano, 18*(9), 6863–6886. https://doi.org/10.1021/acsnano.3c06987.

Zhou, L., Dong, C., Ding, L., Feng, W., Yu, L., Cui, X., & Chen, Yu (2021). Targeting ferroptosis synergistically sensitizes apoptotic sonodynamic anti-tumor nanotherapy. *Nano Today, 39*, 101212. https://doi.org/10.1016/j.nantod.2021.101212.

Zhou, S., Gravekamp, C., Bermudes, D., & Liu, K. (2018). Tumour-targeting bacteria engineered to fight cancer. *Nature Reviews. Cancer, 18*(12), 727–743. https://doi.org/10.1038/s41568-018-0070-z.

Zhou, Y., Yu, L., Dong, C., Liu, J., Yang, B., Chen, Y., & Hu, Z. (2022). Two-dimensional semiconductor heterojunction nanostructure for mutually synergistic sonodynamic and chemoreactive cancer nanotherapy. *Chemical Engineering Journal, 431*, 134017. https://doi.org/10.1016/j.cej.2021.134017.

Zhu, D., Pan, W., Li, H., Hua, J., Zhang, C., & Zhao, K. (2025). Innovative applications of bacteria and their derivatives in targeted tumor therapy. *ACS Nano, 19*(5), 5077–5109. https://doi.org/10.1021/acsnano.4c15237.

Zhu, Y., Chen, P., Hu, B., Zhong, S., Yan, K., Wu, Y., Li, S., Yang, Y., Xu, Z., Lu, Y., Ouyang, Y., Bao, H., Gu, W., Wen, L., & Zhang, Y. (2024). MDSC-targeting gold nanoparticles enhance PD-1 tumor immunotherapy by inhibiting NLRP3 inflammasomes. *Biomaterials, 307*, 122533. https://doi.org/10.1016/j.biomaterials.2024.122533.

SECTION III

Translational research and therapeutic targets

CHAPTER

5

Micro/nanoplatforms for modulating programmed cell death and tumor inflammation

Xilong Wu[1,2], *Huanran Qu*[1,2], *and Yundi Wu*[1,2]

[1]School of Biomedical Engineering, School of Pharmaceutical Sciences, Key Laboratory of Tropical Biological Resources of Ministry of Education, Hainan University, Haikou, P.R. China
[2]State Key Laboratory of Digital Medical Engineering, Hainan Engineering Research Center for Drug Screening and Evaluation, Collaborative Innovation Center of One Health, Hainan University, Haikou, P.R. China

5.1 Overview of programmed cell death and tumor inflammation

The occurrence and development of tumors constitute a multifactorial, multistage, and highly complex process involving genetic mutations, dysregulation of signaling pathways, immune evasion, and dynamic remodeling of the tumor microenvironment (TME) (Gabbutt et al., 2025). In this process, programmed cell death (PCD) and the inflammatory response play a critical role. PCD is not only involved in the elimination of damaged or abnormal cells, but also affects the immune microenvironment of tumors by regulating intercellular signal transduction (An et al., 2025). Meanwhile, the inflammatory response shapes the microenvironment conducive to tumor survival and spread through continuous cytokine release and immune regulation (Wallach et al., 2016).

PCD refers to an orderly death process controlled by the cells' own genes. Different from passive Necrosis, it relies on the activation of specific signaling pathways and the regulation of molecular mechanisms (Liu, He, et al., 2025; Liu, Wu, et al., 2025). According to distinct signaling pathways and morphological characteristics, PCD can be classified into several types, including apoptosis, necroptosis, pyroptosis, autophagy, ferroptosis, cuproptosis, and disulfidptosis, the latter of which has been recently proposed (Fig. 5.1) (Kolb et al., 2017).

Apoptosis is the earliest discovered form of PCD, which was first proposed by Kerr in the 1970s (Kerr et al., 1972). It is characterized by cell shrinkage, nuclear chromatin condensation, DNA fragmentation, and the formation of apoptotic bodies. This process is primarily classified

Inflammation in Tumorigenesis and Cancer Treatment
DOI: https://doi.org/10.1016/B978-0-443-36649-9.00005-0

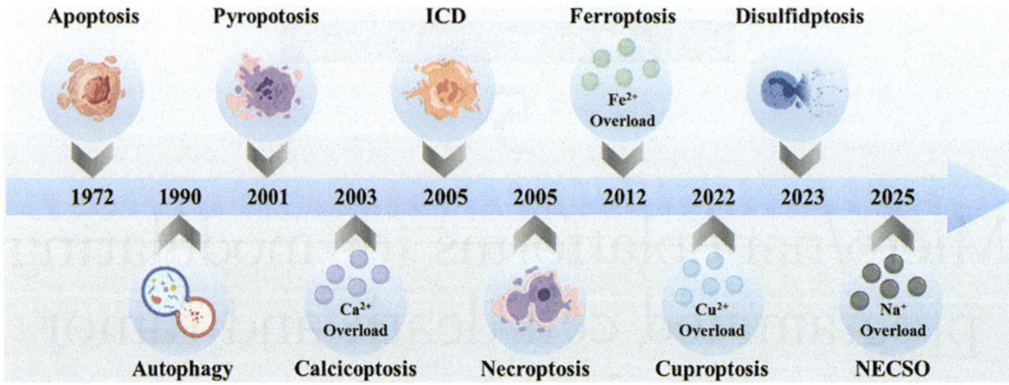

FIGURE 5.1 Chronology of the discovery of various programmed cell death (PCD) types. According to distinct signaling pathways and morphological characteristics, PCD can be classified into several types, including apoptosis, necroptosis, pyroptosis, autophagy, ferroptosis, cuproptosis, and disulfidptosis, the latter of which has been recently proposed. *ICD*, Immunogenic cell death.

into two pathways: the intrinsic pathway (mitochondrial) and the extrinsic pathway (death receptor) (Valentin et al., 2018). The former is based on Bcl-2 family proteins and Caspase-9 (Du, Wang, et al., 2024; Du, Zhao, et al., 2024), while the latter is mediated by receptors such as Fas and tumor necrosis factor receptor (TNFR) to activate Caspase-8 cascade (Di et al., 2023). Both intrinsic and extrinsic pathways activate complex signaling cascades that drive cells to undergo early, middle, and late apoptosis (Meier et al., 2024). The main role of apoptosis in normal physiological state is to maintain tissue homeostasis, but it is often inhibited by p53 mutation or upregulation of antiapoptotic proteins in tumors, thereby promoting the immortalized characteristics of tumor cells (Chen et al., 2019).

Programmed necrosis is a form of cell death between apoptosis and necrosis, which is mediated by key molecules such as RIPK1, RIPK3, and mixed lineage kinase domain-like protein (MLKL). It is characterized by cell swelling and membrane rupture in morphology, and depends on signal regulation in mechanism, and often occurs when the apoptotic pathway is inhibited (Huang et al., 2019). As programmed necrosis can release a large number of intracellular components and trigger immune activation and inflammatory response, it is considered a potential "immunogenic death" pathway in tumor treatment (Zang et al., 2022).

Pyroptosis is a highly inflammatory form of PCD that was first described in 2001 (Cookson & Brennan, 2001). Primarily mediated by proteins of the Gasdermin family, pyroptosis is characterized by progressive cellular swelling culminating in plasma membrane rupture, resulting in the release of intracellular contents and the induction of a robust inflammatory response (Yu et al., 2021). While pyroptosis can enhance tumor immunogenicity, its excessive activation may contribute to chronic inflammation and tumor progression, indicating a dual role in cancer biology (Li, Xi, et al., 2025; Li, Yuan, et al., 2025; Li, Zhang, et al., 2025).

Autophagy is a process in which eukaryotic cells use lysosomes to degrade cytoplasmic proteins and damaged organelles under the regulation of autophagy-related genes (Debnath et al., 2023). According to the different scopes and processes of autophagy, it can be divided into three types: macroautophagy, microautophagy, and chaperone-mediated autophagy

(Assi & Kimmelman, 2023). Autophagy includes basal autophagy under physiological conditions and induced autophagy under stress conditions (Pietrocola et al., 2016). The former is a self-protection mechanism of cells and plays an important role in maintaining cellular homeostasis. However, excessive autophagy may lead to metabolic stress, degradation of cell components, and even cell death (Yamazaki et al., 2021). The role of autophagy in tumors is dual: in the early stage, it may play a tumor suppressor role by eliminating damaged cells, while after the formation of tumors, autophagy is often used to maintain energy supply and promote tumor cell resistance and survival (Weiner & Lotze, 2012).

Ferroptosis is a form of cell death that relies on iron-catalyzed lipid peroxidation, and its core mechanism is the depletion of intracellular glutathione (GSH) and the inactivation of glutathione peroxidase 4 (GPX4), leading to the accumulation of membrane lipid peroxidation (Cui, Tang, et al., 2024; Cui, Wang, et al., 2024). Cells with ferroptosis will show the characteristics of reduced mitochondrial volume, increased density of bilayer membrane structure, decreased or disappeared mitochondrial crista, and their nuclear size will be normal, and there will be no chromatin condensation phenomenon commonly seen in apoptosis (Lei et al., 2024). Cuproptosis is a new form of cell death proposed in 2022, which is caused by the direct binding of mitochondrial tricarboxylic acid cycle proteins and copper ions, leading to protein aggregation and fatty acylation stress, resulting in cell death (Tsvetkov et al., 2022; Xu et al., 2021). Disulfidptosis is the collapse of cytoskeleton and imbalance of energy metabolism caused by excessive accumulation of disulfide bonds in cells (Kang et al., 2023; Zheng et al., 2023).

Inflammatory response is a defensive response of the body to infection, injury, or stimulation, including acute inflammation and chronic inflammation (Denk & Greten, 2022). Acute inflammation usually clears pathogens rapidly through the recruitment of immune cells and the release of cytokines, while chronic inflammation leads to long-term activation of the immune system due to continuous stimulation, which leads to tissue remodeling and abnormal cell proliferation. A large number of epidemiological and pathological studies have shown that about 25% of malignant tumors are closely related to chronic inflammation (Zhao et al., 2021), such as liver cancer caused by hepatitis, gastric cancer caused by gastritis, and colorectal cancer caused by colitis (Manjili et al., 2022). In the early stage of tumor development, chronic inflammation can promote the activation of oncogenes and the inactivation of tumor suppressor genes by inducing DNA damage and gene mutations (Shalapour & Karin, 2019). At the same time, immune cells such as tumor-associated macrophages (TAMs), neutrophils, and myeloid-derived suppressor cells (MDSCs) are reprogrammed in the inflammatory environment to secrete immunosuppressive factors, further weakening the body's antitumor immune response and forming favorable conditions for tumor immune escape (Jayakumar & Bothwell, 2019). However, acute inflammation can inhibit tumor growth through immune cell-mediated clearance (Yang & Karin, 2014). Therefore controlling the type and intensity of inflammatory response is an important direction to achieve balanced regulation in tumor treatment.

In summary, PCD is the core process to maintain cell homeostasis and regulate tumor fate, while inflammation is involved in the occurrence, progression, and immune regulation of tumors through a variety of signaling pathways. Although they are mechanistically independent, they are closely related in time and space in tumor biology (Ritter & Greten, 2019). An in-depth understanding of these biological processes provides a theoretical basis for the functional design of micro/nanoplatforms. By reasonably constructing micro/nanoplatforms with precise targeting and controllable stimulus responses, the induction of PCD, and the effective regulation of inflammatory response in tumors can be realized, thus opening up new strategies and directions for tumor therapy.

5.2 Chemotherapy-induced programmed cell death and tumor inflammatory responses mediated by micro/nanoplatforms

As an important way of tumor treatment, the main mechanism of chemotherapy is to induce cell death by destroying DNA replication of tumor cells, interfering with protein synthesis, or inhibiting the process of cell division (Zhang et al., 2016). Traditional chemotherapy drugs, such as doxorubicin (DOX), cisplatin (CDDP), and paclitaxel (PTX), have achieved remarkable results in the treatment of a variety of cancers, but there are still some problems such as nonspecific drug distribution, high systemic toxicity, and strong drug resistance, which lead to limited efficacy (Browning et al., 2017; Huang et al., 2023; Wang et al., 2017). In recent years, the rapid development of micro/nanotechnology has provided new solutions for the precise delivery of chemotherapeutic drugs.

By loading drugs with micro/nanoplatforms and intelligentized modification, the local enrichment concentration of drugs in tumors can be significantly increased, systemic side effects can be reduced, and specific PCD can be effectively induced, so as to achieve a more efficient and controllable tumor killing effect. Based on the enhanced permeability and retention effect of tumor tissue, nanocarriers can achieve passive enrichment, and by modifying ligands such as folic acid, arginine-glycine-aspartic acid (a tripeptide used for cell adhesion targeting) (RGD) peptide, and specific antibodies on the surface of the carrier, active targeted delivery can be further achieved (Fang et al., 2023; Wang et al., 2018; Yi et al., 2023; Zhang et al., 2018). At the same time, responsive nanoplatforms can take advantage of the special chemical characteristics of the tumor microenvironment (such as pH, high concentration of peroxide, and high concentration of GSH) to achieve precise drug release in specific areas. For example, Tang et al. (2024) constructed a novel RGD-modified micellar RPA@DOX loaded with adriamycin to improve tumor targeting and enhance the effect of chemotherapy against breast cancer. The results showed that the nanoplatform showed outstanding tumor targeting and caused tumor cell apoptosis, thereby producing excellent antitumor effect. Pereira et al. (2023) developed pH/ GSH-responsive tumor-targeting Nanogels, DOX-nanogels, which are efficiently internalized into cells through CD44 receptor-mediated endocytosis. Subsequently, DOX release is triggered in response to the high GSH concentration and acidic environment in the tumor microenvironment, and the released DOX is translocated into the nucleus to induce cytotoxicity. By inhibiting topoisomerase II and damaging the DNA structure, it induces the loss of mitochondrial membrane potential and activation of Caspase cascade, thereby triggering the typical apoptotic response. Zhong et al. (2016) used a novel hyaluronic acid chitoacid-activated PTX prodrug micelle HA-dOG-PTX-PM, which was used to effectively target and treat xenograft human breast cancer in vitro and in vivo. After active targeting of tumors, the nanomicelles release drugs in the tumor acidic microenvironment in a responsive manner, thereby enhancing local killing effect. By stabilizing microtubules and blocking the mitotic cycle,

PTX causes tumor cells to stay in the G_2/M phase for a long time, thereby upregulating the expression of p53 and Bax, and inducing programmed necrosis.

In addition to single drug delivery, researchers have also developed multidrug synergistic nanosystems. For example, Xu et al. (2019) designed a nanomicelle coloaded with DOX and CDDP, and the drugs can be released sequentially at the tumor site. The former disrupts DNA structure to induce apoptosis, and the latter induces ferroptosis through the accumulation of metal ions, thus forming an "apoptosis-ferroptosis" dual-path synergistic effect. Wu, Li, et al. (2024) and Wu, Liu, et al. (2024) employed Schiff base linkages to conjugate oxidized hyaluronic acid (OHA) with primaquine (PQ) and DOX, thereby creating acid-sensitive nanoprodrugs (O@PD). The enhanced drug endocytosis of O@PD via CD44 may potentially augment the accumulation of drugs within tumors. The actively targeted carrier sustains its size under normal pH conditions, yet disintegrates in the acidic tumor microenvironment, thereby facilitating rapid drug release. The incorporation of PQ significantly elevates the efficacy of DOX-induced tumor therapy by suppressing autophagic flux and promoting apoptosis. The synergistic impact of PQ and DOX within O@PD manifests remarkable antitumor characteristics, rendering it a promising platform for the treatment of triple-negative breast cancer through autophagy inhibition and chemotherapy. In addition, the coloading of chemotherapeutic drugs and immunomodulators into the nanoplatform can also promote tumor cell death and regulate the local inflammatory microenvironment. For example, Lan et al. (2020) used a coloading system containing DOX and an indoleamine 2, 3-dioxygenase (IDO) inhibitor to block immunosuppressive pathways while inducing cell death with chemotherapy, thereby further activating $CD8^+$T cell responses. Zhang, Huang, et al. (2024), Zhang, Jiang, et al. (2024), and Zhang, Yang, et al. (2024) designed and fabricated a pH-responsive nanodrug delivery system formed by encapsulating a DOX prodrug and dual hydralazine (HDZ). In this system, the cRGD peptide was introduced to enhance its active targeting ability towards tumors. Moreover, hydrazone bonds were incorporated to endow the system with low-pH-responsive drug release characteristics specific to the tumor stroma microenvironment (TSM). The coloading of dual HDZ and DOX enabled this system to continuously normalize tumor vasculature after each injection. As a result, the penetration of nanodrugs deep into tumors was consistently enhanced. Noticeably, tumor blood vessels dilated significantly. This further facilitated the downregulation of the expression levels of HIF-1α, α-SMA, and fibronectin. These alterations in the TSM not only increased the accumulation and penetration of nanodrugs within tumors but also promoted the infiltration of immune cells into the tumor microenvironment.

In general, the chemotherapy system based on micro/nanoplatforms not only improves drug utilization and efficacy (Akakuru et al., 2022; Kang et al., 2022) but also achieves precise intervention in cell death type and inflammation regulation (Qin et al., 2018; Qin et al., 2025), laying a solid foundation for the development of combined treatment strategies.

5.3 Metal ion-induced programmed cell death and tumor inflammatory responses mediated by micro/nanoplatforms

In recent years, metal ion-mediated tumor therapy has become a research hotspot in the field of nanomedicine (Fig. 5.2). Its unique feature is that it can directly participate in

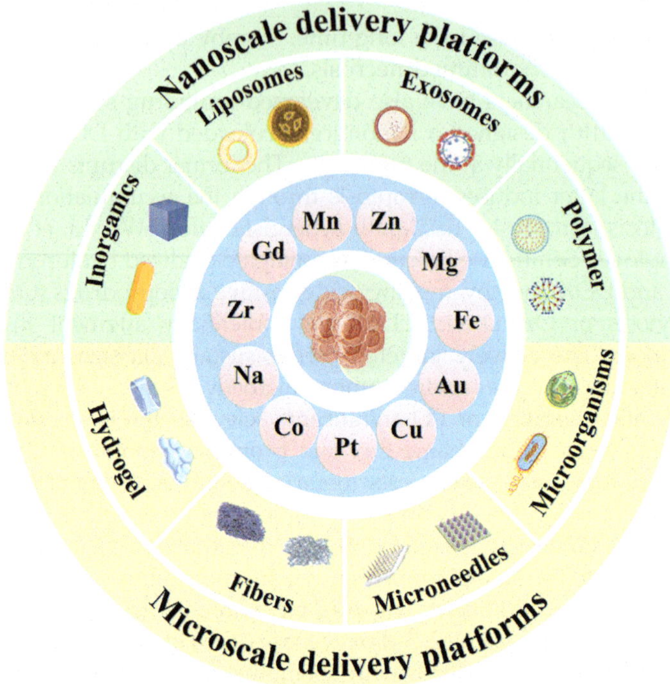

FIGURE 5.2 Micro/nanoplatforms developed for metal ion-induced programmed cell death and tumor inflammatory. In recent years, metal ion-mediated tumor therapy has become a research hotspot in the field of nanomedicine.

intracellular metabolism through redox regulation, thereby triggering a variety of PCD pathways and regulating tumor inflammatory microenvironment (An et al., 2025). Among the many metal ions, Fe, Cu, and other metal elements with valency change ability are widely used in chemodynamic therapy (CDT) due to their excellent chemical catalytic properties and biological activities (Chen et al., 2024). CDT uses the overexpressed H_2O_2 in tumor cells as a reaction substrate to generate •OH through the catalysis of transition metal ions (Fenton or Fenton-like reaction), and then induces lipid peroxidation, DNA damage, and mitochondrial dysfunction. Thus CDT can induce various forms of cell death such as ferroptosis, apoptosis, or pyroptosis (Hao et al., 2023). Compared with chemotherapy, CDT has the advantages of independent stimulation of traditional drugs, high selectivity, and avoiding the development of drug resistance.

Iron-based nanomaterials are the first class of nanomaterials used in CDT. Fe^{2+} reacts with H_2O_2 to form highly reactive •OH via the Fenton reaction, which initiates the ferroptosis process. Yu, He, et al. (2023) and Yu, Jia, et al. (2023) designed a microneedle drug delivery system, which can gradually release Fe^{2+} in the slightly acidic environment of tumors, generate reactive oxygen species (ROS) through the Fenton reaction, destroy cell membrane, and trigger ferroptosis. In addition, synergistic cell death can be achieved by combining Fe-based nanoplatforms with chemotherapeutic drugs. For example, Shi et al. (2025) designed DOX/Zr-MOF/Fe-CDs nanosystem, which, on the one hand, induces ferroptosis through Fe^{2+} catalytic reaction to produce ROS, and on the other hand, adriamycin interferes with DNA replication to trigger apoptosis, forming a synergistic effect of ferroptosis and apoptosis, which significantly enhances the therapeutic effect. Some studies have also found that ROS generated by iron-catalyzed reaction can lead to the decrease of mitochondrial membrane potential and the activation of Caspase, thereby achieving the synergistic effect of ferroptosis and apoptosis to promote tumor cell death (Wang, Jin, et al., 2024; Wang, Ren, et al., 2024; Wang, Yan, et al., 2024). Cu-based nanomaterials have been considered an important alternative system for Fenton-like reaction due to their Cu^{+}/Cu^{2+} cycling reaction in a weak acid environment. Cu^{+} can react with H_2O_2 to form •OH, and Cu^{2+} can be oxidized to form Cu^{2+}, which can be reduced back to Cu^{+} by GSH to achieve continuous ROS generation. This "GSH depletion-ROS amplification" process can effectively induce ferroptosis and necroptosis (Huang et al., 2024; Jia et al., 2022). Huang et al. (Zhu et al., 2023) constructed a hollow nanoshell structure based on CuP, which can rapidly release Cu^{+} in tumor cells, deplete intracellular GSH, and induce oxidative stress imbalance, thereby triggering ferroptosis. Li, Pei, et al. (2024) and Li, Qi, et al. (2024) reported that Cu^{2+} accumulation in mitochondria was promoted by using the copper ionophore Elesclomol, which induced a cuproptosis process related to lipid acylated protein aggregation and mitochondrial stress. This mechanism relies on the disruption of mitochondrial protein homeostasis and energy metabolism disorder, which leads to the selective death of tumor cells. To further enhance the therapeutic effect, some Cu-based platforms have been designed as multifunctional composite systems. For example, Gu and coworkers (Hu et al., 2024) coloaded Cu^{2+} and chemotherapeutic drug CDDP in polymer nanocapillaries. CDDP induced apoptosis through DNA adducts, while Cu^{+} catalyzed reactions enhanced ROS levels and promoted ferroptosis, thus achieving multipathway synergy. In addition, Cu ions can also induce disulfidptosis by promoting mitochondrial respiratory chain disorder and energy depletion. Yu, Jin, et al. (2025) and Yu, Li, et al. (2025) reported that Cu^{2+} can trigger the typical disulfidptosis process by destroying the intracellular redox balance and inhibiting nicotinamide adenine dinucleotide phosphate (NADPH) regeneration, leading to abnormal accumulation of disulfide bonds and cytoskeletal collapse. In this study, Cu Ion-treated cancer cells showed significant F-actin aggregation and decreased adenosine triphosphate (ATP) level, while cell death was significantly inhibited in the presence of NADPH donor or disulfide reducing agent, which further proved the mechanism of Cu^{2+} inducing disulfide bond stress to cause disulfide death.

In addition, the emergence of nanozymes in recent years provides a more controlled catalytic system for metal ion-mediated CDT. Nanozymes are a class of nanomaterials with enzyme-like activity, which can mimic the functions of peroxidase, oxidase, superoxide dismutase, etc. (Gao et al., 2007; Zhang, Huang, et al., 2024; Zhang, Jiang, et al., 2024; Zhang, Yang, et al., 2024). Nanoenzymes represented by Fe_3O_4 can catalyze the decomposition of H_2O_2 or other substrates to produce ROS and other substances in tumor cells, which can trigger tumor cell stress and induce PCD. For example, Fe_3O_4 nanozymes exhibit both peroxidase-like and oxidase-like activities and can efficiently produce ROS under weak acid conditions, leading to lipid peroxidation and membrane structure disruption (An et al., 2025; Chang et al., 2023). Compared with the traditional metal ion release system, the nanoenzyme catalysis system has the advantages of high catalytic efficiency, strong reaction stability, and few side reactions (Jia et al., 2025). It is worth noting that metal ions and their catalytic products also have significant regulatory effects on tumor immune microenvironment (Song et al., 2025; Tang et al., 2021). The production of ROS not only directly causes cell death, but also promotes tumor cells to release damage-associated molecular patterns

(DAMPs), such as ATP and HMGB1, thereby activating macrophages and dendritic cells and enhancing antitumor immune responses (An et al., 2025). Yao et al. (2025) developed a novel metal-organic frameworks (MOFs)-based nanozyme drug delivery system designated as D/P@ZUCO. This system exploited a zinc-doped ferrite core ($ZnFe_2O_4$) and a copper-doped zirconium-based shell [NH_2-UiO66 (Cu/Zr)] to manifest multienzyme activities. Specifically, peroxidase peroxidase (POD)-like, glutathione oxidase GSH-Ox-like, and catalase CAT-like activities were integrated within a single platform. The D/P@ZUCO system effectively catalyzed the generation of ROS, thereby inducing ferroptosis and augmenting the proapoptotic effect of DOX within the tumor microenvironment. Moreover, the inhibition of autophagy by PQ further magnified this effect, facilitating immunogenic cell death (ICD) and triggering a robust antitumor immune response. Fe-mediated ROS production can also upregulate the NF-κB and NLRP3 inflammasome pathways, promote the release of inflammatory factors, regulate the polarization of immune cells, and transform TAMs from M2 to proinflammatory M1, thereby contributing to the recovery of immune responses (An et al., 2025; Zhao et al., 2025).

In general, metal ion-based micro/nanoplatforms achieve in situ ROS amplification and cell death pathway activation in tumors through CDT, showing superior antitumor potential (Wei et al., 2022). They participate in catalytic reactions or nanoenzymatic reactions through Fe and Cu plasma, triggering various forms of programmed death such as ferroptosis, pyroptosis, and apoptosis, accompanied by the release of inflammatory signals and the activation of immune cells. Different from traditional chemotherapy, metal ion-mediated strategies can not only induce cell death at the chemical level, but also achieve immune remodeling and inflammation regulation by regulating the tumor microenvironment, which has become a promising direction in current tumor treatment research (An et al., 2025; Li, Pei, et al., 2024; Li, Qi, et al., 2024).

5.4 Light stimulation-induced programmed cell death and tumor inflammatory responses mediated by micro/nanoplatforms

Phototherapy is one of the important breakthroughs in the field of precision cancer therapy in recent years, which has attracted wide attention due to its advantages of noninvasiveness, strong spatial and temporal control, and precise local effect (Hu et al., 2020). By stimulating specific photosensitive materials with light sources, light energy can be converted into chemical or thermal energy to induce cell membrane damage, mitochondrial dysfunction, and protein denaturation, thereby triggering various forms of PCD (Tang et al., 2022). According to the different modes of energy conversion, phototherapy mainly includes photodynamic therapy (PDT), photothermal therapy (PTT), and photothermoelectric catalysis (PTEC) (Fig. 5.3) (He et al., 2025; Xu et al., 2025).

PDT is a treatment method that uses photosensitizer to transfer energy to oxygen molecules to produce ROS after being excited by specific wavelength light, thus causing oxidative stress damage to cells (Li et al., 2023). Common photosensitizers include porphyrins, phthalocyanine, BODIPY derivatives, etc., which can undergo photochemical reactions under light, resulting in rapid accumulation of intracellular ROS. ROS can attack

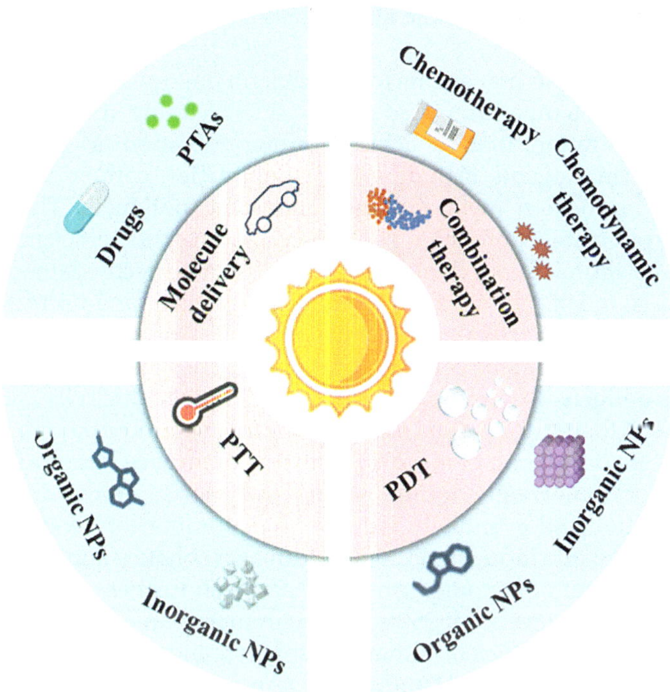

FIGURE 5.3 Micro/nanoplatforms developed for light stimulation -induced programmed cell death and tumor inflammatory. According to the different modes of energy conversion, phototherapy mainly includes photodynamic therapy (PDT), photothermal therapy (PTT), and photothermoelectric catalysis.

cell membrane lipids, proteins, and nucleic acids, leading to mitochondrial membrane potential breakdown and cytochrome C release, thereby activating Caspase signaling pathway and inducing apoptosis (Ji et al., 2018; Wang, Jin, et al., 2024; Wang, Ren, et al., 2024; Wang, Yan, et al., 2024). In addition, excessive ROS can also cause programmed death, such as ferroptosis and pyroptosis. For example, ROS can promote the production of lipid peroxides and inhibit GPX4 activity, leading to ferroptosis (Wang, Qiao, et al., 2023; Wang, Zhang, et al., 2023). Moreover, ROS overload can induce the activation of NLRP3 inflammasome, leading to pyroptosis-related Gasdermin D cleavage and membrane pore formation (Ding et al., 2024). These oxidative stress processes are accompanied by the release of inflammatory signals, such as high mobility group 1 protein (HMGB1) efflux, ATP release, and calretin excretion, which activate dendritic cells and promote antitumor immune responses (Yu, Jin, et al., 2025; Yu, Li, et al., 2025). However, conventional PDT still has the problems of limited light penetration depth and strong oxygen dependence, and the hypoxic environment within the tumor often limits the efficiency of ROS generation. Therefore researchers solve these problems by constructing micro/nanoplatforms. For example, Zhu et al. (2022) designed H-MnO_2@TPyP@Bro composite nanoparticles, which can produce reactive oxygen species under light, while Mn^{2+} can catabolize H_2O_2 overexpressed in the microenvironment to produce O_2, improve local hypoxia, and thus enhance the efficacy of PDT. In addition, upconversion nanoparticles can absorb near-infrared light with stronger tissue penetration ability and emit short-wavelength light to activate surface-modified photosensitizers, thereby breaking the shallow limitation of conventional PDT (Li et al., 2018; Shao et al., 2020).

Different from PDT, PTT utilizes photothermal agents to absorb light energy and convert it into thermal energy, inducing local temperature rise (43°C–50°C), leading to cellular structural damage and protein denaturation, thereby achieving tumor ablation (Melamed et al., 2015). The types of photothermal agents include gold nanoparticles, carbon-based materials (graphene, carbon dots), transition metal sulfides, and some polymers. These materials have excellent light absorption ability and high photothermal conversion efficiency, and can achieve rapid heating under illumination. Photothermal effects can directly damage the cell membrane and mitochondrial membrane structure, leading to apoptosis and necrosis (Peng et al., 2021). In addition, heat stress can activate changes in the expression of heat shock proteins. The exposure of HSP70 and HSP90 on the cell membrane surface not only marks the occurrence of ICD but also acts as antigens to stimulate the activation of dendritic cells and promote cytotoxic T cell response (Huang et al., 2021). For example, the tumor-targeting nanodrug CS-1@PB[HM] NPs designed by Long et al. (2023) can rapidly induce gasdermin E (GSDME)-dependent pyrolysis of tumor cells, induce strong pyroptosis, promote the release of tumor antigens and DAMPs, and eventually induce the maturation of dendritic cells (DCs) and trigger ICD. Therefore while inducing PCD, PTT can also enhance antitumor immune responses. With the development of nanomedicine, PTT has been further extended to PTEC, which significantly increases the level of ROS by locally inducing an electric field with a temperature gradient, thus achieving efficient tumor cell ablation and showing great potential for clinical application (Tang et al., 2018). Yang's team (An et al., 2025) designed a multifunctional nanoparticle, $Cu_5FeS_{3.6}Se_{0.4}$. The nanoparticles exhibit remarkable photothermal, thermoelectric, and chemical kinetic properties. Under near-infrared light irradiation, $Cu_5FeS_{3.6}Se_{0.4}$ nanoparticles can not only directly induce tumor cell ablation but also generate thermoelectric potential to accelerate the Fenton reaction and promote the generation of ROS for chemokinetic therapy. The resulting ROS induces oxidative stress in tumor cells, which promotes the occurrence of cuproptosis and pyroptosis.

The construction of micro/nanoplatforms enables multimode synergism and controlled release of phototherapy. For example, the composite system of photothermal materials and photosensitizers can achieve the combined effects of PDT and PTT under light irradiation: ROS produced by PDT leads to membrane oxidation and mitochondrial damage, while the heat generated by PTT can further accelerate the oxidation reaction and inhibit DNA repair ability, thereby forming an oxidative stress amplification cycle (Ai et al., 2023; Luo et al., 2025). Some studies have also introduced metal ions into the photothermal platform to use the photothermal effect to accelerate the Fenton reaction rate, so as to realize photothermal and chemical dynamic synergistic treatment under light, and significantly improve ROS production and cell death efficiency (An et al., 2025; Wu et al., 2025). In addition, oxidative stress and inflammatory response during photothermal or photodynamic processes can be further amplified by modulators. For example, the loading of immune adjuvants (such as CpG oligonucleotide or R837) in nanosystems can enhance the transmission of ICD signals, promote the activation of dendritic cells and the infiltration of T cells, thereby forming a "light stimulation-cell-death-immune activation" positive feedback loop (An et al., 2025). At the level of inflammation regulation, ROS and heat stress induced by light stimulation can achieve controlled activation of inflammation-related signaling pathways (Cun et al., 2025).

For example, the use of surface-modified antioxidant polymers or loaded antiinflammatory drugs can maintain the cell death effect while avoiding systemic inflammation spreading. On the other hand, the production of ROS and heat can be controlled by adjusting the light intensity and duration, thus achieving a dynamic balance between therapeutic effect and inflammatory response (An et al., 2025).

In summary, light-stimulated micro/nanoplatforms can induce multiple types of PCD through different mechanisms such as PDT, PTT, PTEC, and generate controlled inflammatory responses in the process, which provides a new multidimensional synergistic strategy for tumor treatment.

5.5 Ultrasound stimulation–induced programmed cell death and tumor inflammatory responses mediated by micro/nanoplatforms

Ultrasound (US) stimulation has attracted extensive attention in tumor treatment in recent years due to its strong tissue penetration ability, accurate spatial positioning, noninvasive and controllable characteristics (Liang et al., 2023). Ultrasonic-based tumor therapy mainly includes sonodynamic therapy (SDT) and piezocatalytic therapy (Fig. 5.4). Although they both use US as an external stimulus, the mechanism of action is different: the former relies on US to stimulate sonosensitizers to produce ROS to achieve cell killing.

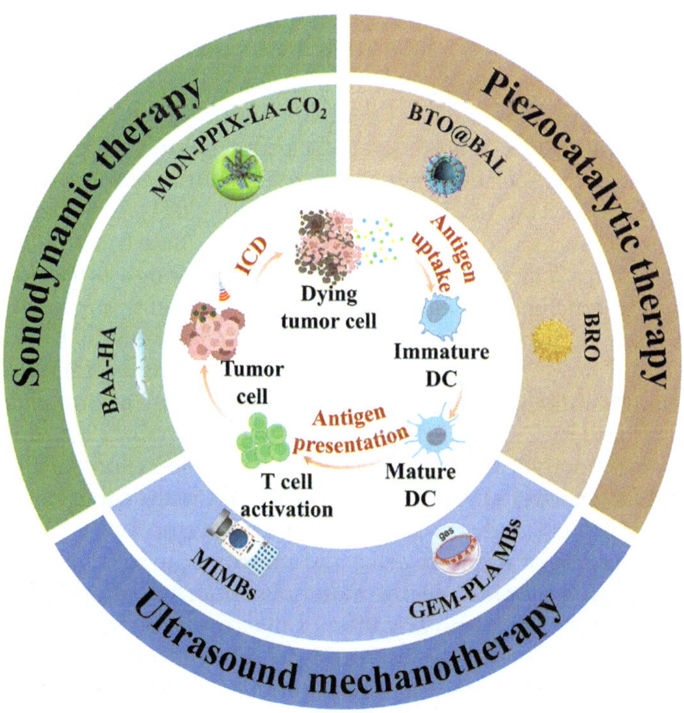

FIGURE 5.4 Micro/nanoplatforms developed for ultrasound stimulation–induced programmed cell death and tumor inflammatory. Ultrasonic-based tumor therapy mainly includes sonodynamic therapy (SDT) and piezocatalytic therapy (PCT).

The latter uses piezoelectric materials to generate an electric field under the action of mechanical force, catalyzing the production of ROS or other products (Chen, Sang, et al., 2025; Chen, Sun, et al., 2025; Cui, Tang, et al., 2024; Cui, Wang, et al., 2024; Liu, Li, et al., 2020; Liu, Yan, et al., 2020).

The core principle of SDT is to use US to excite the sonosensitizer. Through the ultrasonic cavitation effect, that is, the process of the formation and collapse of microbubbles in the liquid medium caused by US, this process will produce a local instantaneous reaction environment of high temperature and high pressure, thereby stimulating the sonosensitizer to produce ROS. ROS can trigger mitochondrial membrane potential loss, cytochrome C release, and Caspase cascade activation, leading to apoptosis (Ren et al., 2025; Xiong et al., 2025; Zhou et al., 2024). When the level of ROS is too high, it can also trigger lipid peroxidation and DNA fragmentation, which further trigger ferroptosis and pyroptosis (Sun et al., 2024; You et al., 2022). Single SDT is limited by problems such as oxygen dependence and limited ROS production, while these limitations can be effectively overcome by constructing multifunctional nanoplatforms. For example, Qu et al. (2025) designed boron nanosheet with in-situ grown gold nanoparticles coated with hyaluronic acid (BAA–HA) nanocomposite, in which Au nanoparticles exhibit the function of catalase to decompose the overexpressed H_2O_2 in the microenvironment to produce O_2 to alleviate hypoxia, while B NSs and Au form heterojunction to enhance the electron–hole separation efficiency and achieve double enhancement of the acoustic force effect. To enhance the ROS level and synergetic PTT to activate tumor immunogenic death. Another type of strategy is the use of nanocellulatory-based acoustic cavitation enhancement, such as the introduction of gas precursors (e.g., C_3F_8, $NH_3 \cdot BH_3$) into the nanosystem to rupture microbubbles and amplify local energy under ultrasonic irradiation, thereby increasing ROS production and cell destruction capacity (Pan et al., 2023; Sun et al., 2022; Ya et al., 2023).

Under the action of the US, piezoelectric materials can generate electric fields, which, in turn, trigger redox reactions to generate ROS. The generated electric fields can also use compounds overexpressed in tumor cells as sacrificial agents to catalyze the decomposition of H_2O_2 into H_2 and O_2 (Deng et al., 2025; Hao et al., 2026; Zhong et al., 2021). Dong et al. (2025) synthesized a nanoheterojunction indocyanine green–zeolitic imidazolate framework-8–hyaluronic acid (IZH), which generates a strong internal electric field through ultrasonic stimulation to enhance the separation efficiency of electrons and holes, thereby improving the generation efficiency of ROS, and then triggering ferroptosis and apoptosis of tumor cells. Under the joint action of US-induced ROS and gas molecules, the tumor immune microenvironment can also be significantly improved. On the one hand, an appropriate amount of ROS can promote the release of DAMPs, stimulate the maturation of DCs, and enhance antigen presentation, thereby activating T cell-mediated immune response (An et al., 2025; Du, Wang, et al., 2024; Du, Zhao, et al., 2024; He et al., 2023). On the other hand, the local mechanical damage caused by US and gas can enhance the permeability of the microenvironment, promote the infiltration of immune cells, and improve the immunosuppressive state. In addition, the gas released by piezoelectric materials under US can regulate the inflammatory signaling pathway, promote the polarization of macrophages from M2 to M1 type, and further enhance the antitumor immune response. This multilevel effect composed of "physical stimulation, chemical catalysis, and immune regulation" makes US-stimulated micro/nanoplatforms not only have cell killing function, but also achieve systemic immune activation through inflammatory regulation (Xie, Guo, et al., 2024; Xie, Zhang, et al., 2024; Yu, He, et al., 2023; Yu, Jia, et al., 2023).

Compared with chemotherapy and phototherapy, the outstanding advantages of US-stimulated micro/nanoplatforms lie in their deep penetration and precise focusing. Through reasonable design of micro/nanoplatforms, PCD induction with multiple mechanisms can be achieved within tumors. At the same time, the mechanical damage and oxidative stress process caused by US stimulation can also activate the inflammatory response and promote the remodeling of the immune system, making US-stimulated micro/nanoplatform one of the ideal strategies for precise killing and immune reversal in tumor treatment in the future.

5.6 Alternating magnetic field stimulation–induced programmed cell death and tumor inflammatory responses mediated by micro/nanoplatforms

Alternating magnetic field (AMF), as a noninvasive and remote adjustable external stimulation method, has shown unique advantages in tumor treatment (An et al., 2025). By combining with magnetic micro/nanomaterials (Fig. 5.5), AMFs can generate heat, mechanical force, electric field, or electrochemical reactions in the local tumor, thereby inducing various forms of PCD and regulating local inflammatory response at the lesion site (Chen, Sang, et al., 2025; Chen, Sun, et al., 2025; Fan & Guo, 2023; Gavilán et al., 2021). There are four main strategies for tumor treatment based on AMFs: magnetic thermal therapy (MHT), magnetothermodynamic (MTD), magnetic-thermo-electric therapy, and magnetoelectric

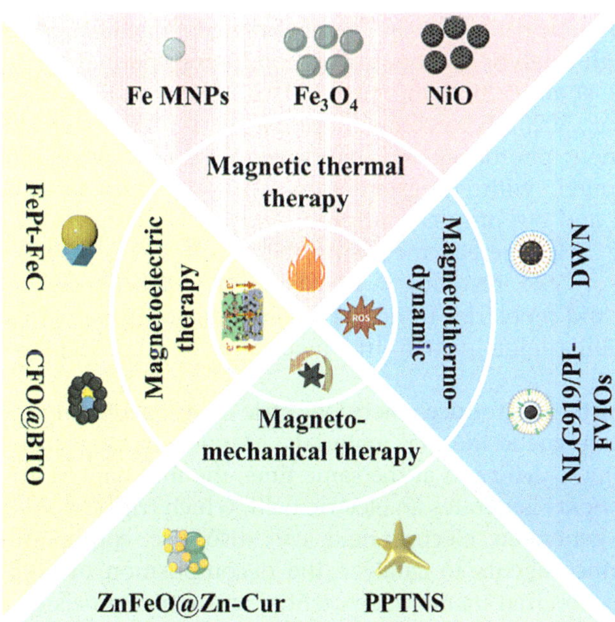

FIGURE 5.5 Micro/nanoplatforms developed for alternating magnetic field (AMF) stimulation–induced programmed cell death and tumor inflammatory. *DWN*, Ddoped rare-earth upconversion nanocomposite integrated with tungsten iron ($FeWO_4$) nanoparticles. AMF, as a noninvasive and remote adjustable external stimulation method, has shown unique advantages in tumor treatment.

therapy. Although these methods all rely on the response of magnetic nanomaterials, their energy conversion mode, ROS generation mechanism, and cell death pathways are different (An et al., 2025; Li et al., 2021; Pan et al., 2021; Zhang et al., 2020; Yu). The design of micro/nanoplatforms can not only optimize the magnetic response performance of magnetic materials but also realize multimode cooperation to improve the efficiency of PCD and regulate the inflammatory response (An et al., 2025; Qi et al., 2024; Wang, Jin, et al., 2024; Wang, Ren, et al., 2024; Wang, Yan, et al., 2024).

MHT uses magnetic nanoparticles to generate heat under the action of AMF, which increases the temperature of tumor tissues to more than 43°C, leading to denaturation of cellular proteins and changes in membrane structure (Xie, Guo, et al., 2024; Xie, Zhang, et al., 2024; Yang et al., 2023). At the same time, magnetic heating therapy can activate immune-related signals, and local high temperature promotes the efflux of heat shock proteins to form ICD signals, thereby enhancing the antigen presentation ability of dendritic cells (Jiang et al., 2022). Zhang's team (Wang, Gu, et al., 2022; Wang, Qi, et al., 2022) constructed Fe_3O_4@PVP@DOX nanoplatform, which can achieve efficient magneto-thermal transformation under AMF, raising the local tumor temperature to about 45°C, inducing cell membrane disruption and mitochondrial membrane potential changes. The magnetothermal effect not only promoted the heat-triggered release of drug DOX, but also promoted the expression of heat shock proteins through heat stress, induced ICD, and activated dendritic cell maturation, and significantly enhanced $CD8^+$ T cell infiltration and tumor suppression effect. Some researchers have proposed the concept of nonmetallic materials as magnetic heating agents. For example, Xie, Guo, et al. (2024) and Xie, Zhang, et al. (2024) found that graphite block showed excellent magnetic heating efficiency, thanks to its excellent eddy current thermal conductivity. This study marks the pioneering application of nonmetallic materials in MHT in vivo and provides a new reference for the design of magnetic heating micro/nanoplatforms. MTD is that magnetic nanoparticles can not only generate heat under an AMF, but also produce ROS through catalytic reactions, thus combining thermal effects with chemical dynamic effects (Liu, Li, et al., 2020; Wang, Jin, et al., 2024; Wang, Ren, et al., 2024; Wang, Yan, et al., 2024; Yan, et al., 2020). For example, Liu, He, et al. (2025) and Liu, Wu, et al. (2025) designed a magnetic-phototriggered nanoenzyme doped rare-earth upconversion nanocomposite integrated with tungsten iron ($FeWO_4$) nanoparticles (DWN). When costimulated by AMF and 808 nm near-infrared laser, DWN nanoenzyme releases multivalent metal ions in the TME, thereby increasing the production of reactive oxygen species and the consumption of GSH, resulting in MTD-enhanced ferroptosis and cell atrophy. These effects trigger ICD and repolarize tumor-associated macrophages, which enhance immune responses and inhibit tumor growth and metastasis of triple-negative breast cancer in mice.

Magnetic-thermo-electric therapy further introduces thermoelectric components into the micro/nanoplatforms on the basis of magnetic thermal materials. Magnetic nanoparticles generate local heat under the action of an AMF, and at the same time, the internal electron migration of the thermoelectric components generates an electric field, which triggers redox reactions and generates ROS. The generated electric field can also use compounds overexpressed in tumor cells as sacrifice agents to catalyze the decomposition of H_2O_2 into H_2, and O_2, which can affect mitochondrial membrane potential and ion channels (Dai et al., 2026; Wang, Qiao, et al., 2023; Wang, Zhang, et al., 2023). This "magnetic-thermoelectric" synergistic effect can enhance the generation of ROS, thereby inducing apoptosis, ferroptosis, and necrosis. Yuan et al. (2025) developed a magnetothermal-thermoelectric heterojunction of cobalt ferrite ($CoFe_2O_4$) (CFO)/strontium titanate ($SrTiO_3$) (STO). The AMF first triggers the CFO to generate heat, which activates the thermoelectric effect of STO, leading to the separation of electrons and holes and the production of $\cdot O_2^-$ and ·OH. It can promote the maturation of DCs and enhance the immune response by upregulating immune molecules (such as VCAM-1 and ICAM-1). Magnetoelectric therapy uses magnetic coupling with piezoelectric materials to convert AMFs directly into electricity, gas, or ion currents, so as to achieve nonthermal and nonchemical cell killing (Zhang et al., 2021). For example, Chen et al. (2017) designed a FeGa@P (VDF-TrFE) linear magnetoelectric nanorobot that can witively and accurately steer to a target location by rotating a magnetic field and perform magnetoelectric-assisted drug release on demand to kill cancer cells. Compared with magnetoelectric therapy alone, magnetoelectric therapy still retains high killing ability in hypoxic or heat-sensitive tumors, and the treatment intensity can be precisely regulated in time and space.

In general, the AMF micro/nanoplatforms can induce PCD through multiple mechanisms such as magnetic heating, magnetic thermal dynamic, magnetic thermoelectric, and magnetic electric, and regulate the inflammatory response in the process. It provides a new noninvasive, efficient, and controllable strategy for the treatment of deep tumors. The design of micro/nanoplatforms can not only optimize the magnetic response performance but also realize the synergistic effect of multiple pathways such as heat, electricity, ROS, and gas, which makes the AMF stimulation show great potential in tumor killing and immune regulation.

5.7 Interaction between programmed cell death and tumor inflammatory response

Traditional cancer therapies, such as chemotherapy and radiotherapy, mainly aim to enhance tumor cell death, but often ignore the complex feedback of inflammation. Chemotherapy drugs induce apoptosis or pyroptosis through DNA damage and protein function disruption, accompanied by the release of local inflammatory factors. These inflammatory signals can enhance the activation of immune cells but may also trigger immunosuppressive or protumor signals. Radiotherapy produces a large number of free radicals, which can induce apoptosis, necrosis, and ferroptosis, and activate the NF-κB pathway, causing the release of IL-6, HMGB1, HSP70, and other molecules. This local inflammation can enhance antitumor immunity, as well as promote tumor progression under long-term low-grade inflammation conditions (Ma et al., 2025; Sabit et al., 2025; Wang, Gu, et al., 2022; Wang, Qi, et al., 2022). Therefore unidirectional induction of PCD cannot fully control the tumor microenvironment, while ignoring the regulation of inflammation may lead to limited efficacy or increased side effects. The introduction of micro/nanoplatforms provides a new strategy for regulating the bidirectional relationship between PCD and tumor inflammation (Zhu et al., 2023). Through the precise design of nanoparticles and external stimulation systems, tumor targeting in space and time-controlled release can be achieved, so that PCD occurs centrally at the tumor site, and the intensity and duration of inflammation can be regulated at the same time (Irvine & Dane, 2020; Zhang, Huang, et al., 2024; Zhang, Jiang, et al., 2024; Zhang, Yang, et al., 2024).

PCD induced by micro/nanoplatforms and tumor inflammation has a close two-way regulation relationship in the tumor microenvironment. When tumor cells undergo different types of PCD after stimulation, they will release a variety of inflammatory signals, including DAMPs, cytokines, and chemokines (Wu, Li, et al., 2024; Wu, Liu, et al., 2024; Yang et al., 2021). These signals can activate TLR, NF-κB, NLRP3, and other inflammatory pathways to induce dendritic cell maturation, macrophage polarization, and T cell recruitment, thereby participating in the regulation of innate and adaptive immunity (Jiang et al., 2017; Li, Yuan, et al., 2025; Li, Zhang, et al., 2025; Xi, et al., 2025). Simultaneously, the inflammatory state in the tumor microenvironment also affects the type and efficiency of PCD in turn: local inflammatory factors such as TNF-α, IL-6, and IL-1β can promote the activation of PCD pathway, and this bidirectional regulation mechanism enables PCD and inflammation to form a complex feedback network in the tumor microenvironment (Fig. 5.6) (Lu et al., 2024).

In summary, the nanoplatform combined with external physical stimulation can not only efficiently induce various types of PCD but also accurately regulate the local inflammatory response to achieve the dynamic regulation of the tumor microenvironment in space and time. This bidirectional regulation strategy makes PCD and inflammatory response to achieve the best balance between killing tumor cells and activating the immune system, which provides a new idea for precise cancer treatment.

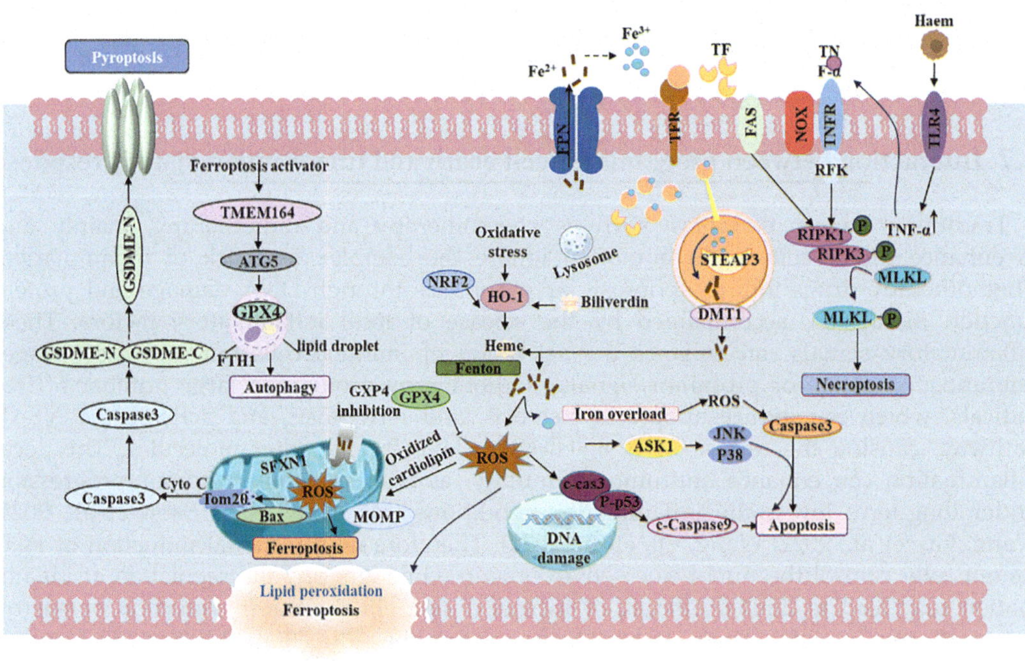

FIGURE 5.6 Interaction between programmed cell death (PCD) and tumor inflammatory response. The inflammatory state in the tumor microenvironment also affects the type and efficiency of PCD. Inturn, local inflammatory factors such as TNF-α, IL-6, and IL-1β can promote the activation of PCD pathway, and this bidirectional regulation mechanism enables PCD and inflammation to form a complex feedback network in the tumor microenvironment.

AI disclosure

During the preparation of this work, the author(s) used the built-in abstracting tool in ELSA. The authors share a single abstract across Chapters 3, 4, and 5, so no independent abstracts are provided. After using this tool/service, the author(s) reviewe(s) and edite(s) the content as needed and take(s) full responsibility for the content of the publication.

References

Ai, Y., He, M. Q., Sun, H., Jia, X., Wu, L., Zhang, X., Sun, H. B., & Liang, Q. (2023). Ultra small high-entropy alloy nanoparticles: Efficient nanozyme for enhancing tumor photothermal therapy. *Advanced Materials, 35*(23). https://doi.org/10.1002/adma.202302335, http://onlinelibrary.wiley.com/journal/10.1002/(ISSN)1521-4095.

Akakuru, O. U., Zhang, Z., Iqbal, M. Z., Zhu, C., Zhang, Y., & Wu, A. (2022). Chemotherapeutic nanomaterials in tumor boundary delineation: Prospects for effective tumor treatment. *Acta Pharmaceutica Sinica B. 12*(6), 2640–2657. https://doi.org/10.1016/j.apsb.2022.02.016, http://www.elsevier.com/wps/find/journaldescription.cws_home/725753/description#description.

An, J., Yang, Y., Feng, Y., Wang, S., Wang, S., Zhang, B., Yan, X., & Jiang, B. (2025). Proton-driven deformability enables nanozyme-integrated vaccine for enhanced tumor immunotherapy. *Advanced Materials*. https://doi.org/10.1002/adma.202509994, http://onlinelibrary.wiley.com/journal/10.1002/(ISSN)1521-4095.

Assi, M., & Kimmelman, A. C. (2023). Impact of context-dependent autophagy states on tumor progression. *Nature Cancer, 4*(5), 596–607. https://doi.org/10.1038/s43018-023-00546-7.

Browning, R. J., Reardon, P. J. T., Parhizkar, M., Pedley, R. B., Edirisinghe, M., Knowles, J. C., & Stride, E. (2017). Drug delivery strategies for platinum-based chemotherapy. *ACS Nano, 11*(9), 8560–8578. https://doi.org/10.1021/acsnano.7b04092, http://pubs.acs.org/journal/ancac3.

Chang, M., Wang, Z., Dong, C., Zhou, R., Chen, L., Huang, H., Feng, W., Wang, Z., Wang, Y., & Chen, Y. (2023). Ultrasound-amplified enzyodynamic tumor therapy by perovskite nanoenzyme-enabled cell pyroptosis and cascade catalysis. *Advanced Materials, 35*(7). https://doi.org/10.1002/adma.202208817, http://onlinelibrary.wiley.com/journal/10.1002/(ISSN)1521-4095.

Chen, K., Zhou, A., Zhou, X., He, J., Xu, Y., & Ning, X. (2024). Cellular Trojan Horse initiates bimetallic Fe-Cu MOF-mediated synergistic cuproptosis and ferroptosis against malignancies. *Science Advances, 10*(15). https://doi.org/10.1126/sciadv.adk3201, https://www.science.org/toc/sciadv/10/15.

Chen, X., Zhu, Q., Xu, X., Shen, S., Zhang, Y., & Mo, R. (2019). Sequentially site-specific delivery of apoptotic protein and tumor-suppressor gene for combination cancer therapy. *Small (Weinheim an der Bergstrasse, Germany), 15*(40). https://doi.org/10.1002/smll.201902998, http://onlinelibrary.wiley.com/journal/10.1002/(ISSN)1613-6829.

Chen, X. Z., Hoop, M., Shamsudhin, N., Huang, T., Özkale, B., Li, Q., Siringil, E., Mushtaq, F., Di Tizio, L., Nelson, B. J., & Pané, S. (2017). Hybrid magnetoelectric nanowires for nanorobotic applications: Fabrication, magnetoelectric coupling, and magnetically assisted in vitro targeted drug delivery. *Advanced Materials, 29*(8). https://doi.org/10.1002/adma.201605458, http://www3.interscience.wiley.com/journal/119030556/issue.

Chen, Y., Sun, H., Li, Y., Han, X., Yang, Y., Chen, Z., Zhao, X., Qian, Y., Liu, X., Zhou, F., Bai, J., & Qiao, Y. (2025). Magnetic nanomaterials for hyperthermia-based therapy and controlled drug delivery. *Bioactive Materials, 53*, 591–629. https://doi.org/10.1016/j.bioactmat.2025.07.033, https://www.sciencedirect.com/science/journal/2452199X.

Chen, Z. G., Sang, L., Liu, Y. J., & Bai, Z. Q. (2025). Sono-piezo dynamic therapy: Utilizing piezoelectric materials as sonosensitizer for sonodynamic therapy. *Advancement of Science, 12*(12), 2417439. https://doi.org/10.1002/advs.202417439.

Cookson, B. T., & Brennan, M. A. (2001). Pro-inflammatory programmed cell death. *Trends in Microbiology, 9*(3), 113–114. https://doi.org/10.1016/s0966-842x(00)01936-3.

Cui, S. K., Wang, K., & Huang, Z. H. (2024). Ferroptosis and the tumor microenvironment. *Journal of Experimental & Clinical Cancer Research: CR, 43*(1), 315. https://doi.org/10.1186/s13046-024-03235-0.

Cui, X., Tang, X., Niu, Y., Tong, L., Zhao, H., Yang, Y., Jin, G., Li, M., & Han, X. (2024). Functional phosphorene: Burgeoning generation, two-dimensional nanotherapeutic platform for oncotherapy. *Coordination Chemistry Reviews, 507*. https://doi.org/10.1016/j.ccr.2024.215744, https://www.sciencedirect.com/science/journal/00108545.

Cun, F., Chen, J., Li, H., Kou, Y., Wang, M., Li, X., Chen, H., & Kong, J. (2025). Mesoporous gold nanospheres confined platinum nanoclusters as robust ROS and oxygen nanogenerators for nir-ii hyperthermia cancer therapy. *Advanced Science, 12*(28). https://doi.org/10.1002/advs.202502688, http://onlinelibrary.wiley.com/journal/10.1002/(ISSN)2198-3844.

Dai, C., He, Y., Lu, H., Feng, X., Long, N., Song, Q., Li, Y., Wang, Y., Martin, L. L., Fan, C., & Sun, D. (2026). Nanoquadruplex-driven hydrogen therapy: NIR-controlled release for targeted cancer ferroptosis. *Biomaterials, 326*. https://doi.org/10.1016/j.biomaterials.2025.123635, https://www.sciencedirect.com/science/journal/01429612.

Debnath, J., Gammoh, N., & Ryan, K. M. (2023). Autophagy and autophagy-related pathways in cancer. *Nature Reviews. Molecular Cell Biology, 24*(8), 560–575. https://doi.org/10.1038/s41580-023-00585-z.

Deng, H., Li, X., Pan, L., Tang, M., Song, P., Long, B., Sun, X., Li, Y., Zhang, H., Wang, S., Wang, Z., & Kong, X. (2025). Single-Atom W anchored hexagonal boron nitride piezoelectric nanosonosensitizer remodels tumor microenvironment for enhanced sonodynamic therapy. *Advanced Functional Materials, 35*(26). https://doi.org/10.1002/adfm.202420974, http://onlinelibrary.wiley.com/journal/10.1002/(ISSN)1616-3028.

Denk, D., & Greten, F. R. (2022). Inflammation: The incubator of the tumor microenvironment. *Trends Cancer, 8*(11), 901–914. https://doi.org/10.1016/j.trecan.2022.07.002.

Di, Y., Shen, Q., Yang, Z., Song, G., Fang, T., Liu, Y., Liu, Y., Luo, Q., Wang, F., Yan, X., Bai, H., Huang, Y., Lv, F., & Wang, S. (2023). Biosynthesis of multifunctional transformable peptides for inducing tumor cell apoptosis. *Small (Weinheim an der Bergstrasse, Germany), 19*(48). https://doi.org/10.1002/smll.202303035, http://onlinelibrary.wiley.com/journal/10.1002/(ISSN)1613-6829.

Ding, F., Liu, J., Ai, K., Xu, C., Mao, X., Liu, Z., & Xiao, H. (2024). Simultaneous activation of pyroptosis and cGAS-STING pathway with epigenetic/ photodynamic nanotheranostic for enhanced tumor Photoimmunotherapy. *Advanced Materials, 36*(7). https://doi.org/10.1002/adma.202306419, http://onlinelibrary.wiley.com/journal/10.1002/(ISSN)1521-4095.

Dong, L. L., Yang, X. J., You, H. P., & Song, S. Y. (2025). Nanoconfined heterojunctions with enhanced piezoelectricity for amplifying reactive oxygen species storms-triggered tumor ferroptosis-like/apoptosis. *Nano Today, 64*, 102785. https://doi.org/10.1016/j.nantod.2025.102785.

Du, F., Zhao, H., Song, Y., Feng, Z., Liu, K., Wang, Z., Guo, R., Qiu, L., Chen, Q., & Zhou, L. (2024). Apoptosis-sensitizing tumor nanomedicine by regulating pyroptosis-associated inflammatory cell death. *Advanced Functional Materials, 34*(44). https://doi.org/10.1002/adfm.202406150, http://onlinelibrary.wiley.com/journal/10.1002/(ISSN)1616-3028.

Du, M., Wang, T., Peng, W. R., Feng, R. J., Goh, M., & Chen, Z. Y. (2024). Bacteria-driven nanosonosensitizer delivery system for enhanced breast cancer treatment through sonodynamic therapy-induced immunogenic cell death. *Journal of Nanobiotechnology, 22*(1), 167. https://doi.org/10.1186/s12951-024-02437-0.

Fan, H. H., & Guo, Z. J. (2023). Tumor microenvironment-responsive manganese-based nanomaterials for cancer treatment. *Coordination Chemistry Reviews, 480*, 215027. https://doi.org/10.1016/j.ccr.2023.215027.

Fang, R. H., Gao, W. W., & Zhang, L. F. (2023). Targeting drugs to tumours using cell membrane-coated nanoparticles. *Nature Reviews Clinical Oncology, 20*(1), 33–48. https://doi.org/10.1038/s41571-022-00699-x.

Gabbutt, C., Duran-Ferrer, M., Grant, H. E., Mallo, D., Nadeu, F., Househam, J., Villamor, N., Müller, M., Heath, S., Raineri, E., Krali, O., Nordlund, J., Zenz, T., Gut, I. G., Campo, E., Lopez-Guillermo, A., Fitzgibbon, J., Barnes, C. P., Shibata, D., ... Graham, T. A. (2025). Fluctuating DNA methylation tracks cancer evolution at clinical scale. *Nature, 645*(8081), 764–773. https://doi.org/10.1038/s41586-025-09374-4, https://www.nature.com/nature/.

Gao, L., Zhuang, J., Nie, L., Zhang, J., Zhang, Y., Gu, N., Wang, T., Feng, J., Yang, D., Perrett, S., & Yan, X. (2007). Intrinsic peroxidase-like activity of ferromagnetic nanoparticles. *Nature Nanotechnology, 2*(9), 577–583. https://doi.org/10.1038/nnano.2007.260.

Gavilán, H., Avugadda, S. K., Fernández-Cabada, T., Soni, N., Cassani, M., Mai, B. T., Chantrell, R., & Pellegrino, T. (2021). Magnetic nanoparticles and clusters for magnetic hyperthermia: Optimizing their heat performance and developing combinatorial therapies to tackle cancer. *Chemical Society Reviews, 50*(20), 11614–11667. https://doi.org/10.1039/d1cs00427a, http://pubs.rsc.org/en/journals/journal/cs.

Hao, J. N., Ge, K., Chen, G., Dai, B., & Li, Y. (2023). Strategies to engineer various nanocarrier-based hybrid catalysts for enhanced chemodynamic cancer therapy. *Chemical Society Reviews, 52*(22), 7707–7736. https://doi.org/10.1039/d3cs00356f, http://pubs.rsc.org/en/journals/journal/cs.

Hao, Z., He, Y., Liu, C., Xue, W., Liu, Z., Li, A., Tu, W., & Zhang, X. (2026). Piezoelectric catalytic activation of cGAS-STING pathway by Ga-based liquid metal nanoparticles for enhanced antitumor immunotherapy.

Biomaterials, 327. https://doi.org/10.1016/j.biomaterials.2025.123745, https://www.sciencedirect.com/science/journal/01429612.

He, M., Wang, M., Xu, T., Zhang, M., Dai, H., Wang, C., Ding, D., & Zhong, Z. (2023). Reactive oxygen species-powered cancer immunotherapy: Current status and challenges. *Journal of Controlled Release, 356*, 623–648. https://doi.org/10.1016/j.jconrel.2023.02.040, www.elsevier.com/locate/jconrel.

He, M., Xiao, M., Wang, R., Fan, J., Peng, X., & Sun, W. (2025). Phototherapeutic nanoagents for cancer immunotherapy. *Progress in Materials Science, 147*. https://doi.org/10.1016/j.pmatsci.2024.101347, https://www.sciencedirect.com/science/journal/00796425.

Hu, G., Cheng, W., Gu, M., Hang, L., Yang, W., Liu, T., Li, W., Shi, X., Liu, M., & Tian, J. (2024). Vitamin e succinate-glycol chitosan modified copper ferrite nanocomposites for lung cancer: Targeted oxidative stress regulation induces cuproptosis and ferroptosis. *Chemical Engineering Journal, 493*. https://doi.org/10.1016/j.cej.2024.152408, https://www.sciencedirect.com/science/journal/13858947.

Hu, J. J., Lei, Q., & Zhang, X. Z. (2020). Recent advances in photonanomedicines for enhanced cancer photodynamic therapy. *Progress in Materials Science, 114*, 100685. https://doi.org/10.1016/j.pmatsci.2020.100685.

Huang, H. J., Huang, S. Y., Wang, T. H., Lin, T. Y., Huang, N. C., Shih, O., Jeng, U. S., Chu, C. Y., & Chiang, W. H. (2023). Clay nanosheets simultaneously intercalated and stabilized by PEGylated chitosan as drug delivery vehicles for cancer chemotherapy. *Carbohydrate Polymers, 302*. https://doi.org/10.1016/j.carbpol.2022.120390, http://www.elsevier.com/wps/find/journaldescription.cws_home/405871/description#description.

Huang, L., Zhu, J., Wu, G., Xiong, W., Feng, J., Yan, C., Yang, J., Li, Z., Fan, Q., Ren, B., Li, Y., Chen, C., Yu, X., & Shen, Z. (2024). A strategy of "adding fuel to the flames" enables a self-accelerating cycle of ferroptosis-cuproptosis for potent antitumor therapy. *Biomaterials, 311*. https://doi.org/10.1016/j.biomaterials.2024.122701, https://www.sciencedirect.com/science/journal/01429612.

Huang, X., Jin, J., Qian, W., & Ye, X. (2019). Shikonin overcomes drug resistance and induces necroptosis by regulating the mir-92a-1-5p/Mlkl axis in chronic myeloid leukemia cells. *Blood, 134*(Supplement_1), 1633. https://doi.org/10.1182/blood-2019-125600.

Huang, X., Lu, Y., Guo, M., Du, S., & Han, N. (2021). Recent strategies for nano-based PTT combined with immunotherapy: From a biomaterial point of view. *Theranostics, 11*(15), 7546–7569. https://doi.org/10.7150/THNO.56482, https://www.thno.org/v11p7546.htm.

Irvine, D. J., & Dane, E. L. (2020). Enhancing cancer immunotherapy with nanomedicine. *Nature Reviews. Immunology, 20*(5), 321–334. https://doi.org/10.1038/s41577-019-0269-6.

Jayakumar, A., & Bothwell, A. L. M. (2019). RIPK3-induced inflammation by I-MDSCs promotes intestinal tumors. *Cancer Research, 79*(7), 1587–1599. https://doi.org/10.1158/0008-5472.Can-18-2153.

Ji, C., Gao, Q., Dong, X., Yin, W., Gu, Z., Gan, Z., Zhao, Y., & Yin, M. (2018). A Size-reducible nanodrug with an aggregation-enhanced photodynamic effect for deep chemo-photodynamic therapy. *Angewandte Chemie - International Edition, 57*(35), 11384–11388. https://doi.org/10.1002/anie.201807602, http://onlinelibrary.wiley.com/journal/10.1002/(ISSN)1521-3773.

Jia, C. Y., Guo, Y. X., & Wu, F. G. (2022). Chemodynamic therapy via fenton and fenton-like nanomaterials: Strategies and recent advances. *Small (Weinheim an der Bergstrasse, Germany), 18*(6), 2103868. https://doi.org/10.1002/smll.202103868.

Jia, X. N., Wang, E. R., & Wang, J. (2025). Rational design of nanozymes for engineered cascade catalytic cancer therapy. *Chemical Reviews, 125*(5), 2908–2952. https://doi.org/10.1021/acs.chemrev.4c00882.

Jiang, H., Fu, H., Guo, Y., Hu, P., & Shi, J. (2022). Evoking tumor associated macrophages by mitochondria-targeted magnetothermal immunogenic cell death for cancer immunotherapy. *Biomaterials, 289*. https://doi.org/10.1016/j.biomaterials.2022.121799, http://www.journals.elsevier.com/biomaterials/.

Jiang, W., Von Roemeling, C. A., Chen, Y., Qie, Y., Liu, X., Chen, J., & Kim, B. Y. S. (2017). Designing nanomedicine for immuno-oncology. *Nature Biomedical Engineering, 1*(2). https://doi.org/10.1038/s41551-017-0029, www.nature.com/natbiomedeng/.

Kang, N., Son, S., Min, S., Hong, H., Kim, C., An, J., Kim, J. S., & Kang, H. (2023). Stimuli-responsive ferroptosis for cancer therapy. *Chemical Society Reviews, 52*(12), 3955–3972. https://doi.org/10.1039/d3cs00001j, http://pubs.rsc.org/en/journals/journal/cs.

Kang, N. W., Lee, J. Y., & Kim, D. D. (2022). Hydroxyapatite-binding albumin nanoclusters for enhancing bone tumor chemotherapy. *Journal of Controlled Release: Official Journal of the Controlled Release Society, 342*, 111–121. https://doi.org/10.1016/j.jconrel.2021.12.039.

Kerr, J. F. R., Wyllie, A. H., & Currie, A. R. (1972). Apoptosis: A basic biological phenomenon with wideranging implications in tissue kinetics. *Brit. J. Cancer, 26*(4), 239–257. https://doi.org/10.1038/bjc.1972.33.

Kolb, J. P., Oguin, T. H., Oberst, A., & Martinez, J. (2017). Programmed cell death and inflammation: Winter is coming. *Trends in Immunology, 38*(10), 705–718. https://doi.org/10.1016/j.it.2017.06.009, www.elsevier.com/locate/it.

Lan, Y., Liang, Q., Sun, Y., Cao, A., Liu, L., Yu, S., Zhou, L., Liu, J., Zhu, R., & Liu, Y. (2020). Codelivered chemotherapeutic doxorubicin via a dual-functional immunostimulatory polymeric prodrug for breast cancer immunochemotherapy. *ACS Applied Materials and Interfaces, 12*(28), 31904–31921. https://doi.org/10.1021/acsami.0c06120, http://pubs.acs.org/journal/aamick.

Lei, G., Zhuang, L., & Gan, B. Y. (2024). The roles of ferroptosis in cancer: Tumor suppression, tumor microenvironment, and therapeutic interventions. *Cancer Cell, 42*(4), 513–534. https://doi.org/10.1016/j.ccell.2024.03.011.

Li, F., Du, Y., Liu, J., Sun, H., Wang, J., Li, R., Kim, D., Hyeon, T., & Ling, D. (2018). Responsive assembly of upconversion nanoparticles for pH-activated and near-infrared-triggered photodynamic therapy of deep tumors. *Advanced Materials, 30*(35). https://doi.org/10.1002/adma.201802808, http://onlinelibrary.wiley.com/journal/10.1002/(ISSN)1521-4095.

Li, H., Pei, P., He, Q., Dong, X., Zhang, C., Shen, W., Chen, H., Hu, L., Tao, Y., & Yang, K. (2024). Nanozyme-coated bacteria hitchhike on CD11b+ immune cells to boost tumor radioimmunotherapy. *John Wiley and Sons Inc, China Advanced Materials, 36*(8). https://doi.org/10.1002/adma.202309332, http://onlinelibrary.wiley.com/journal/10.1002/(ISSN)1521-4095.

Li, Z., Zhou, Z., Wang, Y., Wang, J., Zhou, L., Cheng, H. B., & Yoon, J. (2023). Activatable nano-photosensitizers for precise photodynamic cancer therapy. *Coordination Chemistry Reviews, 493*. https://doi.org/10.1016/j.ccr.2023.215324, http://www.journals.elsevier.com/coordination-chemistry-reviews/.

Li, H. Z., Xi, Z. Y., Fan, C. Y., Xi, X. R., Zhou, Y., Zhao, M., & Xu, L. (2025). Nanomaterials evoke pyroptosis boosting cancer immunotherapy. *Acta Pharmaceutica Sinica B, 15*(2), 852–875. http://doi.org/10.1016/j.apsb.2024.11.011.

Li, J. C., Luo, Y., & Pu, K. Y. (2021). Electromagnetic nanomedicines for combinational cancer immunotherapy. *Angewandte Chemie-International Edition, 60*(23), 12682–12705. https://doi.org/10.1002/anie.202008386.

Li, Y. N., Qi, H. L., Geng, Y. J., Li, L. J., & Cai, X. Q. (2024). Research progress of organic photothermal agents delivery and synergistic therapy systems. *Colloid Surf. B-Biointerfaces, 234*, 113743. https://doi.org/10.1016/j.colsurfb.2024.113743.

Li, Z. L., Zhang, H. B., Gong, Q. Y., & Luo, K. (2025). Biomaterials nanoplatform-based tumor vaccines for immunotherapy. *Bioactive Materials, 51*, 924–961. https://doi.org/10.1016/j.bioactmat.2025.06.038.

Li, Z., Yuan, M., Liu, H. R., Liu, C., Zhang, J. H., Guo, Y. F., Li, Y. F., He, Y. C., Zhang, X. W., & Gao, D. W. (2025). Piezo-STING agonists enhance tumor penetration and catalytic-immunotherapy. *Advanced Functional Materials, 35*(32), 2419032. https://doi.org/10.1002/adfm.202419032.

Liang, S., Yao, J., Liu, D., Rao, L., Chen, X., & Wang, Z. (2023). Harnessing nanomaterials for cancer sonodynamic immunotherapy. *Advanced Materials, 35*(33). https://doi.org/10.1002/adma.202211130, http://onlinelibrary.wiley.com/journal/10.1002/(ISSN)1521-4095.

Liu, X., Yan, B., Li, Y., Ma, X., Jiao, W., Shi, K., Zhang, T., Chen, S., He, Y., Liang, X. J., & Fan, H. (2020). Graphene oxide-grafted magnetic nanorings mediated magnetothermodynamic therapy favoring reactive oxygen species-related immune response for enhanced antitumor efficacy. *ACS Nano, 14*(2), 1936–1950. https://doi.org/10.1021/acsnano.9b08320, http://pubs.acs.org/journal/ancac3.

Liu, Y., He, J., Chen, J., Chen, T., Li, W., Yang, Z., & Zeng, F. (2025). Programmed cell death in triple-negative breast cancer. *Cellular and Molecular Biology Letters, 30*(1). https://doi.org/10.1186/s11658-025-00789-5, https://cmbl.biomedcentral.com.

Liu, R. C., Wu, Y. D., Qu, H. R., & Wu, X. L. (2025). Magnetically and optically powered nanozymes: Boosting breast cancer therapy with magnetothermodynamic-enhanced ferroptosis and apoptosis. *Chemical Engineering Journal, 509*, 161353. https://doi.org/10.1016/j.cej.2025.161353.

Liu, Z., Li, J. P., Chen, W. E., Liu, L., & Yu, F. F. (2020). Light and sound to trigger the Pandora's box against breast cancer: A combination strategy of sonodynamic, photodynamic and photothermal therapies. *BioMaterials, 232*, 119685. https://doi.org/10.1016/j.biomaterials.2019.119685.

Long, Y., Fan, J., Zhou, N., Liang, J., Xiao, C., Tong, C., Wang, W., & Liu, B. (2023). Biomimetic Prussian blue nanocomplexes for chemo-photothermal treatment of triple-negative breast cancer by enhancing ICD.

BioMaterials, 303. https://doi.org/10.1016/j.biomaterials.2023.122369, http://www.journals.elsevier.com/biomaterials/.

Lu, Q., Kou, D., Lou, S., Ashrafizadeh, M., Aref, A. R., Canadas, I., Tian, Y., Niu, X., Wang, Y., Torabian, P., Wang, L., Sethi, G., Tergaonkar, V., Tay, F., Yuan, Z., & Han, P. (2024). Nanoparticles in tumor microenvironment remodeling and cancer immunotherapy. *Journal of Hematology and Oncology, 17*(1). https://doi.org/10.1186/s13045-024-01535-8, https://jhoonline.biomedcentral.com.

Luo, T., Zhang, M., Xu, J., Yuan, D., Yin, B., Zhu, Y., Yan, S., Pan, M., Mo, D., Li, X., Liang, X., Qin, Z., Deng, H., & Qian, Z. (2025). Jahn-Teller distortion-engineered self-propelled nanorobots for mitochondrial targeting and bioenergetic disruption in tumor therapy. *Bioactive Materials, 54*, 273–290. https://doi.org/10.1016/j.bioactmat.2025.08.021, https://www.sciencedirect.com/science/journal/2452199X.

Ma, M., Zhang, Y., Pu, K., & Tang, W. (2025). Nanomaterial-enabled metabolic reprogramming strategies for boosting antitumor immunity. *Chemical Society Reviews, 54*(2), 653–714. https://doi.org/10.1039/d4cs00679h.

Manjili, S. H., Isbell, M., Ghochaghi, N., Perkinson, T., & Manjili, M. H. (2022). Multifaceted functions of chronic inflammation in regulating tumor dormancy and relapse. *Seminars in Cancer Biology, 78*, 17–22. https://doi.org/10.1016/j.semcancer.2021.03.023, http://www.elsevier.com/inca/publications/store/6/2/2/9/4/3/index.htt.

Meier, P., Legrand, A. J., Adam, D., & Silke, J. (2024). Immunogenic cell death in cancer: Targeting necroptosis to induce antitumour immunity. *Nature Reviews. Cancer, 24*(5), 299–315. https://doi.org/10.1038/s41568-024-00674-x, https://www.nature.com/cancer/.

Melamed, J. R., Edelstein, R. S., & Day, E. S. (2015). Elucidating the fundamental mechanisms of cell death triggered by photothermal therapy. *ACS Nano, 9*(1), 6–11. https://doi.org/10.1021/acsnano.5b00021.

Pan, J., Xu, Y., Wu, Q., Hu, P., & Shi, J. (2021). Mild magnetic hyperthermia-activated innate immunity for liver cancer therapy. *Journal of the American Chemical Society, 143*(21), 8116–8128. https://doi.org/10.1021/jacs.1c02537, http://pubs.acs.org/journal/jacsat.

Pan, M., Hu, D., Yuan, L., Yu, Y., Li, Y., & Qian, Z. (2023). Newly developed gas-assisted sonodynamic therapy in cancer treatment. *Acta Pharmaceutica Sinica B, 13*(7), 2926–2954. https://doi.org/10.1016/j.apsb.2022.12.021, http://www.elsevier.com/wps/find/journaldescription.cws_home/725753/description#description.

Peng, Z., Yuan, L., XuHong, J., Tian, H., Zhang, Y., Deng, J., & Qi, X. (2021). Chiral nanomaterials for tumor therapy: Autophagy, apoptosis, and photothermal ablation. *Journal of Nanobiotechnology, 19*(1). https://doi.org/10.1186/s12951-021-00965-7, http://www.jnanobiotechnology.com/start.asp.

Pereira, T. A., Ramos, D. N., Sobral, L. M., Martins, Y. A., Petrilli, R., Fantini, M. D. A. C., Leopoldino, A. M., & Lopez, R. F. V. (2023). Liquid crystalline nanogel targets skin cancer via low-frequency ultrasound treatment. *International Journal of Pharmaceutics, 646*. https://doi.org/10.1016/j.ijpharm.2023.123431, www.elsevier.com/locate/ijpharm.

Pietrocola, F., Pol, J., Vacchelli, E., Baracco, E. E., Levesque, S., Castoldi, F., Maiuri, M. C., Madeo, F., & Kroemer, G. (2016). Autophagy induction for the treatment of cancer. *Autophagy, 12*(10), 1962–1964. https://doi.org/10.1080/15548627.2016.1214778, http://www.tandfonline.com/toc/kaup20/current.

Qi, F., Bao, Q., Hu, P., Guo, Y., Yan, Y., Yao, X., & Shi, J. (2024). Mild magnetic hyperthermia-activated immunoresponses for primary bladder cancer therapy. *BioMaterials, 307*. https://doi.org/10.1016/j.biomaterials.2024.122514, https://www.sciencedirect.com/science/journal/01429612.

Qin, Y. T., Rao, Z. Y., An, J. X., Zhang, S. M., Wang, Y. Z., Pan, T., & Zhang, X. Z. (2025). Inhibiting Chemotherapy Immune Tolerance and Reversing Tumor Microenvironment by Macrophage-Targeted Nanohybrid Systems for Enhancing Tumor Chemo-Immunotherapy. *Advanced Functional Materials, 35*(37). https://doi.org/10.1002/adfm.202501954, http://onlinelibrary.wiley.com/journal/10.1002/(ISSN)1616-3028.

Qin, S. Y., Zhang, A. Q., & Zhang, X. Z. (2018). Recent advances in targeted tumor chemotherapy based on smart nanomedicines. *Small (Weinheim an der Bergstrasse, Germany), 14*(45), 1802417. https://doi.org/10.1002/smll.201802417.

Qu, H., Zhang, Y., Chen, M., Shao, S., Chen, J., Wu, Y., & Wu, X. (2025). NIR-II photo- and sono-responsive hyaluronic acid-capped nanozymes for glioblastoma-targeting theranostics. *International Journal of Biological Macromolecules, 306*. https://doi.org/10.1016/j.ijbiomac.2025.141737, https://www.sciencedirect.com/science/journal/01418130.

Ren, S., Zhang, M., Cai, C., Zhang, N., Wang, Z., Li, G., Liu, Q., Zhu, H., An, H., & Chen, Y. (2025). A carrier-free ultrasound-responsive polyphenol nanonetworks with enhanced sonodynamic-immunotherapy for synergistic therapy of breast cancer. *Biomaterials, 317*. https://doi.org/10.1016/j.biomaterials.2025.123109, https://www.sciencedirect.com/science/journal/01429612.

Ritter, B., & Greten, F. R. (2019). Modulating inflammation for cancer therapy. *The Journal of Experimental Medicine, 216*(6), 1234–1243. https://doi.org/10.1084/jem.20181739.

Sabit, H., Pawlik, T. M., Radwan, F., Abdel-Hakeem, M., Abdel-Ghany, S., Wadan, A. H. S., Elzawahri, M., El-Hashash, A., & Arneth, B. (2025). Precision nanomedicine: Navigating the tumor microenvironment for enhanced cancer immunotherapy and targeted drug delivery. *Molecular Cancer, 24*(1). https://doi.org/10.1186/s12943-025-02357-z, https://molecular-cancer.biomedcentral.com.

Shalapour, S., & Karin, M. (2019). Pas de deux: Control of anti-tumor immunity by cancer-associated inflammation. *Immunity, 51*(1), 15–26. https://doi.org/10.1016/j.immuni.2019.06.021.

Shao, Y., Liu, B., Di, Z., Zhang, G., Sun, L. D., Li, L., & Yan, C. H. (2020). Engineering of Upconverted metal-organic frameworks for near-infrared light-triggered combinational photodynamic/chemo-/immunotherapy against hypoxic tumors. *Journal of the American Chemical Society, 142*(8), 3939–3946. https://doi.org/10.1021/jacs.9b12788, http://pubs.acs.org/journal/jacsat.

Shi, W., Li, C., Wang, N., Lu, H., Miao, G., Cai, M., Yang, J., Zhang, Y., Qu, Y., Tang, Y., Wang, Y., & Shen, H. (2025). Fe-doped carbon dots control the biodegradation behaviors of Zr-based metal–Organic framework for tumor-specific chemotherapy and ferroptosis enhanced sono-chemodynamic therapy. *Small (Weinheim an der Bergstrasse, Germany), 21*(32). https://doi.org/10.1002/smll.202502028, http://onlinelibrary.wiley.com/journal/10.1002/(ISSN)1613-6829.

Song, J., Zhao, X. Q., Wang, K. Y., Liang, Y. Y., Zhang, L., Guo, B. F., & Jiang, W. (2025). Mito-nanozyme: Mitochondria-targeted nanozyme for cancer therapy. *Coordination Chemistry Reviews, 542*, 216899. https://doi.org/10.1016/j.ccr.2025.216899.

Sun, L., Zhou, J. E., Luo, T., Wang, J., Kang, L., Wang, Y., Luo, S., Wang, Z., Zhou, Z., Zhu, J., Yu, J., Yu, L., & Yan, Z. (2022). Nanoengineered neutrophils as a cellular sonosensitizer for visual sonodynamic therapy of malignant tumors. *Advanced Materials, 34*(15). https://doi.org/10.1002/adma.202109969, http://onlinelibrary.wiley.com/journal/10.1002/(ISSN)1521-4095.

Sun, S., Huang, X., Yang, N., Lei, H., Pei, Z., Han, Z., Liu, L., Gong, F., Yu, Q., Li, J., Chen, Y., & Cheng, L. (2024). Fluorinated titanium oxide (TiO_2-xFx) nanospindles as ultrasound-triggered pyroptosis inducers to boost sonodynamic immunotherapy. *ACS Nano*. https://doi.org/10.1021/acsnano.4c05448, http://pubs.acs.org/journal/ancac3.

Tang, G., He, J., Liu, J., Yan, X., & Fan, K. (2021). Nanozyme for tumor therapy: Surface modification matters. *Exploration, 1*(1), 75–89. https://doi.org/10.1002/exp.20210005.

Tang, L., Zhang, A., Zhang, Z., Zhao, Q., Li, J., Mei, Y., Yin, Y., & Wang, W. (2022). Multifunctional inorganic nanomaterials for cancer photoimmunotherapy. *Cancer Communications, 42*(2), 141–163. https://doi.org/10.1002/cac2.12255, https://onlinelibrary.wiley.com/journal/25233548.

Tang, X., Gao, D., Liu, X., Liu, J., Chen, T., & He, J. (2024). Novel RGD-decorated micelles loaded with doxorubicin for targeted breast cancer chemotherapy. *Biomedicine and Pharmacotherapy, 180*. https://doi.org/10.1016/j.biopha.2024.117460, https://www.sciencedirect.com/science/journal/07533322.

Tang, Z., Zhao, P., Ni, D., Liu, Y., Zhang, M., Wang, H., Zhang, H., Gao, H., Yao, Z., & Bu, W. (2018). Pyroelectric nanoplatform for NIR-II-triggered photothermal therapy with simultaneous pyroelectric dynamic therapy. *Materials Horizons, 5*(5), 946–952. https://doi.org/10.1039/c8mh00627j, http://pubs.rsc.org/en/journals/journal/mh.

Tsvetkov, P., Coy, S., Petrova, B., Dreishpoon, M., Verma, A., Abdusamad, M., Rossen, J., Joesch-Cohen, L., Humeidi, R., Spangler, R. D., Eaton, J. K., Frenkel, E., Kocak, M., Corsello, S. M., Lutsenko, S., Kanarek, N., Santagata, S., & Golub, T. R. (2022). Copper induces cell death by targeting lipoylated TCA cycle proteins. *Science (New York, N.Y.), 375*(6586), 1254–1261. https://doi.org/10.1126/science.abf0529, https://www.science.org/doi/10.1126/science.abf0529.

Valentin, R., Grabow, S., & Davids, M. S. (2018). The rise of apoptosis: Targeting apoptosis in hematologic malignancies. *Blood, 132*(12), 1248–1264. https://doi.org/10.1182/blood-2018-02-791350.

Wallach, D., Kang, T. B., Dillon, C. P., & Green, D. R. (2016). Programmed necrosis in inflammation: Toward identification of the effector molecules. *Science (New York, N.Y.), 352*(6281). https://doi.org/10.1126/science.aaf2154, http://science.sciencemag.org/content/sci/352/6281/aaf2154.full.pdf.

Wang, D., Gu, W., Chen, W., Zhou, J., Yu, L., Kook Kim, B., Zhang, X., & Seung Kim, J. (2022). Advanced nanovaccines based on engineering nanomaterials for accurately enhanced cancer immunotherapy.

Coordination Chemistry Reviews, 472. https://doi.org/10.1016/j.ccr.2022.214788, http://www.journals.elsevier.com/coordination-chemistry-reviews/.

Wang, H., Qiao, C., Guan, Q., Wei, M., & Li, Z. (2023). Nanoparticle-mediated synergistic anticancer effect of ferroptosis and photodynamic therapy: Novel insights and perspectives. *Asian Journal of Pharmaceutical Sciences, 18*(4). https://doi.org/10.1016/j.ajps.2023.100829, http://www.journals.elsevier.com/asian-journal-of-pharmaceutical-sciences/recent-articles/.

Wang, X., Liu, X., Li, Y., Wang, P., Feng, X., Liu, Q., Yan, F., & Zheng, H. (2017). Sensitivity to antitubulin chemotherapeutics is potentiated by a photoactivable nanoliposome. *Biomaterials, 141*, 50–62. https://doi.org/10.1016/j.biomaterials.2017.06.034, http://www.journals.elsevier.com/biomaterials/.

Wang, Y., Chen, X., He, D., Zhou, Y., & Qin, L. (2018). Surface-modified nanoerythrocyte loading DOX for targeted liver cancer chemotherapy. *Molecular Pharmaceutics, 15*(12), 5728–5740. https://doi.org/10.1021/acs.molpharmaceut.8b00881, http://pubs.acs.org/journal/mpohbp.

Wang, S. Y., Jing, H. Q., Yang, R., Heger, Z., Krizkova, S., Zhou, Y., Liang, X. Y., Adam, V., & Li, N. (2024). Magnetocaloric-responsive hydrogel nanoarchitectonics for pyroptosis-relay-immunotherapy to suppress post-operation tumor recurrence and metastasis. *Advanced Functional Materials, 34*(22), 2314194. https://doi.org/10.1002/adfm.202314194.

Wang, X., Qi, Y. Y., Hu, Z. R., Jiang, L. J., Pan, F., Xiang, Z., Xiong, Z. Q., Jia, W. W., Hu, J. Z., & Lu, W. (2022). Fe_3O_4@PVP@DOX magnetic vortex hybrid nanostructures with magnetic-responsive heating and controlled drug delivery functions for precise medicine of cancers. *Advanced Composites and Hybrid Materials, 5*(3), 1786–1798. https://doi.org/10.1007/s42114-022-00433-2.

Wang, X., Yan, B., Li, H. G., Yuan, J. L., Guo, J. Y., Wang, S. Y., Dai, P. G., & Liu, X. L. (2024). Reprogrammed IDO-induced immunosuppressive microenvironment synergizes with immunogenic magnetothermodynamics for improved cancer therapy. *ACS Applied Materials & Interfaces, 16*(24), 30671–30684. https://doi.org/10.1021/acsami.4c02740.

Wang, Y. J., Zhang, Y. Z., Xin, X., Yang, J. B., Wang, M. H., Wang, R. L., Guo, P., Huang, W. J., Sobrido, A. J., Wei, B. Q., & Li, X. H. (2023). In situ photocatalytically enhanced thermogalvanic cells for electricity and hydrogen production. *Science (New York, N.Y.), 381*(6655), 291–296. https://doi.org/10.1126/science.adg0164.

Wang, Z., Ren, X. J., Li, Y. F., Qiu, L., Wang, D. Z., Liu, A. N., Liang, H., Li, L., Yang, B., Whittaker, A. K., Liu, Z. S., Jin, S. Z., Lin, Q., & Wang, T. J. (2024). Reactive oxygen species amplifier for apoptosis-ferroptosis mediated high-efficiency radiosensitization of tumors. *ACS Nano, 18*(14), 10288–10301. https://doi.org/10.1021/acsnano.4c01625.

Wei, Y., Wu, S., Liu, Z., Niu, J., Zhou, Y., Ren, J., & Qu, X. (2022). Tumor associated macrophages reprogrammed by targeted bifunctional bioorthogonal nanozymes for enhanced tumor immunotherapy. *Materials Today, 56*, 16–28. https://doi.org/10.1016/j.mattod.2022.01.024, http://www.journals.elsevier.com/materials-today/.

Weiner, L. M., & Lotze, M. T. (2012). Tumor-cell death, autophagy, and immunity. *The New England Journal of Medicine, 366*(12), 1156–1158. https://doi.org/10.1056/NEJMcibr1114526.

Wu, X., Li, Y., Wen, M., Xie, Y., Zeng, K., Liu, Y. N., Chen, W., & Zhao, Y. (2024). Nanocatalysts for modulating antitumor immunity: Fabrication, mechanisms and applications. *Chemical Society Reviews, 53*(5), 2643–2692. https://doi.org/10.1039/d3cs00673e, http://pubs.rsc.org/en/journals/journal/cs.

Wu, Y., Zhang, Y., Han, J., Jiang, Y., Chen, M., Gu, X., Jiang, W., Fan, K., & Liu, B. (2025). Nanozyme-based biomimetic intelligent immune organelles for the treatment of bladder-metastasized tumors. *Advanced Materials, 37*(43). https://doi.org/10.1002/adma.202511181, http://onlinelibrary.wiley.com/journal/10.1002/(ISSN)1521-4095.

Wu, Y. D., Liu, X. D., Yao, C., Chen, J. Q., Wu, X. L., & Zhu, M. Q. (2024). Fluorescent hyaluronic acid nanoprodrug: A tumor-activated autophagy inhibitor for synergistic cancer therapy. *International Journal of Biological Macromolecules, 274*(1), 133360. https://doi.org/10.1016/j.ijbiomac.2024.133360.

Xie, G., Guo, S., Li, B., Hou, W., Zhang, Y., Pan, J., Wei, X., & Sun, S. K. (2024). Nonmetallic graphite for tumor magnetic hyperthermia therapy. *Biomaterials, 306*. https://doi.org/10.1016/j.biomaterials.2024.122498, https://www.sciencedirect.com/science/journal/01429612.

Xie, X. X., Zhang, J. X., Wang, Y., Shi, W. R., Tang, R., Tang, Q. S., Sun, S. H., Wu, R. Q., Xu, S. Y., Wang, M. X., Liang, X. L., & Cui, L. G. (2024). Nanomaterials augmented bioeffects of ultrasound in cancer immunotherapy. *Materials Today Bio, 24*, 100926. https://doi.org/10.1016/j.mtbio.2023.100926.

Xiong, B., Yu, J., Wen, C., Li, S., Zhang, S., Fang, Y., Cao, Y., Guan, X., Shen, Y., Zhu, M., Li, X., Zhu, Y., Guo, L., Xu, H., & Yin, H. (2025). Antisense oligonucleotide-loaded nanozyme reverses tumor immune suppression through sonogenetic metabolic therapy. *Journal of Controlled Release, 387*. https://doi.org/10.1016/j.jconrel.2025.114236, https://www.sciencedirect.com/science/journal/01683659.

Xu, C., Wang, Y., Guo, Z., Chen, J., Lin, L., Wu, J., Tian, H., & Chen, X. (2019). Pulmonary delivery by exploiting doxorubicin and cisplatin co-loaded nanoparticles for metastatic lung cancer therapy. *Journal of Controlled Release, 295*, 153–163. https://doi.org/10.1016/j.jconrel.2018.12.013, www.elsevier.com/locate/jconrel.

Xu, H., Ye, D., Ren, M., Zhang, H., & Bi, F. (2021). Ferroptosis in the tumor microenvironment: Perspectives for immunotherapy. *Trends in Molecular Medicine, 27*(9), 856–867. https://doi.org/10.1016/j.molmed.2021.06.014, www.elsevier.com/locate/molmed.

Xu, M., Liu, J., Feng, L., Hu, J., Guo, W., Lin, H., Liu, B., Zhu, Y., Li, S., Berdimurodov, E., Sharipov, A., & Yang, P. (2025). Designing a sulfur vacancy redox disruptor for photothermoelectric and cascade-catalytic-driven cuproptosis–Ferroptosis–Apoptosis therapy. *Nano-Micro Letters, 17*(1). https://doi.org/10.1007/s40820-025-01828-8, https://www.springer.com/journal/40820.

Ya, Z., Guo, S., Li, Y., Zhu, M., Zhang, L., Zong, Y., & Wan, M. (2023). Focused acoustic vortex-mediated sonochemotherapy for the amplification of immunogenic cell death combined with checkpoint blockade to potentiate cancer immunotherapy. *Biomaterials, 301*. https://doi.org/10.1016/j.biomaterials.2023.122278, http://www.journals.elsevier.com/biomaterials/.

Yamazaki, T., Bravo-San Pedro, J. M., Galluzzi, L., Kroemer, G., & Pietrocola, F. (2021). Autophagy in the cancer-immunity dialogue. *Advanced Drug Delivery Reviews, 169*, 40–50. https://doi.org/10.1016/j.addr.2020.12.003, www.elsevier.com/locate/drugdeliv.

Yang, M., Li, J., Gu, P., & Fan, X. (2021). The application of nanoparticles in cancer immunotherapy: Targeting tumor microenvironment. *Bioactive Materials, 6*(7), 1973–1987. https://doi.org/10.1016/j.bioactmat.2020.12.010, http://www.keaipublishing.com/en/journals/bioactive-materials/.

Yang, N., Sun, X., Zhou, Y., Yang, X., You, J., Yu, Z., Ge, J., Gong, F., Xiao, Z., Jin, Y., Liu, Z., & Cheng, L. (2023). Liquid metal microspheres with an eddy-thermal effect for magnetic hyperthermia-enhanced cancer embolization-immunotherapy. *Science Bulletin, 68*(16), 1772–1783. https://doi.org/10.1016/j.scib.2023.07.025, https://www.sciencedirect.com/journal/science-bulletin.

Yang, L., & Karin, M. (2014). Roles of tumor suppressors in regulating tumor-associated inflammation. *Cell Death and Differentiation, 21*(11), 1677–1686. https://doi.org/10.1038/cdd.2014.131.

Yao, C., Zhang, R., Xie, Z., Wu, Y., & Wu, X. (2025). A magnetically actuated MOF-based nanozyme for intensified induction of ferroptosis and immunogenic cell death via autophagy blockade. *Small (Weinheim an der Bergstrasse, Germany), 21*(5). https://doi.org/10.1002/smll.202409026, http://onlinelibrary.wiley.com/journal/10.1002/(ISSN)1613-6829.

Yi, Y., Yu, M., Li, W., Zhu, D., Mei, L., & Ou, M. (2023). Vaccine-like nanomedicine for cancer immunotherapy. *Journal of Controlled Release, 355*, 760–778. https://doi.org/10.1016/j.jconrel.2023.02.015, www.elsevier.com/locate/jconrel.

You, C., Li, X., Wang, D., Chen, H., Liang, L., Chen, Y., Zhao, Y., & Xiang, H. (2022). Self-assembled Aza-boron-dipyrromethene for ferroptosis-boosted sonodynamic therapy. *Angewandte Chemie - International Edition, 61*(41). https://doi.org/10.1002/anie.202210174, http://onlinelibrary.wiley.com/journal/10.1002/(ISSN)1521-3773.

Yu, J., He, S., Zhang, C., Xu, C., Huang, J., Xu, M., & Pu, K. (2023). Polymeric STING pro-agonists for tumor-specific sonodynamic immunotherapy. *Angewandte Chemie - International Edition, 62*(32). https://doi.org/10.1002/anie.202307272, http://onlinelibrary.wiley.com/journal/10.1002/(ISSN)1521-3773.

Yu, L., Li, W., Cao, J., Miao, R., Fu, Y., Wang, X., Xie, J., Zhang, W., Mao, Z., Zhang, H., Zhang, Y., Ou, M., & Mei, L. (2025). Remodeling tumor metabolism via self-amplifying energy-depleting nanocomplexes for effective photodynamic-immunotherapy. *Advanced Functional Materials, 35*(28). https://doi.org/10.1002/adfm.202425831, http://onlinelibrary.wiley.com/journal/10.1002/(ISSN)1616-3028.

Yu, P., Zhang, X., Liu, N., Tang, L., Peng, C., & Chen, X. (2021). Pyroptosis: Mechanisms and diseases. *Signal Transduction and Targeted Therapy, 6*(1). https://doi.org/10.1038/s41392-021-00507-5.

Yu, W. J., Jia, F., Fu, J. Z., Chen, Y. H., Huang, Y., Jin, Q., Wang, Y. X., & Ji, J. (2023). Enhanced transcutaneous chemodynamic therapy for melanoma treatment through cascaded fenton-like reactions and nitric oxide delivery. *ACS Nano, 17*(16), 15713–15723. https://doi.org/10.1021/acsnano.3c02964.

Yu, W. X., Jin, D., Zhang, Y. J., Wang, S. H., Yu, J. J., Liu, M. M., Dai, Y., Yin, Y. C., Cheng, J. J., & Liu, Y. Z. (2025). Provoking tumor disulfidptosis by single-atom nanozyme via regulating cellular energy supply and reducing power. *Nat. Commun. 16*(1), 4877. https://doi.org/10.1038/s41467-025-60015-w.

Zang, X., Song, J., Li, Y., & Han, Y. (2022). Targeting necroptosis as an alternative strategy in tumor treatment: From drugs to nanoparticles. *Journal of Controlled Release, 349*, 213–226. https://doi.org/10.1016/j.jconrel.2022.06.060, www.elsevier.com/locate/jconrel.

Zhang, H., Li, J., Chen, Y., Wu, J., Wang, K., Chen, L., Wang, Y., Jiang, X., Liu, Y., Wu, Y., Jin, D., & Bu, W. (2021). Magneto-electrically enhanced intracellular catalysis of fept-fec heterostructures for chemodynamic therapy. *Advanced Materials, 33*(17). https://doi.org/10.1002/adma.202100472, http://onlinelibrary.wiley.com/journal/10.1002/(ISSN)1521-4095.

Zhang, L., Huang, J., Buratto, D., Han, P., Yang, Z., & Zhou, R. (2024). A pH-responsive nanoparticle delivery system containing dihydralazine and doxorubicin-based prodrug for enhancing antitumor efficacy. *Aggregate, 5*(1). https://doi.org/10.1002/agt2.434, https://onlinelibrary.wiley.com/journal/26924560.

Zhang, X., Li, C. F., Zhang, L., Wu, C. Y., Han, L., Jin, G., Rezaeian, A. H., Han, F., Liu, C., Xu, C., Xu, X., Huang, C. Y., Tsai, F. J., Tsai, C. H., Watabe, K., & Lin, H. K. (2016). TRAF6 Restricts p53 mitochondrial translocation, apoptosis, and tumor suppression. *Molecular Cell, 64*(4), 803–814. https://doi.org/10.1016/j.molcel.2016.10.002, www.molecule.org.

Zhang, Y., Cai, K., Li, C., Guo, Q., Chen, Q., He, X., Liu, L., Zhang, Y., Lu, Y., Chen, X., Sun, T., Huang, Y., Cheng, J., & Jiang, C. (2018). Macrophage-membrane-coated nanoparticles for tumor-targeted chemotherapy. *Nano Letters, 18*(3), 1908–1915. https://doi.org/10.1021/acs.nanolett.7b05263, http://pubs.acs.org/journal/nalefd

Zhang, Y., Wang, X., Chu, C., Zhou, Z., Chen, B., Pang, X., Lin, G., Lin, H., Guo, Y., Ren, E., Lv, P., Shi, Y., Zheng, Q., Yan, X., Chen, X., & Liu, G. (2020). Genetically engineered magnetic nanocages for cancer magneto-catalytic theranostics. *Nature Communications, 11*(1). https://doi.org/10.1038/s41467-020-19061-9, http://www.nature.com/ncomms/index.html.

Zhang, H., Yang, L., Wang, T. T., & Li, Z. (2024). NK cell-based tumor immunotherapy. *Bioactive Materials, 31*, 63–86. https://doi.org/10.1016/j.bioactmat.2023.08.001.

Zhang, R., Jiang, B., Fan, K., Gao, L., & Yan, X. (2024). Designing nanozymes for in vivo applications. *Nature Reviews Bioengineering, 2*(10), 849–868. https://doi.org/10.1038/s44222-024-00205-1.

Zhao, H., Wu, L., Yan, G., Chen, Y., Zhou, M., Wu, Y., & Li, Y. (2021). Inflammation and tumor progression: Signaling pathways and targeted intervention. *Signal Transduction and Targeted Therapy, 6*(1). https://doi.org/10.1038/s41392-021-00658-5, www.nature.com/sigtrans.

Zhao, S., Hou, J., Deng, L., Qi, Z., Tao, N., Ruan, W., Zheng, J., Wang, W., Xu, Q., Saiding, Q., Kong, N., Liu, Y. N., & Tao, W. (2025). Lactate-modulating nanozyme-mediated mitochondrial respiration block for tumor immunosuppression remodeling. *Angewandte Chemie - International Edition, 64*(17). https://doi.org/10.1002/anie.202422203, http://onlinelibrary.wiley.com/journal/10.1002/(ISSN)1521-3773.

Zheng, T., Liu, Q., Xing, F., Zeng, C., & Wang, W. (2023). Disulfidptosis: A new form of programmed cell death. *Journal of Experimental and Clinical Cancer Research, 42*(1). https://doi.org/10.1186/s13046-023-02712-2, https://jeccr.biomedcentral.com.

Zhong, X., Wang, X., Li, J., Hu, J., Cheng, L., & Yang, X. (2021). ROS-based dynamic therapy synergy with modulating tumor cell-microenvironment mediated by inorganic nanomedicine. *Coordination Chemistry Reviews, 437*. https://doi.org/10.1016/j.ccr.2021.213828, http://www.journals.elsevier.com/coordination-chemistry-reviews/.

Zhong, Y., Goltsche, K., Cheng, L., Xie, F., Meng, F., Deng, C., Zhong, Z., & Haag, R. (2016). Hyaluronic acid-shelled acid-activatable paclitaxel prodrug micelles effectively target and treat CD44-overexpressing human breast tumor xenografts in vivo. *Biomaterials, 84*, 250–261. https://doi.org/10.1016/j.biomaterials.2016.01.049, http://www.journals.elsevier.com/biomaterials/.

Zhou, Z., Wang, T., Hu, T., Xu, H., Cui, L., Xue, B., Zhao, X., Pan, X., Yu, S., Li, H., Qin, Y., Zhang, J., Ma, L., Liang, R., & Tan, C. (2024). Synergistic interaction between metal single-atoms and defective WO3–x nanosheets for enhanced sonodynamic cancer therapy. *Advanced Materials, 36*(23). https://doi.org/10.1002/adma.202311002, http://onlinelibrary.wiley.com/journal/10.1002/(ISSN)1521-4095.

Zhu, X., Wang, M., Wang, H., Ding, Y., Liu, Y., Fu, Z., Lin, D., Lu, C., & Tu, X. (2022). Multifunctional hollow MnO_2@Porphyrin@bromelain nanoplatform for enhanced photodynamic therapy. *Small (Weinheim an der Bergstrasse, Germany), 18*(52). https://doi.org/10.1002/smll.202204951, http://onlinelibrary.wiley.com/journal/10.1002/(ISSN)1613-6829.

Zhu, J. Y., Xiong, W., Feng, J., Yang, J., Lu, X. Y., Lu, Y. D., Zhang, Q. Q., Yi, P. W., Feng, Y. Q., Guo, S., Qiu, X. Z., Xu, Y. K., & Shen, Z. Y. (2023). Tumor-generated reactive oxygen species storm for high-performance ferroptosis therapy. *ACS Nano, 17*(12), 11492–11506. https://doi.org/10.1021/acsnano.3c01369.

CHAPTER

6

Micro/nano-enabled immunometabolic regulation in inflammatory tumors

Xilong Wu[1,2], *Ruocan Liu*[1,2], *and Yundi Wu*[1,2]

[1]School of Biomedical Engineering, School of Pharmaceutical Sciences, Key Laboratory of Tropical Biological Resources of Ministry of Education, Hainan University, Haikou, P.R. China
[2]State Key Laboratory of Digital Medical Engineering, Hainan Engineering Research Center for Drug Screening and Evaluation, Collaborative Innovation Center of One Health, Hainan University, Haikou, P.R. China

6.1 Introduction

Interactions between metabolic regulation and immune mechanisms in malignancies have rapidly emerged as a dynamic and developing area of research, offering novel insights into tumor metabolic reprogramming and antitumor immunity (Kapnick et al., 2024). This immunometabolic interaction critically influences tumor progression, immune evasion, and resistance to conventional therapies. Within the hypoxic, nutrient-limited, and inflammatory tumor microenvironment (TME), cancer cells adapt their metabolism to support accelerated proliferation and ensure survival (Chen et al., 2025; Han et al., 2024). Beyond influencing tumor cells, these changes have notable consequences for immune cells inhabiting the TME. The immune cells embedded in the TME typically consist of various cell types, which encompass T lymphocytes, B lymphocytes, tumor-associated macrophages (TAMs), natural killer (NK) cells, dendritic cells (DCs), neutrophils, and myeloid-derived suppressor cells (MDSCs) (Chen et al., 2023; Kaymak et al., 2021; Lian et al., 2022; Wu et al., 2025). Similar to tumor cells, these immune cells adapt their metabolism in response to activation, differentiation, and effector activities, ensuring adequate energy production and biosynthesis (Li et al., 2019; Schild et al., 2025). Actually, the TME, characterized by ionic imbalance, acidity, hypoxia, reduced glucose concentration, nutrient competition, and altered secretory profiles, changes the inherent function of immune cells, leading to either diminished inflammatory responses or enhanced suppressive functions, which in turn enable tumors to evade immune detection (Dong et al., 2023; Jiao et al., 2024; Wang et al., 2025).

Inflammation in Tumorigenesis and Cancer Treatment
DOI: https://doi.org/10.1016/B978-0-443-36649-9.00011-6

Moreover, tumor cells secrete various metabolites such as lactate, prostaglandin E_2, and arginine, which can directly modulate immune cell function (Ma et al., 2024, 2025; Patterson et al., 2024).

In recent years, micro/nanoplatforms have emerged as promising tools to boost tumor-directed immunity by reprogramming metabolic pathways in both cancer and immune cells of the TME, ultimately reshaping the tumor immunosuppressive state (Wang et al., 2025; Yang & Zhang, 2020). This approach effectively mitigates the adverse effects associated with standard treatments while promoting immune microenvironment reprogramming via metabolic intervention and immune pathway modulation. On the one hand, micro/nanomedicines accumulate passively at tumor sites through enhanced permeability and retention (EPR) effects (Ravi Kiran et al., 2021; Zi et al., 2022). Surface-modified nanoparticles can actively target tumor cells, various immune cell subpopulations, and organelle-level structures, including endoplasmic reticulum and Golgi apparatus (Ma et al., 2025; Martin et al., 2020; Zhou et al., 2024). The integration of responsive-release devices also enhances specificity, allowing accurate metabolic regulation, minimizing systemic toxicity, and improving therapeutic efficacy. On the other hand, these micro/nanoplatforms can also carry multiple therapeutic agents, enabling simultaneous metabolic regulation and inducing immune responses through chemotherapy, radiotherapy, photodynamic therapy (PDT), photothermal therapy (PTT), and sonodynamic therapy (SDT) (Hu et al., 2024; Liu et al., 2023; Lu et al., 2023; Wu et al., 2024; Yu et al., 2021). Multifunctional micro/nanoplatforms both reshape the tumor immune microenvironment (TIME) and enhance the antitumor potency of these therapeutic modalities, strengthening the tumor–immunity axis and fostering strong antitumor immune activity.

This chapter delivers an extensive overview of the complex interplay relationship the interplay of immunometabolism with tumor progression, focusing on how metabolic reprogramming within the TME influences immunocyte function and antitumor immune mechanisms (Fig. 6.1). It further delves into the role of micro/nanoplatforms in achieving precise immunometabolic regulation, showcasing cutting-edge research and developments, with the aim of enhancing cancer immunotherapy. By comprehensively addressing the intersection of metabolism, immune regulation, and micro/nano technology, this chapter seeks to inspire the development of next-generation therapeutic strategies that could transform cancer treatment. Ultimately, it emphasizes how micro/nano-enabled immunometabolic regulation may become a cornerstone of future tumor therapies, enabling the development of more potent and personalized treatment paradigms.

6.2 Micro/nano-enabled metabolic reprogramming in tumor cells

Tumor cells display extensive metabolic adaptation to fuel rapid expansion, survival, and resistance to therapies (Ji et al., 2024). The TME is a crucial factor influencing this metabolic shift, as it imposes stress conditions such as hypoxia, nutrient deprivation, and inflammation (Li et al., 2025; Wang et al., 2024; Yang et al., 2025). This altered metabolism not only helps tumor cells to proliferate but also creates an immunosuppressive environment, impairing immune cell functions. Tumor cells consume glucose, amino acids, and lipids at an accelerated rate, disrupting the normal balance of metabolites and toxic metabolite

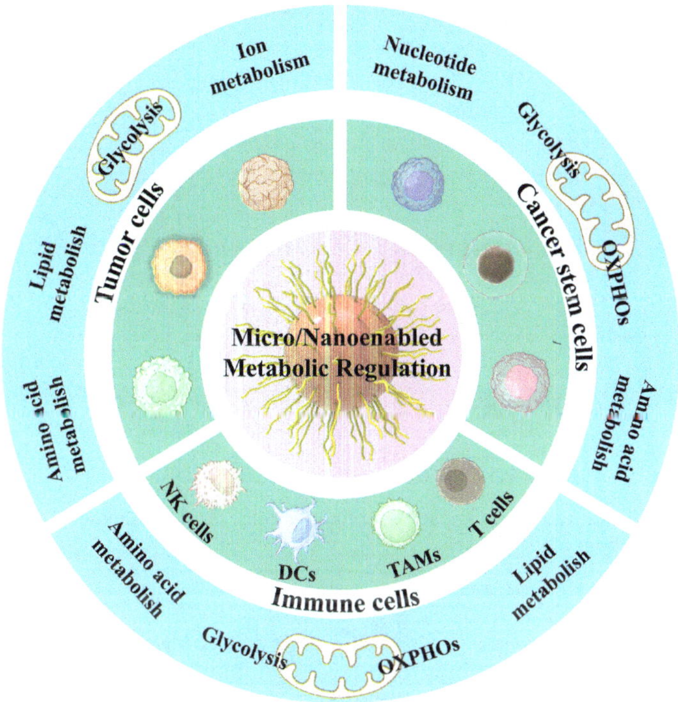

FIGURE 6.1 Schematic diagram of micro/nano-enabled immunometabolic regulation in inflammatory tumors.

accumulation in the TME (Wan et al., 2022). These changes can influence immune cells within the TME, including T cells, TAMs, and DCs, either by directly altering their metabolic pathways or by creating competition for essential nutrients, resulting in immune dysfunction (Cognet & Muir, 2024; Ngwa et al., 2019) (Fig. 6.2). Understanding the metabolic pathways in tumor cells and their impact on immune responses is critical to developing new therapeutic strategies that target both tumor metabolism and the immune system.

6.2.1 Perturbation of glucose metabolism

A hallmark of tumor-associated metabolic alterations is the Warburg effect, in which tumor cells predominantly employ glycolysis to generate energy even with the presence of sufficient oxygen (Hamanaka & Chandel, 2012; Tang et al., 2021). Glucose metabolism reprogramming facilitates accelerated cell proliferation and survival, while concurrently regulating immune responses through multiple mechanisms (Han et al., 2024). By efficiently obtaining energy, tumor cells generate metabolic intermediates that fuel biosynthetic pathways, including nucleotide and lipid synthesis (Fig. 6.3). Compared with normal cells, tumor cells exhibit elevated expression of glucose transporters (Song et al., 2025; Zhou et al., 2024). Among them, GLUT1 (glucose transporter 1) acts as a major facilitator of glucose translocation through cell membranes, with minimal expression observed in mammalian embryos and mature tissues under physiological conditions (Zhou et al., 2025).

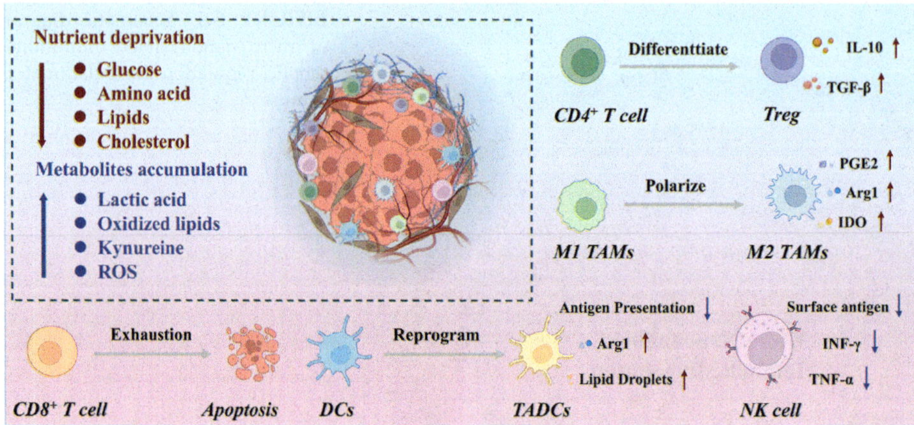

FIGURE 6.2 Tumor metabolic characteristics and their impact on immune cells. *Arg1*, Arginase 1; *IDO*, indoleamine 2,3-dioxygenase; *PEG2*, prostaglandin E2.

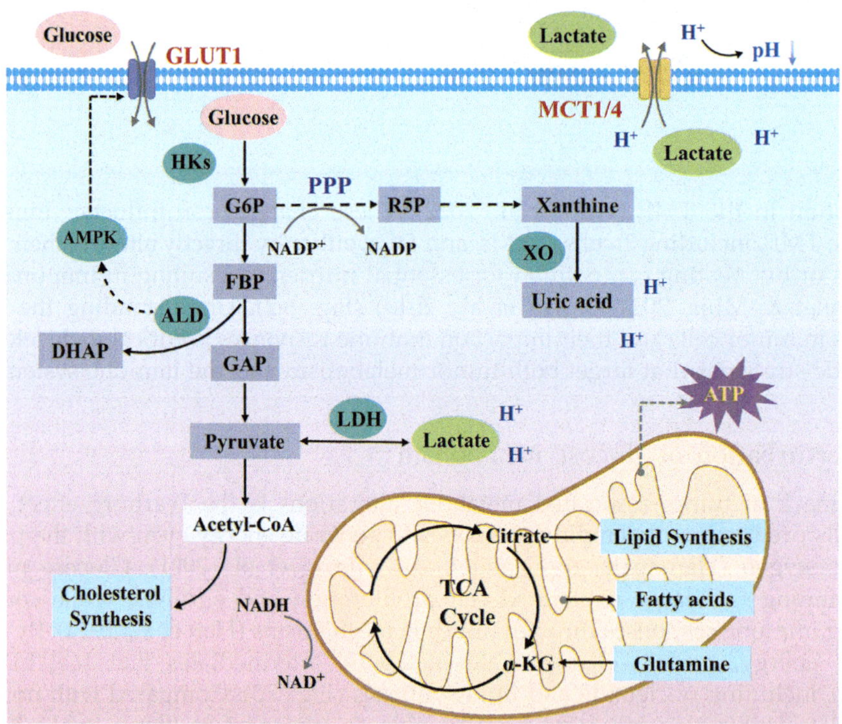

FIGURE 6.3 Schematic diagram of glucose metabolism in tumor cells. *GLUT1*, glucose transporter 1; *G6P*, glucose-6-phosphate; *R5P*, ribose-5-phosphate, *HKs*, hexokinases; *AMPK*, AMP-activated protein kinase; *GAP*, glyceraldehyde 3-phosphate; *PPP*, pentose phosphate pathway; *LDH*, lactate dehydrogenase; *ALD*: aldolase; *XO*: xanthine oxidase; *α-KG*: α-ketoglutarate; *Acetyl-CoA*: acetoacetyl-CoA; *MCT1/4*, monocarboxylate transporters; *FBP*, fructose-1,6-biphosphate.

Importantly, activation triggers a substantial glucose requirement in effector T lymphocytes and NK cells, ensuring adequate energy production and anabolic support needed for their cytotoxic responses (Chen et al., 2025; Jiang et al., 2025). When tumor cells overexpress GLUT1 and efficiently absorb glucose, they create a locally glucose-deprived microenvironment, and hence amplifying the competition for essential nutrients against immune cells, impairing the growth and effector functions of these antitumor lymphocytes (De Leo et al., 2024; Shi et al., 2022; Yan et al., 2022). Enhanced glycolytic activity in tumor cells produces excessive amounts of lactate, pyruvate, and other acidic metabolites, leading to a reduction in intracellular pH (Pérez-Herrero & Fernández-Medarde, 2021). The accumulation of acidic products causes acidification of the TME, which inhibits cell growth and can even trigger apoptosis in some contexts. To maintain pH homeostasis, tumor cells utilize monocarboxylate transporters (MCT1/4) to export lactate into the TME, preventing feedback inhibition of glycolysis (Han et al., 2024; Zhang et al., 2023). These transporters not only facilitate lactate efflux to sustain high glycolytic flux and metabolic symbiosis among heterogeneous tumor regions but are also closely associated with tumor progression, metastasis, and recurrence. Increasing evidence indicates that lactate produced through tumor glycolysis promotes the reprogramming of TAMs toward an immunosuppressive M2-like phenotype, thereby inhibiting the activation and proliferation of tumor-infiltrating immune cells, including cytotoxic T lymphocytes (CTLs), DCs, and NK cells (Li et al., 2025; Ma et al., 2024; Watson et al., 2021).

Overall, inhibiting tumor glucose metabolism and eliminating immunosuppressive lactate in the TME have emerged as effective therapeutic strategies to enhance antitumor immunity. Xie et al. (2019) designed a biomimetic nanosystem (core–shell mesoporous silica nanoparticles–glucose oxidase [CMSN–GOx]) composed of mesoporous SiO_2 loaded with GOx and cloaked with tumor cell membranes. This CMSN–GOx system induces glucose starvation, leading to tumor metabolic ablation and promoting DCs maturation to activate antitumor immune responses. However, the oxygen-dependent catalytic activity of GOx can limit its efficacy in hypoxic tumors (Fu et al., 2018). For it, Chen et al. (Zhang et al., 2022) prepared a biomineralization-inspired cascade nanomaterials (GOx–Mn/hyaluronic acid [HA]) that integrates GOx with manganese-based nanozymes and HA surface modification. The HA coating enables active targeting to CD44-overexpressing tumor cells, while Mn nanozymes catalyze the conversion of H_2O_2 (a byproduct of glucose oxidation) into O_2, establishing a self-sustaining catalytic cycle that amplifies glucose consumption. Blocking key glycolytic enzymes, especially hexokinase 2 (HK2), phosphofructokinase 1 (PFK1), 6-phosphofructo-2-kinase/fructose-2,6-bisphosphatase 3 (PFKFB3), pyruvate kinase, and lactate dehydrogenase A, also provides promising avenues to suppress glycolytic flux (Chen et al., 2025; De Jesus et al., 2022; Shin & Koo, 2021; Zhang et al., 2020). For instance, Yang et al. (2025) designed a lipid-polymer hybrid nanoplatform (2-pN@LNPs) with dual functions of mitochondrial targeting (triphenylphosphine, TPP modification) and tumor targeting (arginine-glycine-aspartic acid [RGD] peptide modification). This platform codelivers mitochondrial uncoupler nicotinamide (Nic) and glycolysis inhibitor 2-deoxy-D-glucose (2-DG), targeting and regulating mitochondrial energy metabolism and glycolysis pathways through a synergistic effect to induce pyroptosis in tumor cells and reshape the TIME. This study found that the nanoparticles could promote proton leakage across the mitochondrial inner membrane, leading to uncoupling of oxidative phosphorylation and entry into futile cycles, and taking advantage of the high glucose dependence of tumor cells,

2-DG was targeted for delivery, thereby causing the collapse of the glycolysis pathway. In vitro cell models and three-dimensional tumor spheroid models, 2-pN@LNPs exhibited significant synergistic antitumor effects, resulting in mitochondrial dysfunction, massive accumulation of reactive oxygen species (ROS), and a significant decrease in adenosine triphosphate (ATP) levels, ultimately triggering pyroptosis-like cell death. Additionally, this therapeutic strategy can enhance the recruitment of CTLs in tumor tissues and induce M1-type macrophage polarization, effectively eliciting durable immunological memory responses to inhibit tumor recurrence and metastasis.

Directly degrading lactate via lactate oxidase (LOx) has proven to be an attractive therapeutic approach. Various micro/nanoplatforms exhibiting LOx-like catalytic activity have been developed, including Cu_3N-C nanozyme (Zhao et al., 2025), LDH/MgO_2 nanoplatform (Sun et al., 2022), Co_4N/C nanocomposites (Zhao et al., 2023), and LOx-loaded nanocarriers/hydrogel (Chen et al., 2024; Wu et al., 2023; Xia et al., 2021). The described micro/nanoplatforms effectively deplete lactate within tumor cells, remodel the TIME, and trigger strong antitumor immune reactions. Given that the monocarboxylate transporters MCT1/4, characterized by high surface expression in tumor cells, serve an essential role in mediating the efflux of lactic acid produced by glycolysis, inhibiting their function has become an important strategy for reshaping the TIME and triggering antitumor immune activity. For this, Li et al. (2025) developed a glucose-modified cationic dendritic lysine (DGL) polymer micelle (GDLAI) for the codelivery of oxaliplatin and MCT4 siRNA. This micelle can achieve targeted delivery to hypoxic tumor cells, where the released oxaliplatin not only exerts chemotherapeutic effects but also induces ICD, and siRNA effectively silences MCT4 expression, blocking the efflux of lactic acid. By regulating the lactic acid-mediated metabolic interplay involving heterogeneous cancer subpopulations and immune cells, this system significantly greatly augments of NK cells ingress and restores the effector function of CTLs.

The abovementioned research reports highlight the crucial role of micro/nanoplatforms in regulating tumor glucose metabolism. Although such platforms have demonstrated significant effects in inhibiting glucose uptake by tumor cells and reducing lactate excretion, their insufficient targeting may cause nonspecific damage to the functions of immune cells or normal tissue cells in the TME. Therefore, in the design of micro/nanoplatforms based on glucose metabolism regulation, it is essential to prioritize enhancing tumor targeting, minimize off-target toxicity, and maintain the integrity of antitumor immune function while achieving effective metabolic intervention, achieving a balance between therapeutic efficacy and safety.

6.2.2 Regulation of amino acid metabolism

Essential for tumor survival and immune modulation, amino acids act as key providers of carbon and nitrogen for biosynthesis, redox balance, and energy production (Chen et al., 2024; Lin et al., 2023). Within the TME, tumor cells exhibit a heightened demand for amino acids, including glutamine, serine, tryptophan, and L-cysteine (Lieu et al., 2020; Zhou et al., 2025). These metabolic dependence fuels tumor progression while intensifying nutrient competition with immune cells, thereby suppressing T cell activation, DC maturation, and macrophage polarization (Jiang et al., 2025). The depletion or altered catabolism of these amino acids further establishes an immunosuppressive milieu characterized by the accumulation of regulatory T cells (Tregs), MDSCs, and M2-like TAMs (Chen et al., 2025;

Han et al., 2024). Hence employing micro/nanotechnology to target amino acid metabolism offers an innovative approach to reprogram both tumor and immune metabolism, restoring effective antitumor immunity.

Glutamine, a plasma amino acid of notably high abundance, functions as a key nutrient in tumor metabolism (Leone et al., 2019). It functions as a carbon and nitrogen donor for nucleotide, lipid, and amino acid biosynthesis and replenishes the TCA cycle through its conversion into glutamate and α-ketoglutarate (α-KG) (Jain et al., 2012; Lv et al., 2025). Cancer cells upregulate glutamine transporters, including alanine-serine-cysteine transporter 2 (SLC1A5) and the enzyme glutaminase (GLS), to sustain proliferation (Hassanein et al., 2013; Yoo et al., 2020). However, excessive glutamine consumption by cancer cells leads to local glutamine deprivation, impairing effector T cell proliferation and DC antigen presentation (Zhang et al., 2025). Additionally, α-KG derived from glutamine contributes to the epigenetic regulation of immunosuppressive genes and promotes M2 macrophage polarization (Liu et al., 2017). Nanotechnology provides precise means to interfere with tumor glutamine metabolism while preserving immune functionality. Li et al. (2025) reported a microacid-responsive bimetallic metal-phenolic nanocapsule (CG@Cap) for the delivery of the aminoamide metabolism inhibitor Telaglenastat (CB839) and glucose oxidase (GOD). Inside tumor cells, GOD oxidizes glucose to gluconic acid and hydrogen peroxide, depleting glucose and increasing ROS production, while CB839 blocks glutamine metabolism. This dual starvation effect disrupts tumor energy supply and remodels the TIME, involving enhanced infiltration of $CD4^+$ and $CD8^+$ T cells, M1 macrophage polarization, and DCs maturation. The growth of squamous cell carcinoma was significantly inhibited after CG@Cap treatment, demonstrating its strong antitumor efficacy. In another study, Chen et al. (2022) developed a nanoparticle platform (Pt–Pd@DON) based on porous platinum–palladium nanoflowers for glutamine antagonist 6-diazo-5-oxo-L-norleucine (DON) delivery. The Pt–Pd component in this platform can generate excessive ROS through mediating electrodynamic therapy (EDT), effectively producing robust tumoricidal effects and precipitating ICD. DON interferes with glutamine metabolism in malignant cells, not only restoring the immune performance of $CD8^+$ T cells and DCs, but also further enhancing the EDT effect of Pt–Pd. The combination of EDT and glutamine metabolism inhibition strategy demonstrated significant antitumor effects, effectively preventing tumor recurrence and metastasis by activating protective immune responses. This study reveals the potential advantages of the synergistic activation of antitumor immunity by exogenous stimulus field-activated ROS therapy and amino acid depletion in tumor cells, providing an important theoretical basis and development direction for glutamine metabolism intervention strategies based on micro/nanoplatforms.

Serine serves a pivotal function in one-carbon metabolism by providing carbon units for nucleotide synthesis and methylation reactions (Zhou et al., 2023). Tumor cells frequently overexpress phosphoglycerate dehydrogenase (PHGDH), the rate-limiting enzyme in the serine synthesis pathway (SSP), allowing them to synthesize serine de novo from glycolytic intermediates (Li et al., 2023; Pacold et al., 2016). This pathway yields glycine and formate, both vital for redox regulation and DNA synthesis. Overexpression of PHGDH correlates with tumor aggressiveness and immune evasion (Shunxi et al., 2023). Competition for serine restricts CTLs cells expansion and cytokine production in TME, while upregulated serine metabolism fortifies tumor antioxidant defenses, reducing immune-mediated oxidative stress (Chen et al., 2025). Nanotechnology-based approaches aim to inhibit tumor SSP activity or adjust serine supply for immune cells. Ma et al. (2025) designed and synthesized a pH-responsive nanoplatform (NCT-503@copper ion-doped hollow Prussian blue [Cu-HMPB]), which is composed of Cu-HMPB loaded with the PHGDH inhibitor NCT-503. In the weakly acidic TME, the framework of NCT-503@Cu-HMPB degrades, continuously releasing NCT-503 and Cu^{2+}. After that, Cu^{2+} can be reduced to cytotoxic cuprous ions through the iron–sulfur cluster formation process mediated by FDX1 in mitochondria, which initiates the lipidation and multimerization of mitochondrial dihydrolipoamide acetyltransferase protein, ultimately triggering cuproptosis in tumor cells. Meanwhile, NCT-503 inhibits the endogenous metabolism of serine and the synthesis of its downstream GSH, weakening the ability of tumor cells to clear copper ions and disrupting the intracellular ROS homeostasis. The abovementioned synergistic mechanism significantly enhances the cuproptosis effect and achieves efficient killing of tumor cells. Saha et al. (2024) indicates that serine deprivation can effectively inhibit tumor growth, accompanied by the activation of type I interferon signaling pathways and enhanced infiltration of immune effector cells in tumor tissues. Additionally, serine depletion can increase the sensitivity of tumors to immune checkpoint inhibitors targeting PD-1. However, current studies based on micro/nanotechnology platforms to regulate serine metabolism to reshape the TME and activate antitumor immune responses are still quite limited.

Tryptophan metabolism in tumor is predominantly regulated by indoleamine 2,3-dioxygenase (IDO1/2) and tryptophan 2,3-dioxygenase (TDO2), enzymes that convert tryptophan into kynurenine (Kyn) (Liu et al., 2023; Oweira et al., 2022). Elevated Kyn levels activate the aryl hydrocarbon receptor (AhR) pathway, leading to Treg expansion and suppression of CTL and NK cell activity (Sheng et al., 2025). Tryptophan depletion in the TME further triggers general control nonderepressible 2 (GCN2) stress signaling in effector T cells, inducing cell cycle arrest and immune exhaustion. The IDO–Kyn–AhR axis therefore constitutes a central metabolic mechanism of immune suppression in tumor (Nguyen et al., 2021). To address this, micro/nanocarriers have been engineered to inhibit IDO and TDO activity and mitigate Kyn accumulation. Zdioruk et al. (2023) synthesized a nanoparticle formulation (PPRX-1701), composed of poly(lactic-co-glycolic acid) and submicron 6-bromo-gallium-3-oxime (BiA) particles. After intravenous administration, BiA can enhance T cell-mediated tumor cell killing by blocking IFNγ-induced DO1 protein expression. In a glioblastoma (GBM) mouse model, the coapplication of BiA with immune checkpoint blockade (ICB) therapy increased the immune activity of the antibody, thus improving a notable rise in survival rate.

Cysteine, a sulfur-containing amino acid, is vital for GSH synthesis and redox equilibrium (Zdioruk et al., 2023). Tumor cells enhance cysteine uptake via xCT (SLC7A11) transporters and increase cystine reduction to maintain elevated GSH levels, enabling resistance to oxidative stress and ROS-triggered apoptosis (Wang et al., 2025). This excessive cysteine consumption depletes extracellular cysteine pools, weakening the capacity of T cells and DCs to synthesize GSH and diminishing their activation and antigen presentation functions (Xu et al., 2025). Moreover, surplus GSH in tumors neutralizes ROS and RNS, conferring resistance to chemo- and immune-therapies. Micro/nanoplatforms targeting cysteine metabolism primarily focus on inhibiting xCT activity or perturbing redox balance to sensitize tumors to immune attack. Sulfur-deficient nanoplatforms, such as Fe-doped metal–organic frameworks (MOFs) or Cu_2O-based nanoparticles (Bai et al., 2024; Li et al., 2025), oxidize cysteine and deplete intracellular GSH, inducing ferroptosis and promoting antigen release and DCs activation. Nanozymes with GSHOx activity, including $Bi_2Fe_4O_9$ nanosheets (Zou et al., 2022), Mn/Fe-MOFs (Zheng et al., 2024), Au-ZrFeMOF system (Li et al., 2025), and Mn-PDA (Lin et al., 2024), catalyze GSH oxidation to disrupt the cysteine–GSH–ROS axis, thereby enhancing immune-mediated cytotoxicity when combined with checkpoint inhibitors. Considering the high complexity of amino acid metabolism, the regulation of a single type of amino acid metabolism is difficult to achieve effective tumor treatment fundamentally. For this reason, Xie et al. (2024) developed a lactate/cysteine dual-consumption probiotic-nanomedicine biohybrid system to enhance the efficacy of cancer chemoimmunotherapy. This system consists of the anaerobic probiotic *Veillonella parvula* (*Vei*) and DOX-loaded MnS-NH_2 nanoparticles (DMnSH). *Vei* can reverse the immunosuppressive state by consuming lactate in TME and deplete cysteine, ultimately restraining the GSH biosynthesis. DMnSH continuously releases DOX and Mn^{2+} in tumor cells, effectively inducing ICD through the cooperative interplay of chemotherapy and CDT, promoting the maturation of DCs, and activating T cells to trigger an antitumor immune response. Since the reversal of the TIME mediated by *Vei*, antitumor immunity can be further amplified. This adaptive immune activation scheme combining dual metabolic intervention strategies with conventional treatment methods effectively inhibited tumor growth (inhibition rate: 82%).

In addition to the aforementioned micro/nanoplatform-mediated amino acid metabolic pathways, these systems can also be engineered to deliver metabolic modulators or specific enzyme inhibitors targeting L-arginine, leucine, methionine (Met), etc. (Qi et al., 2020, 2025; Su et al., 2025; Wang et al., 2025). Notably, the hypoxic state within the TME provides a stable and ideal niche for various anaerobic and facultative anaerobic bacteria (Sun et al., 2023). These bacteria and their metabolites possess inherent bioactivity, enabling precise localization within tumor tissues and sustained biotransformation, offering long-lasting and highly specific driving effects for metabolic regulation. Through integration with micro/nanoplatforms, bacteria can be reprogrammed into carriers or bioreactors that, under localized hypoxic conditions, release amino acid-degrading enzymes or inhibitors to achieve more efficient nutrient deprivation. At the same time, they can produce active molecules such as ROS, reactive nitrogen species (RNS), or immune-stimulatory metabolites to enhance ICD and further remodel the TIME. Compared with conventional chemical or physical metabolic interventions, this approach that leverages the natural metabolic advantages of bacteria in combination with programmable nanocarriers not only improves spatial specificity and the depth of metabolic suppression but may also overcome the limitations of traditional therapies that are often offset by tumor metabolic reprogramming. This could open a safer, more precise, and longer lasting avenue for antitumor immunometabolic modulation. As synthetic biology and nanomedicine continue to converge, micro/nanoplatform-based, bacterially comediated amino acid depletion therapy is expected to become an important future paradigm for tumor immunometabolic intervention, simultaneously targeting tumor metabolic dependencies and immune evasion mechanisms, thereby offering a highly promising strategy for achieving systemic activation of antitumor immunity.

6.2.3 Disruption of lipid metabolism

Lipids are indispensable components of cellular function, encompassing fats, phospholipids, cholesterol, and glycolipids (Yan et al., 2023). They serve as both structural elements of membranes and signaling intermediates regulating energy storage and redox homeostasis (Yu et al., 2021). In tumor cells, abnormal lipid metabolism is recognized as a hallmark of metabolic reprogramming. As opposed to normal cells, cancer cells enhance de novo lipogenesis and fatty acid oxidation (FAO) to adapt to the hypoxic and nutrient-deficient TME (Jin et al., 2023). This reprogramming supplies essential materials for rapid proliferation and produces lipid-derived signaling molecules, including PGE2 and lysophosphatidic acid, which suppress immune activation and promote tumor immune evasion. Fatty acids serve as critical intermediates for energy generation and signaling regulation (Hoy et al., 2021). Tumor cells acquire exogenous fatty acids via transporters such as CD36 and fatty acid transport protein (FATP), while acetyl-CoA carboxylase (ACC) and fatty acid synthase (FASN) mediate endogenous synthesis (Jiang et al., 2021). These lipids support membrane biosynthesis, signaling, or mitochondrial FAO to sustain ATP production. The altered fatty acid flux intensifies nutrient competition, impairing effector T cell function within the TME, whereas Tregs exploit FAO to preserve their suppressive phenotype. Moreover, MDSCs and TAMs accumulate lipid droplets (LDs) and activate PPAR signaling, establishing an immunosuppressive milieu that dampens antitumor immunity (Tu et al., 2022).

Micro/nanotechnology provides precision tools to modulate tumor fatty acid metabolism. ORL (orlistat) and C75 (α-methylene-γ-butyrolactone) are typical FASN inhibitors, often used for the reprogramming of fatty acid metabolism in tumor cells (Tadros et al., 2017). For example, Li et al. (2025) developed a GSH-responsive nanomedicine (ORL@-Cu–MOF) for the delivery of Cu^{2+} and ORL. ORL@Cu–MOF can target tumors and metastases and lymph node metastases (LNM) in mice carrying oral squamous cell carcinoma (OSCC). Cu^{2+} released in mitochondria induces the generation of ROS, leading to morphological and structural changes in mitochondria and endoplasmic reticulum, and induces ferroptosis in OSCC cells. Furthermore, ORL further downregulate the expression of FASN in tumor cells and suppresses lipid uptake and LD formation in OSCC cells, inhibiting the reprogramming of lipid metabolism in OSCC, which promotes ferroptosis in OSCC cells and produces a synergistic therapeutic effect. In addition, ORL@Cu–MOF enhances DC maturation, which in turn facilitates $CD4^{+}/CD8^{+}$ T cells ingress into the TME, thereby remodeling cold tumor into an immunologically active phenotype. Another approach targets mitochondrial FAO to remodel the TIME. Obesity downregulates prolyl hydroxylase 3 (PHD3), promoting FAO and immune suppression (Ringel et al., 2020). Polyethyleneimine-based nanoparticles delivering PHD3 plasmids restore PHD3 expression, inhibit FAO, and reactivate $CD8^{+}$ T cells (Fang et al., 2023). Similarly, carnitine palmitoyl transferase 1 (CPT1) inhibitors such as Etomoxir, when encapsulated in tumor-targeted nanosystems, effectively block fatty acid utilization and sensitize tumors to immunotherapy (Zhang et al., 2022).

Cholesterol constitutes a prerequisite for membrane integrity and signal regulation (Liu et al., 2023). Tumor cells enhance cholesterol synthesis and uptake through lipoprotein receptors (LDL) and the mevalonate (MVA) pathway, stabilizing PD-L1 expression and supporting immune evasion (Wang et al., 2025). To counter this, a multifunctional nanoplatform (MnOxChP) with multiple catalytic activities was developed to potentiate STING-mediated tumor immunotherapy (Liu et al., 2026). The nanoplatform was achieved by modifying MnOx with polyethylenimine (PEI) and coupling cholesterol oxidase (ChOx). MnOx possesses multiple enzymatic catalytic activities similar to POD-like, GSHOx, CAT, and NADPH oxidase (NADPHOx), which can effectively consume GSH and NADPH in TME, increase ROS concentration, and trigger cGAS-STING signaling pathway. Additionally, ChOx catalyzes the oxidation of cholesterol to generate additional H_2O_2, further enhancing the oxidative stress effect mediated by MnOx. Importantly, the cholesterol consumption induced by ChOx can inhibit the PD-1/PD-L1 immune checkpoint axis, thereby alleviating the functional exhaustion of CLTs. This strategy, through the intervention of cholesterol metabolism and the synergy of multienzyme cascade catalysis, activates augments tumor-specific immunity, thereby attenuating distal tumor progression and diminishing pulmonary metastatic burden in 4T1-bearing mice.

Regulating polyunsaturated fatty acids (PUFAs) enhances membrane fragility and facilitates lipid peroxidation (Zhou et al., 2023). As an important PUFAAs, arachidonic acid (AA) regulates the functions of immune cells and tumor immune escape through lipid mediators derived from different metabolic pathways, such as prostaglandins and leukotrienes (Gao et al., 2025). Liu et al. (Liu et al., 2023) constructed a bimetallic composite nanozyme (FeCo/Fe-Co DAzyme) and loaded it with phospholipase A2 (PLA2) and lipoxygenase (LOX). This composite nanozyme possesses multiple enzyme-like catalytic activities, can efficiently generate ROS and deplete GSH, inducing LPO and immunogenic ferroptosis in tumor cells. Meanwhile, PLA2 catalyzes the hydrolysis of membrane phospholipids to release free AA, which is then converted to AA–OOH by LOX and further generates a large amount of $^1O_2$ through the Russell mechanism, significantly promoting the accumulation of LPO. Importantly, IFN-γ released from $CD8^+$ T cells can synergize with AA to regulate phospholipid remodeling mediated by acyl-CoA synthetase long-chain family member 4 (ACSL4), amplifying the lipid peroxidation cascade and achieving efficient and cascade-amplified immunogenic ferroptosis, thereby augmenting antitumor immunity. Cheng and co-worker (Chen et al., 2025) reported a biomimetic nanovesicle (FiFe@red blood cell membrane [RBM]) system that encapsulates the FASN inhibitor (IPI-9119) and iron oxide nanoparticles for the synergistic treatment and metastasis inhibition of castration-resistant prostate cancer (CRPC). The RBM modified on the surface of FiFe@RBM carries CD47 recognition antibodies, which can effectively evade immune clearance, reduce macrophage phagocytosis, and achieve specific targeting of tumor cells. After entering tumor cells, the Fe ions released by FiFe@RBM induce the massive generation of ROS and cause mitochondrial dysfunction, while IPI-9119 inhibits the AKT–mTOR signaling pathway, which synergistically promoting cell apoptosis and enhancing ferroptosis by increasing PUFAs, PUFA-enriched phosphatidylcholine (PUFA-PC), PUFA-enriched phosphatidylethanolamine (PUFA-PE). In the PC-3 xenograft tumor model, FiFe@RBM achieved precise diagnosis and treatment guided by T_1/T_2-weighted MRI, effectively eradicating the primary tumor through the synergistic mediation of magnetic hyperthermia therapy (MHT), apoptosis, and ferroptosis, and significantly inhibiting liver metastasis in nude mouse models by activating and recruiting a large number of NK cells.

As center of lipid metabolism, LDs buffer metabolic stress in tumors by storing neutral lipids and furnishing cellular energy (Jin et al., 2023; Mehta et al., 2023). Dynamic changes in LD levels and proteomic composition have been implicated as key determinants of antitumor immune activation and are closely related to antigen cross-presentation, activation of IFN signaling, production of inflammatory mediators, and pathogen clearance (He et al., 2024). Therefore disruption of LDs formation in tumor cells is a highly promising immunotherapy strategy. To this end, Zhang et al. (2023) developed an ROS-responsive nanocomponent, which enhances the dose deposition of high-energy ionizing radiation (IR) at the tumor site and blocks the generation of LDs, thereby achieving low-dose radiotherapy (LDRT)-driven ferroptosis immunotherapy. This nanocomponent uses an ROS-cleavable thioether bond (TK) linker to connect tetra(4-carboxyphenyl)porphyrin (TCPP) with cationic dendritic polyamidoamine (PAMAM), and folic acid is conjugated at the end of PAMAM for specific targeted delivery toward folate receptor–overexpressing tumor cells. The TCPP part can chelate hafnium ions (Hf^{4+}) through coordination, while the positively charged PAMAM can load negatively charged HIF-1α inhibitory siRNA (siHIF-1α). Inside tumor cells, high levels of ROS can cleave the TK linker, continuously releasing Hf^{4+} and siHIF-1α. Among them, siHIF-1α effectively blocks the endogenous biogenesis of LDs in tumor cells by inhibiting the HIF-1α-FABP3/7 signaling axis, significantly increasing the sensitivity of biofilms to peroxidation; at the same time, Hf^{4+} can enhance the local energy deposition of IR, promoting significant ferroptosis-related lipid peroxidation of membrane phospholipids. Besides, tumor cells undergoing ferroptosis treated with radiotherapy can disrupt the structural integrity of biomembranes to promote tumor-associated antigens (TAAs) and damage-associated molecular patterns (DAMPs) expulsion, which, in turn, initiates inflammatory antitumor immunity, elicits robust T cell-mediated responses and immune memory, and ultimately activates systemic antitumor immunity.

Lipid metabolism serves as both an energy foundation for tumor growth and a key regulator of immune dynamics. Micro/nanoengineered interventions can reprogram this balance, simultaneously impairing tumor metabolic resilience and revitalizing immune metabolism. The integration of multiomics metabolic profiling, stimuli-responsive nanocarriers, and immunometabolic design principles will pave the way for precision, personalized nanotherapeutic strategies targeting lipid metabolism in cancer immunotherapy.

6.2.4 Intervention of nucleotide metabolism pathways in tumors

Nucleotide metabolism constitutes the biochemical foundation of cell proliferation, energy transfer, and genetic information maintenance (Dong et al., 2023; Madsen et al., 2023). It encompasses the synthesis and recycling of purine and pyrimidine nucleotides, which provide essential precursors in DNA and RNA replication as well as intermediates in signaling and epigenetic regulation (Chen et al., 2023). In tumor cells, these metabolic pathways are extensively reprogrammed to sustain uncontrolled proliferation and survival. Key enzymes, such as phosphoribosyl pyrophosphate synthetase, dihydroorotate dehydrogenase (DHODH), and ribonucleotide reductase (RNR), are upregulated, ensuring a constant supply of nucleotides even under hypoxia or nutrient deprivation (Chen et al., 2024; Shi et al., 2023). Meanwhile, purine metabolites (ATP and adenosine) in TME act as extracellular signaling and can activate immunity, which links metabolic activity to immune regulation (Ji et al., 2022). In tumors heightened purine flux via the CD39/CD73 enzymatic axis dephosphorylates ATP to adenosine, driving overaccumulation of this nucleoside in TME (Jeffrey et al., 2020). Adenosine engages A2A and A2B receptors on T cells and NK cells, suppressing their cytotoxic functions while enhancing the immunosuppressive activity of Tregs (Yu et al., 2020). Similarly, enhanced pyrimidine biosynthesis via DHODH supports both tumor DNA replication and immune evasion through the expansion of myeloid-derived suppressor cells (MDSCs) (Dong et al., 2023; Qiu et al., 2021). Additionally, RNR-driven nucleotide reduction maintains the redox balance of tumor cells, indirectly impairing DCs' maturation and antigen presentation. Collectively, dysregulated nucleotide metabolism serves as both a metabolic engine and an immune checkpoint within tumors.

Micro/nanoengineered therapeutics have emerged as powerful tools to selectively target these pathways. Methotrexate (MTX) is a widely used anticancer drug in clinical practice, mainly inhibiting the biosynthesis of DNA and RNA by interfering with one-carbon metabolism and de novo synthesis of purines and pyrimidines (Vander Heiden, 2011). Wan et al. (2022) developed a metal-chelated histidine nanoparticle (FHM) generated through coordination of F^{2+} ions, histidine, and MTX. After entering tumor cells, this nanoparticle can simultaneously inhibit the activities of dihydrofolate reductase, adenosine triphosphate amidotransferase, and thymidylate synthase, thereby blocking one-carbon metabolism, purine production, and pyrimidine biosynthesis, respectively. Additionally, the consumption of histidine metabolism reduces intracellular tetrahydrofolate, intensifying the suppression of one-carbon metabolism. Combining FHM with radiotherapy markedly suppressed tumor growth across various malignancies. As reported in another study, Xiong et al. (2025) engineered a Ru-MOF-based sonodynamic immunotherapy system and functionalized it with mPEG-d-PEI to achieve efficient delivery of antisense oligonucleotides (ASOs) targeting CD73 mRNA. The ROS-mediated endosomal membrane disruption and the "proton sponge effect" of mPEG-d-PEI synergistically promote the endosomal escape of ASOs, effectively silencing CD73 expression and reducing adenosine production. Moreover, this system can autonomously produce oxygen, alleviate tumor hypoxia, and inhibit the hypoxia-HIF-1α-adenosine signaling axis, further reducing adenosine accumulation. This dual-track adenosine inhibition strategy achieved through a cascade mechanism not only potentiates apoptosis-mediated ICD but also activates DCs and CTLs and reduces the infiltration of Tregs in the TME. Notably, this sonodynamic metabolic therapy successfully induced a strong antitumor immunity and lasting immune memory in Hepa1–6 tumor-bearing mouse model, markedly restraining primary tumor progression and curtailing pulmonary metastases

Nicotinamide adenine dinucleotide phosphate (NADPH), in its reduced form, a key coenzyme widely distributed in the cytoplasm, participates in nucleic acid synthesis. In tumor cells, elevated NADPH levels not only serve as precursors for biosynthesis to generate plasma membrane components but also promote the repair of damaged DNA and inhibit ICD and the upregulation of PD-L1 (Binnewies et al., 2018). For this, Wang et al. (2023) reported a nanomedicine (BMS202@HZP NPs) capable of depleting NADPH within tumor cells. This system is composed of polyacrylonitrile-*co*-acrylamide-*co*-*N*-(2-(2-nitro-1*H*-imidazol-1-yl)ethyl)acrylamide (PAAN) loaded with BMS202, an antagonist of PD-1/PD-L1 interaction. The nanomedicine can be targeted to tumor cells via CD44 receptors and carbonic anhydrase IX (CA IX), and under the catalysis of nitroreductase (NTR), which is highly expressed in hypoxic tumor cells, the nitroimidazole groups in the PAAN copolymer are reduced using NADPH as an electron donor, thereby efficiently depleting intracellular NADPH. The depletion of NADPH enhances the sensitivity of LDRT, fixes DNA damage in tumor cells, and promotes the upregulation of PD-L1 expression and the occurrence of ICD. Additionally, as TAMs hardly express NTR, their intracellular NADPH levels remain unaffected, maintaining a high reducing power that helps polarize TAMs toward an M1-like phenotype, thereby alleviating the immunosuppressive state of the TME. After the nitroimidazole groups are reduced to hydrophilic aminimidazole groups by NADPH within tumor cells, the hydrophilic–lipophilic balance of the PAAN copolymer shifts, causing its upper critical solution temperature to automatically drop below physiological temperature, thereby triggering the rapid disintegration of the nanomedicine and the on-demand release of BMS202. BMS202@HZP NPs enhance the response to anti-PD-L1 therapy through LDRT-induced upregulation of PD-L1, while reshaping the immunometabolic landscape of the TME, effectively reversing immunosuppression and synergistically activating antitumor immunity.

Xanthine, as a key intermediate product in the purine metabolic pathway, is critically involved in immune regulation. Its conversion to uric acid (UA) by xanthine oxidoreductase (XOR) constitutes a critical bridge between metabolic and immune processes (Lu et al., 2023). Inspired by the natural XOR, Hu et al. (2024) designed and constructed a novel artificial metabolic enzyme, $FeMoO_4$, which possesses a catalytic domain similar to that of XOR. Within tumor cells rich in xanthine, $FeMoO_4$ can efficiently catalyze the conversion of xanthine into excessive UA, thereby inducing TAMs to release IL-1β and promoting their repolarization to M1 type, while also activating the functions of DCs and CTLs. This metabolic intervention strategy, by promoting metabolic crosstalk among immune cells and synergizing with ICB therapy, significantly inhibits tumor growth in B16 tumor-bearing mouse models, improves the TME, and ultimately effectively activates antitumor immune responses.

Overall, dysregulated nucleotide metabolism supports tumor proliferation and immune escape through intricate metabolic–immune cross-talk. Micro/nano-enabled interventions disrupt this balance via targeted enzyme inhibition, redox modulation, nucleotide depletion, and gene silencing. By coupling metabolic collapse with immune activation, these micro/nanoplatforms reprogram the TME into an immune-responsive state. Future directions will likely integrate metabolic profiling with multifunctional nanoplatforms to achieve personalized, metabolism-based cancer immunotherapy—transforming nucleotide metabolism from a tumor-supportive mechanism into a therapeutic vulnerability.

6.2.5 Regulation of other associated pathways in tumors

Ion and mitochondrial metabolism are two central metabolic pathways that promote tumor growth and survival, while also influencing immune evasion. These metabolic alterations enable tumors to withstand hypoxia, nutrient deprivation, and oxidative stress (Li et al., 2024; Valcarcel-Jimenez et al., 2017). Micro/nanotechnology represents a cutting-edge modality for modulating these metabolic pathways, enhancing antitumor immunity, and improving therapeutic outcomes.

Ion metabolism in tumor cells is characterized by the dysregulated transport and accumulation of essential metal ions, including Ca^{2+}, Na^{+}, Zn^{2+}, $Fe^{2+}/Fe^{3+}$and Mg^{2+} (Gong et al., 2025; He et al., 2023; Xu et al., 2024). These ions play crucial roles across diverse cellular processes, including signal transduction, membrane integrity, and mitochondrial function. In particular, Ca^{2+} ions have been shown to regulate tumor cell signaling and energy metabolism (Chen et al., 2025), while Na^{+} ions contribute to cell membrane stability and metastatic potential (Zhu et al., 2012). Disruption of ion homeostasis can lead to cell death or altered immune responses, facilitating immune evasion in tumors (Gong et al., 2025).

Micro/nanoplatforms, through targeted modulation of ion metabolism, have the potential to improve cancer treatment by disrupting ion homeostasis and enhancing immune cell activation in the TME. For example, nanoparticles targeting Ca channels or K transporters have been developed to regulate ion influx in tumor cells, leading to altered cellular processes (pyroptosis) (Qi et al., 2025; Zhu et al., 2025). Fe ions are a key element in tumor cells and an important component of the active centers of many proteins and enzymes (Zhang et al., 2022). Ferroptosis, a recently recognized programmed cell death (PCD) modality driven by the excessive buildup of Fe ions and lipid peroxidation (LPO) within cells, holds promise for overcoming drug resistance issues associated with traditional therapies that rely on the apoptotic pathway (Lin et al., 2023). However, tumor cells can maintain iron ion levels by regulating iron homeostasis, resisting ferroptosis. Additionally, the limited catalytic Fe ions available from the unstable soluble iron pool within tumor cells further restrict the therapeutic efficacy of ferroptosis. To address this, Zhang et al. (2022) reported a dual-pathway targeting nanoparticle (MOF@GOx@MnO_2@PEG, abbreviated as magnetic-guided micro/nanoplatform [MGMP]) for enhancing ferroptosis and synergistically promoting immunotherapy. This nanoplatform is constructed from Fe-MOF, GOx, MnO_2, and PEG. In the TME, high concentrations of GSH are effectively consumed by MnO_2, disrupting the cellular redox balance and inhibiting the clearance of ROS. Simultaneously, GOx catalyzes the oxidation of glucose to generate H_2O_2, which is then converted into highly toxic OH under the Fenton catalysis of Fe–MOF, and downregulates the expression of ferroportin 1 (FPN1), leading to intracellular iron accumulation. This dual-pathway regulatory strategy efficiently induces ferroptosis and releases TAAs, when combined with ICB therapy, significantly enhances immune cell penetration into tumor tissue. As an efficient dual-homeostasis disruptor, MGMP simultaneously disrupts the redox balance and iron homeostasis within tumor cells, providing an innovative and synergistic therapeutic paradigm for ferroptosis-based cancer immunotherapy. These ion-targeting nanoparticles can enhance and strengthen anticancer therapeutic performance through immune activation and suppressing tumor progression. By carefully controlling ion concentrations, these nanomedicines can also influence the immune response, shifting the TME toward a more favorable state for antitumor immunity.

Mitochondrial metabolism, another vital process in tumor cells, is closely linked to cellular energy production, oxidative stress management, and immune modulation (Kopecka et al., 2020). Tumor cells often exhibit mitochondrial dysfunction, characterized by altered oxidative phosphorylation and increased production of ROS. This dysfunction facilitates tumor growth together with the promotion of immune evasion by suppressing the activation of DCs and T cells (Chen et al., 2023; Wang et al., 2024). By targeting mitochondrial metabolism, nanomedicine can enhance ROS production within tumor cells, thereby inducing ICD and eliciting robust antitumor immunity (Yan et al., 2023).

Nanomedicines that modulate mitochondrial metabolism achieve this by disrupting mitochondrial function and enhancing oxidative stress in tumor cells (Sabatino et al., 2018). For instance, metal-based nanoparticles can generate ROS through the Fenton reaction or other redox pathways, which leads to mitochondrial damage and initiation of immune responses (Wang et al., 2024). These nanoparticles drive tumor cytotoxicity as well as activate immune cells (DCs and CTLs) by triggering ICD. As a result, mitochondrial-targeting nanomedicines can enhance both the direct killing of tumor cells and the reprogramming of TIME to boost antitumor immunity. Furthermore, combining ion metabolism regulation with mitochondrial targeting through nanotechnology offers a powerful strategy for cancer immunotherapy. By modulating ion homeostasis and mitochondrial function simultaneously, these therapies can enhance ROS accumulation and facilitate ferroptosis or other forms of cell death (Cun et al., 2025; Zhang et al., 2025). The synergistic effects of such nanomedicines not only disrupt tumor cell metabolism but also reprogram the TIME, resulting in superior antitumor efficacy. It is worth noting that issues such as rapid clearance in the bloodstream, protease degradation, and insufficient targeting selectivity for tumor cells have led to off-target effects in micro/nanoplatforms based on mitochondrial regulation, thereby posing potential safety risks. For this, Wang et al. (2024) developed an in situ self-assembling nanosystems with mitochondrial targeting ability, which is composed of hydrophobic mitochondrial targeting peptides, hydrophilic PEG, and an NTR-activated prodrug. The PEG shell endows the nanosystems with prolonged systemic circulation while also effectively protecting the mitochondrial targeting peptides from protease degradation. After entering tumor cells, in a high concentration GSH environment, the carrier is reduced and broken, releasing free mitochondrial targeting peptide molecules. These molecules accumulate on the mitochondrial membrane and self-assemble in situ within the subcellular organelle to form stable nanofiber structures. The nanofibers located in the mitochondria significantly enhance the damage efficiency of the loaded drug to the mitochondria, induce severe mitochondrial dysfunction, and trigger lethal mitophagy. This intense mitophagy further disrupts the contact interface homeostasis between mitochondria and the endoplasmic reticulum to activate the ICD pathway, driving the maturation of DCs and facilitating CTL activation and infiltration. Additionally, mitochondrial dysfunction simultaneously inhibits the bidirectional metabolic process of oxidative phosphorylation (OXPHOS) and glycolysis, manifested as lowered oxygen utilization and reduced lactate secretion, thereby reshaping the metabolic characteristics of the TME and fostering TAMs polarization toward the antitumor M1 type. This mitochondrial-targeting in situ self-assembly strategy successfully transforms immune-rejecting cold tumors into immune-responsive hot tumors through multimechanism synergy, significantly enhancing their sensitivity to radiotherapy and ICB therapy.

In conclusion, micro/nano-enabled modulation of ion and mitochondrial metabolism holds great promise in cancer therapy. These strategies, particularly those involving the use of nanomedicines, provide new avenues for overcoming tumor resistance to treatment and enhancing antitumor immune responses. By targeting specific metabolic pathways, such as ion transport and mitochondrial function, these nanomedicines can improve the efficacy of cancer treatments and help overcome the challenges posed by the TME. The ongoing advancement of nanotechnology-driven therapeutic strategies will strengthen our capacity to accurately regulate tumor metabolic pathways and immune dynamics, opening new avenues for more efficient and individualized cancer therapies.

6.2.6 Rewriting immune metabolic in cancer stem cells

Cancer stem cells (CSCs) represent a subset of tumor-initiating cells characterized by their capacity for self-renewal and the potential to differentiate into multiple cell lineages (Han et al., 2024). Due to their capabilities in tumor initiation, metastasis, relapse, and drug resistance, they have become a current research hotspot (Ahmed et al., 2018; Li et al., 2023). Compared with tumor cells of higher undifferentiation degree, CSCs exhibit significantly different metabolic phenotypes, can flexibly switch energy supply modes, and promote immune suppression and immune escape by remodeling the TME (Thomas & Yu, 2017). For instance, CSCs regulate the plasticity of glucose metabolism through the HIF-1α/mTOR dual pathways. In hypoxic microenvironments, they preferentially enhance glycolysis, while in oxygen-rich conditions, they switch to mitochondrial OXPHOS to maintain stem cell characteristics (Milella et al., 2025). In addition, CSCs promote LD accumulation by upregulating FAO and enhancing lipid uptake, and activate the MVA pathway and its downstream cholesterol synthesis pathway (Wang et al., 2023). CSCs exhibit a stronger metabolic dependence on glutamine and branched-chain amino acids to replenish tricarboxylic acid cycle (TCA) intermediates and participate in epigenetic regulation. They also maintain the antioxidant defense system by enhancing the cystine/cysteine–glutathione axis (Wang et al., 2023). Meanwhile, tryptophan activates the AhR signaling pathway via the kynurenine pathway, promoting the formation of an immunosuppressive microenvironment (Chen et al., 2020). In TME, CSCs promote TIME and tumor immune escape through the abovementioned metabolic adaptation characteristics that are different from those of normal tumor cells. Therefore targeting the metabolism of CSCs has become a new strategy to improve tumor treatment, although exploration in this field is not yet fully developed.

Given the high dependence of CSCs on glycolysis and mitochondrial OXPHOS, Pan et al. (2022) designed a mitochondria-targeted nanoplatform (GNSs-dPG-3BP) for the synergistic intervention of metabolic inhibition and PTT in CSCs. This platform is constructed by hexokinase 2 (HK2) inhibitor 3-bromopyruvate (3BP), mitochondrial targeting group TPP, gold nanostars (GNSs), and CSCs-targeting ligand HA. GNSs-dPG-3BP selectively targets mitochondrial HK2 via 3BP, leading to substantial suppression of glycolytic activity, triggering cytochrome c release, promoting apoptotic cell death, and improving the therapeutic outcomes of photothermal treatment in breast cancer. Although this nanosystem effectively eliminates CSCs through the combined inhibition of glycolysis and photothermal ablation, its impact on modulating the TIME has not yet been evaluated. Yao et al. (2025) developed an LDRT-triggered biogenerator (RTB) by coassembling a radiation-responsive iNOS expression gene circuit (pDNAiNOS) with β-lapachone (LAP) in a supramolecular form and integrating it into cationic liposomes targeting CSCs. After administration of RTB and subsequent LDRT, the level of nuclear factor erythroid 2-related factor 2 (Nrf2) in CSCs was upregulated, remotely activating RIGC-dependent iNOS expression, leading to arginine depletion and substantial nitric oxide production. The synergistic effect of LDRT and RTB treatment significantly enhanced the combined cytotoxic effect of LDR and LAP through spontaneous NO generation and upregulation of NQO1. Additionally, the arginine deprivation induced by RTB, in combination with high levels of NO and ROS stress, led to severe mitochondrial dysfunction in CSCs, which not only inhibited OXPHOS activity, drove their transition to a differentiated state, weakening self-renewal ability and drug resistance, but also promoted more immunogenic necroptosis, stimulating adaptive antitumor immune responses.

In the TME, the bidirectional communication between CSCs and immune cells significantly promotes tumor progression and the formation of treatment resistance (Malanchi et al., 2012). Research indicates that CSCs can recruit monocytes/macrophages by secreting chemokines such as CCL2 and CSF1, and promote their polarization to M2-type TAMs, while M2-type TAMs enhance the maintenance of CSC stemness by releasing various bioactive mediators, including IL-6, epidermal growth factor, and WNT ligands (Bayik & Lathia, 2021; Chen et al., 2025; Feng et al., 2023; Raghavan et al., 2019). Feng's team (Li et al., 2024) developed an iron-based aerosolized nanocatalytic drug (DFHC), composed of iron-doped mesoporous silica nanoparticles, with citrate loaded in their pores and modified with dextran on the surface for targeted delivery. DFHC utilizes the specific binding of dextran to the CD206 receptor to efficiently target M2-type TAMs and enter the lysosome, where Fe^{2+} ions and citrate are released under acidic conditions to form in situ citrate-iron complexes, thereby disrupting the iron metabolism homeostasis of TAMs. In the tumor-promoting microenvironment where CSCs and TAMs coexist, the iron metabolism level is significantly elevated. Against this backdrop, DFHC can induce enhanced CD44-mediated iron endocytosis and trigger ferroptosis in CSCs due to the accumulation of glucose-6-phosphate (G6P), causing redox imbalance. In a mouse model of lung cancer, DFHC effectively inhibited the proliferation and stemness characteristics of CSCs by regulating the iron metabolism of TAMs, significantly delaying the progression of early-stage lung cancer. This study proposes a strategy to intervene in the metabolic interaction network between immune cells and CSCs, providing a new therapeutic approach for reshaping the TIME and activating antitumor immune responses.

6.3 Micro/nano-enabled metabolic reprogramming in modulating immune cell

Immune cells are pivotal in orchestrating antitumor immune responses, and their wide-ranging functional capabilities are vital for the body's defense against tumor development (Hu et al., 2022). These cells are broadly divided into innate immune cells, including macrophages, NK cells, DCs, and granulocytes, and adaptive immune cells, such as T and B lymphocytes (Xu et al., 2024; Zhou et al., 2024). Immune cells display significant metabolic flexibility, enabling them to adjust to dynamic environmental conditions and carry out their functional roles effectively. However, within the TME, immune cells often undergo metabolic reprogramming driven by tumor-derived factors and nutrient scarcity (Ma et al., 2025; Mu et al., 2024). This reprogramming, while facilitating the immune cell's rapid activation, proliferation, and differentiation, can also be coopted by tumors to suppress antitumor immune responses and support tumor progression. The ability of immune cells to effectively utilize energy resources such as glucose, amino acids, lipids, and mitochondrial substrates is central to their function (Kapnick et al., 2024; Li et al., 2025). Metabolic alterations in immune cells induced by the TME can promote their polarization toward immunosuppressive phenotypes, thereby facilitating tumor immune evasion. (Nel et al., 2022). Beyond targeting tumor cell metabolism, direct interventions in immune cell metabolism via precise metabolic modulation provide an emerging strategy for reprogramming the immune landscape. Fig. 6.4 summarizes the relevant metabolic characteristics of the major immune cells involved in antitumor immunity in TME, under both the suppressive and activated states. Emerging micro/nanoplatforms have shown the potential to selectively target immune cell metabolism, thereby enhancing antitumor immunity and improving the efficacy of immunotherapies.

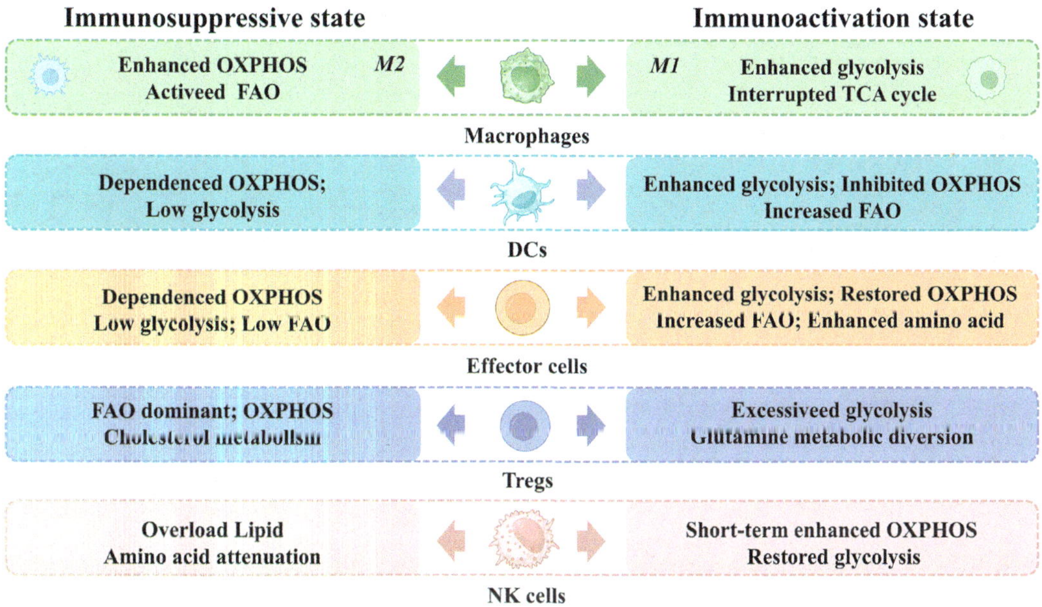

FIGURE 6.4 The metabolic characteristics of main immune cells in tumor microenvironment (TME). *FAO*, Fatty acid oxidation.

6.3.1 Modulation of macrophage metabolism

As the predominant immune cell population in TME, the metabolic signature of TAMs governs their polarization phenotypes and immune functionality (Liu et al., 2024). Functionally polarized into proinflammatory M1 and immunosuppressive M2 subsets, these cells coordinate immune responses through divergent metabolic strategies. M1 macrophages rely on heightened glycolytic flux to fuel rapid energy production, supporting phagocytosis, ROS generation, and proinflammatory cytokine secretion, thereby directly eliminating tumor cells and activating T cell–mediated adaptive immunity (Li et al., 2025). In contrast, M2 macrophages leverage mitochondrial OXPHOS and FAO for efficient energy generation, preferentially localizing to hypoxic, acidic niches within the TME (Karimova et al., 2025; Xu et al., 2025). These M2-polarized cells secrete immunosuppressive factors such as IL-10 and TGF-β to promote angiogenesis, matrix remodeling, and metastatic dissemination, while simultaneously suppressing DC antigen presentation and $CD8^+$ T cell activity. This functional polarization fundamentally arises from a comprehensive remodeling of metabolic networks (Fan et al., 2025). M1 polarization employs a Warburg-like metabolic reprogramming strategy, leveraging the TCA cycle to prioritize citrate and succinate accumulation. These metabolites drive epigenetic modifications to activate proinflammatory gene expression while also supplying substrates for synthesizing effector molecules like ROS and NO (Fig. 6.5) (Kim & Bae, 2018). Conversely, M2 polarization establishes metabolic symbiosis with tumor cells through CD36-mediated lipid scavenging and cholesterol efflux activation. M2 macrophages scavenge oxidized lipids released by tumors to sustain their survival while reciprocally secreting proangiogenic factors and

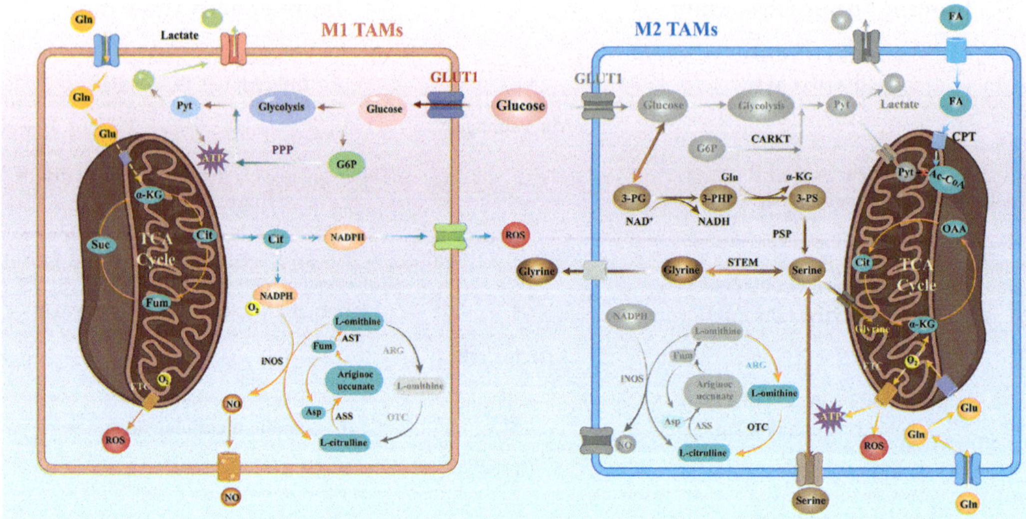

FIGURE 6.5 Metabolic reprogramming of TAMs. *ARG*, arginase; *Asp*, aspartate; *ASS*, argininosuccinate synthase; *AST*, aspartate aminotransferase; *Cir*, citrate; *Fum*, fumarate; *Gla*, glutamine; *HK2*, hexokinase 2; *OTC*, ornithine transcarbamylase; *PSP*, phosphoserine phosphatase; *Pyt*, pyruvic acid; *Suc*, succinate; *α-KG*, α-ketoglutarate.

immunosuppressive signals. Critically, pathological features of TME persistently reinforce M2 metabolic adaptation via stress sensors such as HIF-1α and AMPK, transforming macrophages from immune sentinels into accomplices of immune evasion (Vitale et al., 2019).

Boosting glycolysis pathway in TAMs has become a potential approach to advance tumor immunotherapy. As an upstream inhibitor of mTOR, Redd1 restricts glycolytic flux in macrophages. Guo et al. (2021) developed an innovative mannose-modified outer membrane vesicle micro/nanodelivery system that selectively targets CD206 high M2-like TAMs. This system achieves dual functionality by delivering Redd1 siRNA to silence metabolic checkpoints while synchronously releasing paclitaxel via acid-sensitive bonds to generate on-site inflammatory signaling and ICD. In the 4T1 murine model, this combined strategy upregulates glycolysis and induces M1 repolarization of macrophages, driving concomitant tumor suppression and metastasis inhibition. By integrating receptor-targeted recognition with metabolic gene silencing (Redd1 knockdown), this work demonstrates precise cellularly specific metabolic remodeling capabilities, highlighting a dual-targeting strategy (receptor-locking plus metabolic silencing) to reconfigure immunosuppressive TAMs for enhanced antitumor immunity. However, Hypoxia in TME critically impedes M1-like TAM differentiation. To counteract hypoxia-imposed metabolic constraints, Jiang et al. (2021) engineered a nanoemulsion (α-T-K) coencapsulating KIRA6 (endoplasmic reticulum stress inhibitor) and α-tocopherol (oxidative stress scavenger). This dual-pathway inhibitor system synergistically attenuates ER stress and oxidative stress cascades, thereby reprogramming TAM metabolism through glycolytic potentiation concurrent with FAO suppression. The metabolic rewiring notably enhances M2-to-M1 repolarization efficiency under hypoxic conditions, while concomitantly improving the infiltration and effector function of cytotoxic $CD8^+$ T cells within tumor lesions.

Lipid metabolic reprogramming has been demonstrated to be one of the most important hallmarks of TAMs, exerting a decisive influence on macrophage phenotype and function and driving tumorigenesis as well as resistance to immunotherapy (Wu et al., 2024). Accordingly, targeting lipid metabolism in TAMs may offer a promising avenue for antitumor strategies. For this, Ma et al. (2023) developed an ROS-responsive composite hydrogel incorporating hollow mesoporous CuS nanoparticles (iF-CuS-M) encapsulating FSP1 inhibitors, surface-coated with tumor cell membranes, and integrated with sulfosuccinimidyl oleate (SSO). This composite hydrogel can respond and release therapeutic agents under the action of abundant ROS in the TME. Thereinto, SSO could target the CD36 receptors on the surface of MDSCs, M2-TAMs, and Treg cells, blocking lipid uptake and reprogramming lipid metabolism, thereby alleviating their immunosuppressive phenotype and promoting the infiltration of CTLs. Meanwhile, the released iF-CuS-M homotypically targets tumor cells, inhibits the intrinsic ability of GPX4, and works in parallel with iFSP1-mediated FSP1 inactivation to enhance lipid peroxidation and achieve tumor-specific T cell immunity through ICD. In another study, Peng et al. (2025) engineered two mitochondria-targeted liposomes with MST@A/C for M2 TAMs and BST@2-DG liposomes for tumor cells. After mitochondrial localization in M2 TAMs, MST@A/C releases atractyloside (ATR), a high-affinity specific inhibitor of mitochondrial ADP/ATP exchange, which effectively suppresses OXPHOS metabolism and reduces cellular oxygen consumption. Concurrently, curcumin released from this system significantly downregulates CD36 expression in TAMs, blocking lipid uptake and reprogramming lipid metabolism to eliminate M2 TAMs while inducing their repolarization into the M1 phenotype, thereby ameliorating the immunosuppressive microenvironment and enhancing antitumor efficacy. Meanwhile, BST@2-DG delivers 2-DG to 4T1 cell mitochondria, where it inhibits glycolysis to reduce glucose consumption. This metabolic rewiring promotes nutrient uptake and glucose metabolism in TAMs, coordinating enhanced M2-to-M1 phenotypic conversion to synergistically enhance antitumor effects. This study demonstrates that combined metabolic intervention exhibits superior efficacy in macrophage reprogramming and tumor suppression compared to single-target metabolic modulation.

Beyond lipid metabolism and glycolysis, amino acid metabolism has also been identified as a potential therapeutic target for TAMs. Within the TME, TAMs exploit amino acid metabolic pathways to potentiate their protumorigenic polarization and functional transformation (Jiang et al., 2022). Postpolarization, TAMs demonstrate pronounced metabolic competency in tryptophan and arginine uptake/utilization, which manifests the prototypical phenotypic and functional hallmarks of immunosuppressive macrophages (Chen et al., 2025). Mechanistically, amino acid metabolic cascades in TAMs orchestrate bidirectional exchanges of cytokines, oncometabolites, and signaling molecules with neighboring cellular constituents, dynamically reshaping the immunological landscape of the TME. Emerging therapeutic strategies leveraging micro/nanoplatforms have been developed to target amino acid transporters and rate-limiting enzymes within these metabolic pathways. These innovative formulations exhibit substantial promise in reprogramming TAMs toward antitumor phenotypes while synergistically enhancing systemic antitumor immunity. Although M2-like TAMs constitute the predominant antigen-presenting cells (APCs) population within tumors, their heightened lysosomal cathepsin activity compromises antigen cross-presentation efficiency, thereby impeding $CD8^+$ T cell activation (Cui et al., 2021).

To overcome this, Qiao et al. (2024) engineered a biomimetic nanoplatform (MSN-E64@CM) that integrates the galactose ligand-functionalized cancer cell membrane-coated mesoporous silica carrying the cysteine protease inhibitor E64. This nanoplatform could selectively target and suppress cysteine proteases in the lysosomes of M2-like TAMs. The consequent metabolic reprogramming synergistically enhances antigen cross-presentation capacity while directly priming $CD8^{+}$ CTLs.

It is crucial to emphasize that the therapeutic potential of macrophage metabolic remodeling extends beyond targeting singular pathways. By using micro/nanoplatforms to enhance glycolysis, inhibit fatty acid uptake and FAO, and regulate lysosomal function or other mechanisms in a spatiotemporal coordinated manner, it is possible to elevate macrophage inflammatory set-points at the metabolic level, enhance DAMPs and antigen cross-presentation at the antigen level, and relieve T-cell suppression at the signaling level. This approach can effectively transform the immune-cold TME into an immune-hot one. As programmable micro/nanoplatforms, membrane biomimicry, and subcellular targeting technologies continue to mature, macrophage-centered metabolic immunotherapies are emerging as a key strategy to enhance immune therapy, achieving higher response rates and more durable remissions.

6.3.2 Modulation of dendritic cell metabolism

DCs, as central elements of the immune system, are crucial for initiating and modulating immune responses, especially in antitumor immunity. As professional APCs, DCs can efficiently capture, process, and present TAAs to T cells, thereby activating adaptive immune responses (Del Prete et al., 2023). However, due to the metabolic reprogramming of tumor leading to intensified nutrient competition and the accumulation of immunosuppressive metabolic products, DCs often exhibit metabolic dysfunction, characterized by impaired maturation, reduced antigen-presenting capacity, and weakened costimulatory signals, which in turn weakens their ability to activate T cells and promotes tumor immune escape (O'neill & Pearce, 2015; Vitale et al., 2019). Therefore the use of innovative micro/nanoplatforms to target and regulate the metabolic state of DCs has become an important strategy to enhance their immune activation potential, restore their functional homeostasis, and improve the efficacy of tumor immunotherapy.

Glycolysis is one critical metabolic pathway, which is vital for their activation and subsequent T cell priming (Lawless et al., 2017). Upon encountering pathogens or tumor antigens, DCs undergo metabolic reprogramming, notably shifting from oxidative phosphorylation OXPHOS to glycolysis, a process that provides the rapid ATP and metabolic intermediates necessary for DC activation and cytokine production. This metabolic shift supports the increased energy demand associated with antigen presentation and T-cell activation (Dong et al., 2023; Peng et al., 2021). However, in the TME, excessive lactate production increased glycolytic activity by tumor cells can create a hostile environment for DCs. Therefore increasing the glycolytic level of DCs is of great significance for the restoration of their antigen-presenting function and the enhancement of antitumor immune responses. Inamdar et al. (2023) developed a calcium phosphate microparticle vaccine formulation (F16BP MPs) loaded with fructose-1,6-bisphosphate (F16BP) and PFK15. PFK15 is an inhibitor targeting PFKFB3, which can suppress glycolytic flux in tumor cells; while

F16BP, as the catalytic product of the downstream enzyme of PFKFB3, phosphofructokinase, can specifically relieve the glycolytic inhibition on DCs. Notably, even in the presence of PFK15, this nanovaccine can effectively restore the glycolytic activity of DCs, thereby inducing strong induction of innate and adaptive immune reactions in a melanoma-bearing mouse model. This strategy of combining a glycolytic inhibitor with a key glycolytic metabolite provides an innovative research idea for improving the metabolic function of DCs and enhancing their immune activation ability.

Recent research has demonstrated that dysregulated lipid accumulation is one of the key mechanisms leading to the decline in cross-presentation ability of DCs (Qin et al., 2023; Yin et al., 2020). Thus reshaping the lipid metabolism of DCs has become an important strategy to restore their immune function. The high expression of the lipid transport receptor Msr1 on the surface of DCs promotes their lipid uptake in TME, thereby causing abnormal enrichment of lipid metabolites (Herber et al., 2010). Although Msr1 is also expressed in TAMs, the lipid uptake of these cells mainly depends on the CD36 receptor rather than Msr1, suggesting that Msr1 can be a potential target for DC-specific intervention (Su et al., 2020). To achieve this, Xu et al. (2023) designed and developed a multilevel lipid reprogramming nanoparticle TS-PP@FU for DCs functional regeneration. This system is constructed through the self-assembly of the amphiphilic poly(ε-caprolactone)-block-polyethyleneimine copolymer with the ACC inhibitor 5-(tetradecanoyloxy)-2-furoic acid (TOFA), the XBP1 mRNA splicing inhibitor STF-083010 (STF), and the Msr1 antagonist fucoidan (FU). FU can block the recognition and uptake of extracellular lipids by competitively binding to Msr1, thereby achieving targeted intervention of tumor-associated dendritic cells and inhibiting their exogenous lipid intake. The internalized nanoparticles can synergistically regulate endogenous lipid synthesis at two levels: on the one hand, TOFA inhibits the de novo synthesis pathway of fatty acids; on the other hand, STF inhibits the transcriptional activity of lipid synthesis-related genes. Therefore the administration of TS-PP@FU achieves multilevel and multitarget lipid metabolism reprogramming, effectively reversing the functional disorder phenotype of CDs. This strategy can be further combined with αPD-1 to significantly enhance CTLs activation and achieve effective tumor growth inhibition in TNBC models.

DCs in tumor typically exhibit highly activated MVA pathways, which are key to cholesterol metabolism (Mullen et al., 2016). Dysregulated activation of the metabolism signaling can compromise antigen-presenting function of DCs (Mullen et al., 2016; Xia et al., 2018). To reverse this immunosuppressive state, Yan et al. (2022) developed a multifunctional hydrogel delivery system (Gel@NPs), designed to reshape the immune function of DCs by regulating their cholesterol metabolism. This system integrates graphene oxide (GO), metformin hydrochloride (MET), and mannosylated nanoparticles (Man-OVA) loaded with rosuvastatin (RSV). The hydrogel can continuously release Man-OVA at the tumor site, and the mannose ligands on its surface demonstrate specific recognition of the highly expressed mannose receptors on DCs, thus ensuring targeted delivery. RSV can inhibit the MVA pathway, thereby reprogramming the cholesterol metabolism of DCs and restoring their maturation and antigen-presenting capabilities. Meanwhile, GO generates a photothermal effect under near-infrared light irradiation, eliciting ICD of tumor cells and yielding high levels of TAAs, which can be readily internalized, processed, and subsequently displayed by activated DCs to T lymphocytes. Additionally, MET is capable of the suppressing PD-L1 expression on tumor cell membranes, mitigating the TIME and further promoting T cell-mediated immune activation. This study reveals the critical connection between cholesterol metabolism regulation and the functional state of DCs and demonstrates that the hydrogel-based delivery system, as an immunometabolic intervention agent, holds significant application prospects in DC-mediated cancer immunotherapy.

6.3.3 Modulation of T cell metabolism

T cells, as key components of the adaptive immune system, play an essential role in maintaining the balance of cellular and humoral immune responses (Kishton et al., 2017). Typically, naive T cells recognize cytokines and tumor antigens through T cell receptor (TCR) and differentiate into T cell subsets ($CD8^+$ and $CD4^+$ T cells) to initiate antitumor immune responses (Viel et al., 2025). T cells are subject to strict metabolic regulation during proliferation and differentiation to maintain a balance between nutrient supply and energy demand (Chen et al., 2025). For instance, naive T cells generate ATP through OXPHOS, while activated T cells shift their metabolic mode to glycolysis, accompanied by the catabolism of glutamine and branched-chain amino acids, enhancing the uptake of glucose and amino acids to replenish intermediates for the TCA cycle and support the synthesis of lipids, nucleic acids, and proteins (Huang et al., 2024; Wang et al., 2011; Zou et al., 2025). Research has demonstrated that the activation of PI3K/Akt signaling pathway increases the expression of nutrient transporters (GLUT-1 or SLC1a5) by enhancing mTOR signaling, further promoting glycolysis, and improving glucose utilization (Wilfahrt & Delgoffe, 2024; Yin et al., 2019). Notably, Tregs with immunosuppressive properties maintain a high OXPHOS state through lipid metabolism remodeling, dominated by FAO (Beckermann et al., 2017; Han et al., 2024; Yan et al., 2023). This metabolic characteristic gives Tregs a survival advantage in the low-glucose TME. Additionally, Tregs rely on the uptake of large amounts of lactate to promote Foxp3-dependent RNA splicing-mediated expression of CTLs-associated protein 4 (CTLA-4), thereby enhancing their immunosuppressive function (Ma et al., 2025; Watson et al., 2021). To address the challenges posed by metabolic dysregulation in TME to T cell function, in addition to targeting tumor cell metabolic reprogramming, the direct regulation of key nodes in T cell metabolism (such as glycolysis rate-limiting enzymes, GLS, etc.) using nanomedicines has shown therapeutic potential in enhancing T cell immune surveillance capabilities.

Tumor cells exhibit a predatory glucose consumption behavior that drives T cell exhaustion, a dysfunctional state characterized by mitochondrial metabolic impairment. Therefore restoring mitochondrial biosynthesis and function can help break this immunosuppressive predicament. Currently, strategies to eto improve mitochondrial flexibility in T cells primarily involve peroxisome proliferator-activated receptor (PPAR) agonists, anti-4-1BB stimulation, and alternative nutrient supply.Chen et al. (2025) developed a lipid nanoparticle factory (L@Mn@SPD) coloaded with spermidine (SPD), Mn^{2+}, and $MnO(OH)_2$ to alleviate T cell exhaustion in tumor immunotherapy. SPD is a nitrogen-containing, low-molecular-weight alkaline compound that has been proven to enhance mitochondrial function in the heart, nervous system, liver, and immune system. This nanoliposome achieves a four-stage immune therapy cascade reaction: (1) ROS generated by the synergy of Mn^{2+} and SPD can directly kill tumor cells and enhance their immunogenicity; (2) Mn^{2+}

further activates DCs, promoting antigen presentation through the STING signaling pathway and effectively activating $CD8^+$ T cells; (3) SPD can repair mitochondrial dysfunction and alleviate $CD8^+$ T cell exhaustion; (4) $MnO(OH)_2$ releases O_2 under the action of intracellular H_2O_2, reducing the expression of HIF-1α and further improving the exhausted state of $CD8^+$ T cells. This combined treatment strategy, based on restoring T cell mitochondrial function, achieved a 74.7% tumor inhibition rate in the 4T1 tumor-bearing mouse, significantly increased the number of $CD8^+$ T cells in the spleen, and successfully induced a systemic antitumor immunity.

Cholesterol on the T cell membrane is a key factor in regulating TCR clustering and the formation of the immunological synapse. Studies have shown that after $CD8^+$ T cells are activated, the expression of acetyl-CoA acetyltransferase-1 (ACAT-1) is upregulated, and this enzyme can convert free cholesterol into cholesterol esters and store them in intracellular LDs. Avasimibe (AVA), an ACAT-1 inhibitor, can promote TCR clustering by increasing the enrichment of free cholesterol on the cell membrane, thereby enhancing the tumor-killing activity of $CD8^+$ T cells. Li et al. (2018) designed and synthesized a pH-responsive liposome (PTX/αGC-TH-Lip) coloaded with paclitaxel, the immune adjuvant α-galactosylceramide (αGC), and AVA for the chemo-immunotherapy of melanoma. In the B16F10 tumor-bearing mouse xenograft and lung metastasis models, the combination of AVA and this liposome significantly increased the level of free cholesterol in the T cell membrane, enhanced the CTL response, and achieved a stronger antitumor effect. However, the reprogramming effect of AVA on T cell lipid metabolism is often limited by the penetration efficiency of the drug carrier in tumor tissues. To address this, Liu et al. (2023) developed a matrix metalloproteinase-2 (MMP-2)-sensitive tumor-penetrating nanovesicle (EALP) for regulating the cholesterol metabolic pathway to enhance PDT-mediated cancer immunotherapy. After enrichment at the tumor site, this nanovesicle releases internalized RGD peptides through MMP-2-responsive cleavage, promoting its penetration into deep tumor tissues. Subsequently, the released AVA can simultaneously block the cholesterol esterification process in $CD8^+$ T cells and tumor cells. On one hand, it restores the activation function of T cells, and on the other hand, it inhibits the migration ability of tumor cells. Moreover, the immune response triggered by PDT-induced ICD is further amplified under the background of inhibited cholesterol metabolism. Compared with PDT alone, this nanovesicle showed a more significant tumor growth inhibition effect in the B16F10 mouse tumor model. This strategy provides a new idea for enhancing the efficacy of photodynamic cancer immunotherapy by interfering with the cholesterol metabolic pathway.

6.3.4 Modulation of natural killer cell metabolism

NK cells play a critical role in the immune system by acting as frontline defenders against tumors and pathogens through their ability to identify and eliminate infected or malignant cells (Chen et al., 2025; Raza et al., 2023). NK cells identify and destroy tumor cells by releasing cytotoxic granules containing perforin and granzymes and by producing cytokines (IFN-γ, TNF-α, TNF-β, and IL-6) (Li et al., 2025; Myers & Miller, 2021). The activation of these cells is regulated by a complex interplay of activating and inhibitory receptors. The metabolic programming of NK cells is crucial for their function in immune surveillance and antitumor responses. Under normal circumstances, NK cells rely on glycolysis and

OXPHOS to generate the energy required for activation and cytotoxic functions (Choi et al., 2020). During activation, NK cells undergo metabolic reprogramming, primarily characterized by an increase in glycolysis, which is vital for their fast proliferation and efficient immune activation. Glycolysis provides the necessary energy and metabolic intermediates for the production of proinflammatory cytokines and the execution of cytotoxic responses. However, in the TME, the acidic and hypoxic conditions intensify the competition for nutrients between tumor cells and immune cells, often limiting the energy supply to NK cells and thereby affecting their function (Jin et al., 2025; Wang et al., 2025). To enhance NK cell-mediated antitumor immunity, increasing evidence suggests that directly targeting the metabolism of NK cells is an effective strategy.

In this context, He et al. (2023) designed and synthesized biocompatible black phosphorus quantum dots encapsulated by human serum albumin (BPQDs@HSA) as an immune-sensitizer, aiming to enhance the cytotoxic activity of NK cells against tumor cells and achieve synergistic tumor suppression. The study demonstrated that BPQDs@HSA could interact with TLRs on the surface of NK cells, activate the downstream NF-κB signaling pathway, regulate cytokine secretion, and promote Th1-type immune responses. Notably, as a phosphate group donor, BPQDs@HSA could specifically bind to phosphatidylinositol 4-phosphate 5-kinase type 1 gamma (PIP5K1A), thereby activating the PI3K-Akt-mTOR signaling pathway, reprogramming cellular glycolytic metabolism, promoting oxidative phosphorylation, and effectively maintaining the metabolic homeostasis, survival ability, and immune function of NK cells. Emerging evidence highlights the dual role of IL-21 in driving NK cell proliferation/differentiation and augmenting their functional maturation alongside sustained in vivo persistence (Chen et al., 2023). Given this feature, Meng et al. (2022) researchers developed a bioorthogonal targeting live cell nanocarrier (N3-NK-NPs). This system modifies NK cells and tumor cells through metabolic glycoengineering (MGE) to express azide groups on their surfaces, which then undergo bioorthogonal reactions with protein nanogels carrying IL-21 to achieve cross-linking. MGE serves as an artificial ligand–receptor recognition mechanism here, effectively mediating the specific binding between the two types of cells and thereby enhancing the infiltration ability of NK cells into tumor tissues. Meanwhile, a redox-responsive nanoparticle (ILNPs) formed by the self-assembly of the cytokine IL-21 is in situ anchored on the surface of NK cells, continuously releasing IL-21 in physiological environments to long-term promote the proliferation, activation, and functional maintenance of NK cells, simulating a cell-autocrine effect. This multifunctional nanoplatform that integrates bioorthogonal metabolic labeling and "hitchhiking" delivery strategies provides an innovative and reliable solution for enhancing the targeting, stability, and safety of NK cell therapy.

Current research emphasizes the critical role of NK cell metabolic reprogramming, primarily focusing on enhancing glycolysis and OXPHOS to sustain cytotoxic functions under nutrient-deprived TME conditions (Chen et al., 2025; Miao et al., 2024). Metabolic modulation through micro/nano platform-based approaches significantly improves NK cell persistence, cytokine production, and tumor-killing efficacy, highlighting promising strategies to refine NK cell-based immunotherapies. Further exploration of alternative metabolic pathways, including lipid, nucleotide, and ion metabolism, is expected to inspire innovative nanotherapeutic designs for amplifying NK cell-mediated antitumor immunity.

6.4 Conclusion and perspective

Micro/nano-enabled modulation of tumor metabolism has matured into a versatile framework for strengthening antitumor immunity in inflammatory tumors. Engineered micro/nanoplatforms can rewire metabolic circuits in tumor site, such as glucose utilization, amino acid flux, lipid synthesis and oxidation, nucleotide biosynthesis, and mitochondrial respiratory inhibition, to deprive malignant cells of key fuels while restoring the bioenergetic capacity of tumor-infiltrating immune cells. By improving pharmacokinetics and pharmacodynamics, protecting labile biologics, and enabling delivery across physiological barriers and into specific cell populations or organelles, micro/nanoplatforms provide control over when and where metabolic regulators act. Designs that respond to endogenous or exogenous cues permit on-demand drug release within malignant TIME, and combinations with PDT, MHT, CDT, and SDT modalities trigger immunogenic cell death and increase tumor immunogenicity, thereby amplifying the tumor-immunity cycle.

Notwithstanding these advances, translation is challenged by the profound adaptability of tumor metabolism. When a single pathway is inhibited, tumors often compensate by shunting flux through alternative routes, weakening durable responses.

Besides, precision remains one of the key challenges in the regulation of inflammatory tumor immunity and metabolism enabled by micro/nanoplatforms. This is primarily attributed to the fact that activated lymphocytes and tumor cells share metabolic programs, and indiscriminate inhibition may weaken the immune effector function. The spatial and temporal heterogeneity of metabolic phenotypes across primary lesions and micrometastases further complicates intervention, as oxidative niches may coexist with glycolysis-dominant regions within the same tumor. Delivery barriers, including abnormal vasculature, elevated interstitial pressure, dense extracellular matrix, and solid stress, limit accumulation and uniform distribution of nanomedicines, yielding uneven metabolic modulation. In addition, CSCs, stromal populations, and microbiota critically shape the TIME yet are only sporadically considered in current designs. Finally, complex formulations raise questions about scalability, long-term safety, organ-specific metabolic liabilities, and manufacturing consistency.

Future progress will depend on deeper mapping of patient-specific immunometabolic landscapes and the crosstalk among malignant cells, immune subsets, CSCs, stroma, and resident microbes. Integrating multiomics with functional imaging can identify actionable vulnerabilities and guide rational, individualized designs. Therapeutic platforms should coordinate simultaneous control of complementary pathways, such as constraining glycolysis while blocking lactate export and adjusting FAO or OXPHOS, while differentially augmenting the metabolism of effector T cells and NK cells to avoid collateral suppression. Adaptive, stimuli-responsive carriers capable of sensing local metabolites and redox cues could modulate payload release in real time, matching intratumoral heterogeneity and the evolving course of disease. Strategies that cotarget primary tumors and micrometastatic reservoirs, and that directly address CSC bioenergetics, are likely to prevent relapse and dissemination. Delivery can be improved through stromal remodeling, vascular normalization, size- and shape-optimized carriers, and multistage systems that enhance penetration and achieve more uniform biodistribution. Equally important is rigorous evaluation of safety using standardized assays and computational modeling, coupled with simplification of formulations and preference for clinically compatible components to facilitate reproducible scale-up. As these scientific and engineering threads converge, micro/nano-enabled immunometabolic regulation is poised to shift from experimental promise to clinical utility, transforming the immunosuppressive TME into a therapeutically tractable vulnerability and delivering durable, systemic antitumor immunity for patients.

AI disclosure

During the preparation of this work, the author(s) used ELSA's built-in abstract generation system, the summary for this chapter is the same as the one at the beginning of Chapter 3; there is no separate abstract, so it was generated by AI. After using this tool/service, the author(s) reviewed and edited the content as needed and take(s) full responsibility for the content of the publication.

References

Ahmed, N., Escalona, R., Leung, D., Chan, E., & Kannourakis, G. (2018). Tumour microenvironment and metabolic plasticity in cancer and cancer stem cells: Perspectives on metabolic and immune regulatory signatures in chemoresistant ovarian cancer stem cells. *Seminars in Cancer Biology, 53*, 265–281. https://doi.org/10.1016/j.semcancer.2018.10.002.

Bai, J., Zhang, X., Zhao, Z., Sun, S., Cheng, W., Yu, H., Chang, X., & Wang, B. (2024). CuO nanozymes catalyze cysteine and glutathione depletion induced ferroptosis and cuproptosis for synergistic tumor therapy. *Small (Weinheim an der Bergstrasse, Germany), 20*(40). https://doi.org/10.1002/smll.202400326, http://onlinelibrary.wiley.com/journal/10.1002/(ISSN)1613-6829.

Bayik, D., & Lathia, J. D. (2021). Cancer stem cell–immune cell crosstalk in tumour progression. *Nature Reviews. Cancer, 21*(8), 526–536. https://doi.org/10.1038/s41568-021-00366-w.

Beckermann, K. E., Dudzinski, S. O., & Rathmell, J. C. (2017). Dysfunctional T cell metabolism in the tumor microenvironment. *Cytokine & Growth Factor Reviews, 35*, 7–14. https://doi.org/10.1016/j.cytogfr.2017.04.003.

Binnewies, M., Roberts, E. W., Kersten, K., Chan, V., Fearon, D. F., Merad, M., Coussens, L. M., Gabrilovich, D. I., Ostrand-Rosenberg, S., Hedrick, C. C., Vonderheide, R. H., Pittet, M. J., Jain, R. K., Zou, W., Howcroft, T. K., Woodhouse, E. C., Weinberg, R. A., & Krummel, M. F. (2018). Understanding the tumor immune microenvironment (TIME) for effective therapy. *Nature Medicine, 24*(5), 541–550. https://doi.org/10.1038/s41591-018-0014-x, http://www.nature.com/nm/index.html.

Chen, G., Xu, Q., Feng, Z., Xu, Q., Zhang, X., Yang, Y., Zhang, Y., Liang, X.-J., Yu, Z., & Yu, M. (2022). Glutamine antagonist synergizes with electrodynamic therapy to induce tumor regression and systemic antitumor immunity. *ACS Nano, 16*(1), 951–962. https://doi.org/10.1021/acsnano.1c08544.

Chen, J., Yang, S., Li, Y., Ziwen, X., Zhang, P., Song, Q., Yao, Y., & Pei, H. (2023). De novo nucleotide biosynthetic pathway and cancer. *Genes Dis, 10*(6), 2331–2338. https://doi.org/10.1016/j.gendis.2022.04.018.

Chen, J., Zhu, Y., Wu, C., & Shi, J. (2020). Nanoplatform-based cascade engineering for cancer therapy. *Chemical Society Reviews, 49*(24), 9057–9094. https://doi.org/10.1039/d0cs00607f.

Chen, L., Zhou, Q., Zhang, P., Tan, W., Li, Y., Xu, Z., Ma, J., Kupfer, G. M., Pei, Y., Song, Q., & Pei, H. (2024). Direct stimulation of de novo nucleotide synthesis by O-GlcNAcylation. *Nature Chemical Biology, 20*(1), 19–29. https://doi.org/10.1038/s41589-023-01354-x.

Chen, N., Yang, Y., Fan, L., Cai, Y., Yin, W., Yang, Z., Zhao, Y., Chen, S., Zhi, H., Xue, L., Zhang, X., An, L., Li, Y., & Ren, T. (2025). The STING-activating nanofactory relieves T cell exhaustion in Mn-based tumor immunotherapy by regulating mitochondrial dysfunction. *Journal of Nanobiotechnology, 23*(1). https://doi.org/10.1186/s12951-025-03469-w, https://jnanobiotechnology.biomedcentral.com.

Choi, B. Y., Jeong, J. H., Eom, J. W., Koh, J. Y., Kim, Y. H., & Suh, S. W. (2020). A novel zinc chelator, 1H10, ameliorates experimental autoimmune encephalomyelitis by modulating zinc toxicity and AMPK activation. *International Journal of Molecular Sciences, 21*(9). https://doi.org/10.3390/ijms21093375, https://www.mdpi.com/1422-0067/21/9/3375/pdf.

Cognet, G., & Muir, A. (2024). Identifying metabolic limitations in the tumor microenvironment. *Science Advances, 10*(40), eadq7305. https://doi.org/10.1126/sciadv.adq7305.

Cui, C., Chakraborty, K., Tang, X. A., Schoenfelt, K. Q., Hoffman, A., Blank, A., McBeth, B., Pulliam, N., Reardon, C. A., Kulkarni, S. A., Vaisar, T., Ballabio, A., Krishnan, Y., & Becker, L. (2021). A lysosome-targeted DNA nanodevice selectively targets macrophages to attenuate tumours. *Nature Nanotechnology, 16*(12), 1394–1402. https://doi.org/10.1038/s41565-021-00988-z, http://www.nature.com/nnano/index.html.

Cun, J.-E., He, Z., Fan, X., Pan, Q., Luo, K., He, B., & Pu, Y. (2025). Copper-based bio-coordination nanoparticle for enhanced pyroptosis-cuproptosis cancer immunotherapy through redox modulation and glycolysis inhibition. *Small (Weinheim an der Bergstrasse, Germany), 21*(6). https://doi.org/10.1002/smll.202409875.

De Jesus, A., Keyhani-Nejad, F., Pusec, C. M., Goodman, L., Geier, J. A., Stoolman, J. S., Stanczyk, P. J., Nguyen, T., Xu, K., Suresh, K. V., Chen, Y., Rodriguez, A. E., Shapiro, J. S., Chang, H. C., Chen, C., Shah, K. P., Ben-Sahra, I., Layden, B. T., Chandel, N. S., ... Ardehali, H. (2022). Hexokinase 1 cellular localization regulates the metabolic fate of glucose. *Molecular Cell, 82*(7), 1261. https://doi.org/10.1016/j.molcel.2022.02.028, www.molecule.org.

De Leo, A., Ugolini, A., Yu, X., Scirocchi, F., Scocozza, D., Peixoto, B., Pace, A., D'Angelo, L., Liu, J. K. C., Etame, A. B., Rughetti, A., Nuti, M., Santoro, A., Vogelbaum, M. A., Conejo-Garcia, J. R., Rodriguez, P. C., & Veglia, F. (2024). Glucose-driven histone lactylation promotes the immunosuppressive activity of monocyte-derived macrophages in glioblastoma. *Immunity, 57*(5), 1105. https://doi.org/10.1016/j.immuni.2024.04.006, https://www.sciencedirect.com/science/journal/10747613.

Del Prete, A., Salvi, V., Soriani, A., Laffranchi, M., Sozio, F., Bosisio, D., & Sozzani, S. (2023). Dendritic cell subsets in cancer immunity and tumor antigen sensing. *Cellular & Molecular Immunology, 20*(5), 432–447. https://doi.org/10.1038/s41423-023-00990-6.

Dong, X., Xia, S., Du, S., Zhu, M. H., Lai, X., Yao, S. Q., Chen, H. Z., & Fang, C. (2023). Tumor metabolism-rewriting nanomedicines for cancer immunotherapy. *ACS Central Science, 9*(10), 1864–1893. https://doi.org/10.1021/acscentsci.3c00702, http://pubs.acs.org/journal/acscii.

Fan, H., Lu, D., Yin, X., Sun, H., Wang, Z., Sun, H., Liu, X., Li, Y., Zhou, Z., Chen, L., Wang, Y., & Xin, T. (2025). The metabolic regulation of tumor-associated macrophage reprogramming. *Molecular Immunology, 187*, 198–209. https://doi.org/10.1016/j.molimm.2025.10.006.

Fang, H., Wu, Y., Chen, L., Cao, Z., Deng, Z., Zhao, R., Zhang, L., Yang, Y., Liu, Z., & Chen, Q. (2023). Regulating the obesity-related tumor microenvironment to improve cancer immunotherapy. *ACS Nano, 17*(5), 4748–4763. https://doi.org/10.1021/acsnano.2c11159, http://pubs.acs.org/journal/ancac3.

Feng, Q., Fang, W., Guo, Y., Hu, P., & Shi, J. (2023). Nebulized therapy of early orthotopic lung cancer by iron-based nanoparticles: Macrophage-regulated ferroptosis of cancer stem cells. *Journal of the American Chemical Society, 145*(44), 24153–24165. https://doi.org/10.1021/jacs.3c08032.

Fu, L.-H., Qi, C., Lin, J., & Huang, P. (2018). Catalytic chemistry of glucose oxidase in cancer diagnosis and treatment. *Chemical Society Reviews, 47*(17), 6454–6472. https://doi.org/10.1039/c7cs00891k.

Gao, Y., Xia, Y., Li, J., Lai, Y., Yin, S., Lin, J., Yu, D., Huang, S., Lu, F., Wang, W., & Chu, Q. (2025). Tumoral ALOX5 mediated arachidonic acid metabolism regulates immune response in non-small cell lung cancer. *Cellular Oncology, 48*(6), 2017–2034. https://doi.org/10.1007/s13402-025-01124-y.

Gong, Q., Shi, L., Wen, L., Zhang, Y., Chen, Z., Wei, X., Song, X., Dong, J., & Liang, C. (2025). Recent advances in metal ions overloading for tumors: Mechanisms, nanomaterials, and therapies. *Materials Today Bio, 35*, 102320. https://doi.org/10.1016/j.mtbio.2025.102320.

Guo, Q., Li, X., Zhou, W., Chu, Y., Chen, Q., Zhang, Y., Li, C., Chen, H., Liu, P., Zhao, Z., Wang, Y., zhou, Z., Luo, Y., Li, C., You, H., Song, H., Su, B., Zhang, T., Sun, T., & Jiang, Chen (2021). Sequentially triggered bacterial outer membrane vesicles for macrophage metabolism modulation and tumor metastasis suppression. *ACS Nano, 15*(8), 13826–13838. https://doi.org/10.1021/acsnano.1c05613.

Hamanaka, R. B., & Chandel, N. S. (2012). Targeting glucose metabolism for cancer therapy. *The Journal of Experimental Medicine, 209*(2), 211–215. https://doi.org/10.1084/jem.20120162.

Han, H., He, T., Wu, Y., He, T., & Zhou, W. (2024). Multidimensional analysis of tumor stem cells: From biological properties, metabolic adaptations to immune escape mechanisms. *Frontiers in Cell and Developmental Biology, 12*.

https://doi.org/10.3389/fcell.2024.1441081, https://www.frontiersin.org/journals/cell-and-developmental-biology#.

Hassanein, M., Hoeksema, M. D., Shiota, M., Qian, J., Harris, B. K., Chen, H., Clark, J. E., Alborn, W. E., Eisenberg, R., & Massion, P. P. (2013). SLC1A5 mediates glutamine transport required for lung cancer cell growth and survival. *Clinical Cancer Research, 19*(3), 560–570. https://doi.org/10.1158/1078-0432.CCR-12-2334, http://clincancerres.aacrjournals.org/content/19/3/560.full.pdf+html.

He, L., Zhao, J., Li, H., Xie, B., Xu, L., Huang, G., Liu, T., Gu, Z., & Chen, T. (2023). Metabolic Reprogramming of NK cells by black phosphorus quantum dots potentiates cancer immunotherapy. *Advanced Science, 10*(8). https://doi.org/10.1002/advs.202202519.

He, Y., Liu, L., Dong, Y., Zhang, X., Song, Y., Jing, Y., Ni, Y., Wang, Y., Wang, Z., & Ding, L. (2024). Lipid droplets-related Perilipin-3: Potential immune checkpoint and oncogene in oral squamous cell carcinoma. *Cancer Immunology, Immunotherapy, 73*(5). https://doi.org/10.1007/s00262-024-03659-9.

Herber, D. L., Cao, W., Nefedova, Y., Novitskiy, S. V., Nagaraj, S., Tyurin, V. A., Corzo, A., Cho, H. I., Celis, E., Lennox, B., Knight, S. C., Padhya, T., McCaffrey, T. V., McCaffrey, J. C., Antonia, S., Fishman, M., Ferris, R. L., Kagan, V. E., & Gabrilovich, D. I. (2010). Lipid accumulation and dendritic cell dysfunction in cancer. *Nature Medicine, 16*(8), 880–886. https://doi.org/10.1038/nm.2172.

Hoy, A. J., Nagarajan, S. R., & Butler, L. M. (2021). Tumour fatty acid metabolism in the context of therapy resistance and obesity. *Nature Reviews Cancer, 21*(12), 753–766. https://doi.org/10.1038/s41568-021-00388-4.

Hu, C., Xuan, Y., Zhang, X., Liu, Y., Yang, S., & Yang, K. (2022). Immune cell metabolism and metabolic reprogramming. *Molecular Biology Reports, 49*(10), 9783–9795. https://doi.org/10.1007/s11033-022-07474-2.

Hu, X., Zhang, B., Zhang, M., Liang, W., Hong, B., Ma, Z., Sheng, J., Liu, T., Yang, S., Liang, Z., Zhang, J., Fan, C., Li, F., & Ling, D. (2024). An artificial metabzyme for tumour-cell-specific metabolic therapy. *Nature Nanotechnology, 19*(11), 1712–1722. https://doi.org/10.1038/s41565-024-01733-y.

Huang, L., Li, H., Zhang, C., Chen, Q., Liu, Z., Zhang, J., Luo, P., & Wei, T. (2024). Unlocking the potential of T-cell metabolism reprogramming: Advancing single-cell approaches for precision immunotherapy in tumour immunity. *Clinical and Translational Medicine, 14*(3). https://doi.org/10.1002/ctm2.1620.

Inamdar, S., Suresh, A. P., Mangal, J. L., Ng, N. D., Sundem, A., Wu, C., Lintecum, K., Thumsi, A., Khodaei, T., Halim, M., Appel, N., Jaggarapu, M. M. C. S., Esrafili, A., Yaron, J. R., Curtis, M., & Acharya, A. P. (2023). Rescue of dendritic cells from glycolysis inhibition improves cancer immunotherapy in mice. *Nature Communications, 14*(1). https://doi.org/10.1038/s41467-023-41016-z, https://www.nature.com/ncomms/.

Jain, M., Nilsson, R., Sharma, S., Madhusudhan, N., Kitami, T., Souza, A. L., Kafri, R., Kirschner, M. W., Clish, C. B., & Mootha, V. K. (2012). Metabolite profiling identifies a key role for glycine in rapid cancer cell proliferation. *Science (New York, N.Y.), 336*(6084), 1040–1044. https://doi.org/10.1126/science.1218595, http://www.sciencemag.org/content/336/6084/1040.full.pdf.

Jeffrey, J. L., Lawson, K. V., & Powers, J. P. (2020). Targeting metabolism of extracellular nucleotides via inhibition of ectonucleotidases CD73 and CD39. *Journal of Medicinal Chemistry, 63*(22), 13444–13465. https://doi.org/10.1021/acs.jmedchem.0c01044.

Ji, H., Wang, W., Li, X., Han, X., Zhang, X., Wang, J., Liu, C., Huang, L., & Gao, W. (2022). p53: A double-edged sword in tumor ferroptosis. *Pharmacological Research, 177*, 106013. https://doi.org/10.1016/j.phrs.2021.106013.

Ji, P., Jin, X.-K., Deng, X.-C., Zhang, S.-M., Liang, J.-L., Li, Q.-R., Chen, W.-H., & Zhang, X.-Z. (2024). Metabolic regulation-mediated reversion of the tumor immunosuppressive microenvironment for potentiating cooperative metabolic therapy and immunotherapy. *Nano Letters, 24*(15), 4691–4701. https://doi.org/10.1021/acs.nanolett.4c01307.

Jiang, M., Li, X., Zhang, J., Lu, Y., Shi, Y., Zhu, C., Liu, Y., Qin, B., Luo, Z., Du, Y., Luo, L., Peng, L., & You, J. (2021). Dual inhibition of endoplasmic reticulum stress and oxidation stress manipulates the polarization of macrophages under hypoxia to sensitize immunotherapy. *ACS Nano, 15*(9), 14522–14534. https://doi.org/10.1021/acsnano.1c04068.

Jiang, M., Cui, H., Liu, Z., Zhou, X., Zhang, L., Cao, L., & Wang, M. (2022). The role of amino acid metabolism of tumor associated macrophages in the development of colorectal cancer. *Cells, 11*(24), 4106. https://doi.org/10.3390/cells11244106.

Jiang, Y., Tao, Q., Qiao, X., Yang, Y., Peng, C., Han, M., Dong, K., Zhang, W., Xu, M., Wang, D., Zhu, W., & Li, X. (2025). Targeting amino acid metabolism to inhibit gastric cancer progression and promote anti-tumor immunity: A review. *Frontiers in Immunology, 16*, 1508730. https://doi.org/10.3389/fimmu.2025.1508730.

Jiao, J., Zhao, Y., Li, Q., Jin, S., & Liu, Z. (2024). LncRNAs in tumor metabolic reprogramming and tumor microenvironment remodeling. *Frontiers in Immunology, 15*. https://doi.org/10.3389/fimmu.2024.1467151.

Jin, J., Yan, P., Wang, D., Bai, L., Liang, H., Zhu, X., Zhu, H., Ding, C., Wei, H., & Wang, Y. (2025). Targeting lactylation reinforces NK cell cytotoxicity within the tumor microenvironment. *Nature Immunology, 26*(7), 1099–1112. https://doi.org/10.1038/s41590-025-02178-8.

Jin, Y., Tan, Y., Wu, J., & Ren, Z. (2023). Lipid droplets: A cellular organelle vital in cancer cells. *Cell Death Discover, 9*(1), 254. https://doi.org/10.1038/s41420-023-01493-z.

Kapnick, S. M., Martin, C. A., & Jewell, C. M. (2024). Engineering metabolism to modulate immunity. *Advanced Drug Delivery Reviews, 204*, 115122. https://doi.org/10.1016/j.addr.2023.115122.

Karimova, A. F., Khalitova, A. R., Suezov, R., Markov, N., Mukhamedshina, Y., Rizvanov, A. A., Huber, M., Simon, H. U., & Brichkina, A. (2025). Immunometabolism of tumor-associated macrophages: A therapeutic perspective. *European Journal of Cancer, 220*. https://doi.org/10.1016/j.ejca.2025.115332, https://www.sciencedirect.com/science/journal/09598049.

Kaymak, I., Williams, K. S., Cantor, J. R., & Jones, R. G. (2021). Immunometabolic interplay in the tumor microenvironment. *Cancer Cell, 39*(1), 28–37. https://doi.org/10.1016/j.ccell.2020.09.004, https://www.journals.elsevier.com/cancer-cell.

Kim, J., & Bae, J. (2018). Metabolic regulation of macrophages in tumor microenvironment. *Current Opinion in Hematology, 25*(1), 52–59. https://doi.org/10.1097/moh.0000000000000390.

Kishton, R. J., Sukumar, M., & Restifo, N. P. (2017). Metabolic regulation of t cell longevity and function in tumor immunotherapy. *Cell Metabolism, 26*(1), 94–109. https://doi.org/10.1016/j.cmet.2017.06.016.

Kopecka, J., Gazzano, E., Castella, B., Salaroglio, I. C., Mungo, E., Massaia, M., & Riganti, C. (2020). Mitochondrial metabolism: Inducer or therapeutic target in tumor immune-resistance? *Seminars in Cell and Developmental Biology, 98*, 80–89. https://doi.org/10.1016/j.semcdb.2019.05.008, http://www.elsevier.com/inca/publications/store/6/2/2/9/4/4/index.htt.

Lawless, S. J., Kedia-Mehta, N., Walls, J. F., McGarrigle, R., Convery, O., Sinclair, L. V., Navarro, M. N., Murray, J., & Finlay, D. K. (2017). Glucose represses dendritic cell-induced T cell responses. *Nature Communications, 8*. https://doi.org/10.1038/ncomms15620, http://www.nature.com/ncomms/index.html.

Leone, R. D., Zhao, L., Englert, J. M., Sun, I. M., Oh, M. H., Sun, I. H., Arwood, M. L., Bettencourt, I. A., Patel, C. H., Wen, J., Tam, A., Blosser, R. L., Prchalova, E., Alt, J., Rais, R., Slusher, B. S., & Powell, J. D. (2019). Glutamine blockade induces divergent metabolic programs to overcome tumor immune evasion. *Science (New York, N.Y.), 366*(6468), 1013–1021. https://doi.org/10.1126/science.aav2588, https://science.sciencemag.org/content/366/6468/1013/tab-pdf.

Li, C., Zhou, M., Li, Y., Jia, H., & Huang, L. (2025). Engineered IL-21-expressing nanovesicles for co-delivery of gox and ferrocene to induce synergistic anti-tumor effects. *Advanced Healthcare Materials, 14*(6), 2403477. https://doi.org/10.1002/adhm.202403477.

Li, J., Luo, X., Wei, M., Li, Z., Li, Y., Zhao, H., Miyagishi, M., Kasim, V., & Wu, S. (2023). YY2/PHGDH axis suppresses tumorigenesis by inhibiting tumor cell de novo serine biosynthesis. *Biomedicine & Pharmacotherapy=Biomedecine & Pharmacotherapie, 165*, 115006. https://doi.org/10.1016/j.biopha.2023.115006.

Li, J., Mao, Y., Chen, S., Ye, R., Fei, Y., Li, Y., Tong, S., Yang, H., & He, Y. (2024). The interplay between metal ions and immune cells in glioma: Pathways to immune escape. *Discover Oncology, 15*(1), 348. https://doi.org/10.1007/s12672-024-01229-0.

Li, M., Yang, Y., Wei, J., Cun, X., Lu, Z., Qiu, Y., Zhang, Z., & He, Q. (2018). Enhanced chemo-immunotherapy against melanoma by inhibition of cholesterol esterification in CD8+ T cells. *Nanomedicine: Nanotechnology, Biology and Medicine, 14*(8), 2541–2550. https://doi.org/10.1016/j.nano.2018.08.008.

Li, X., Wenes, M., Romero, P., Huang, S. C.-C., Fendt, S.-M., & Ho, P.-C. (2019). Navigating metabolic pathways to enhance antitumour immunity and immunotherapy. *Nature Reviews Clinical Oncology, 16*(7), 425–441. https://doi.org/10.1038/s41571-019-0203-7.

Lian, X., Yang, K., Li, R., Li, M., Zuo, J., Zheng, B., Wang, W., Wang, P., & Zhou, S. (2022). Immunometabolic rewiring in tumorigenesis and anti-tumor immunotherapy. *Molecular Cancer, 21*(1). https://doi.org/10.1186/s12943-021-01486-5.

Lieu, E. L., Nguyen, T., Rhyne, S., & Kim, J. (2020). Amino acids in cancer. *Experimental and Molecular Medicine, 52*(1), 15–30. https://doi.org/10.1038/s12276-020-0375-3, https://www.nature.com/emm/.

Lin, H., Jiang, C., Wang, B., Wang, Y., Shangguan, Z., Wu, Y., Wang, X., Huang, Y., Wang, L., Chen, P., Li, X., Zhong, Z., & Wu, S. (2024). Glutathione degradable manganese-doped polydopamine nanoparticles for photothermal therapy and cGAS-STING activated immunotherapy of lung tumor. *Journal of Colloid and Interface Science, 663*, 167–176. https://doi.org/10.1016/j.jcis.2024.02.100.

Lin, Y., Chen, X., Yu, C., Xu, G., Nie, X., Cheng, Y., Luan, Y., & Song, Q. (2023). Radiotherapy-mediated redox homeostasis-controllable nanomedicine for enhanced ferroptosis sensitivity in tumor therapy. *Acta Biomaterialia, 159*, 300–311. https://doi.org/10.1016/j.actbio.2023.01.022.

Liu, J., Ma, Z., Jia, W., & Lan, P. (2024). Targeting macrophage metabolism to enhance tumor immunotherapy. *Cellular & Molecular Immunology, 21*(5), 530–532. https://doi.org/10.1038/s41423-024-01149-7.

Liu, P.-S., Wang, H., Li, X., Chao, T., Teav, T., Christen, S., Di Conza, G., Cheng, W.-C., Chou, C.-H., Vavakova, M., Muret, C., Debackere, K., Mazzone, M., Huang, H.-D., Fendt, S.-M., Ivanisevic, J., & Ho, P.-C. (2017). α-ketoglutarate orchestrates macrophage activation through metabolic and epigenetic reprogramming. *Nature Immunology, 18*(9), 985–994. https://doi.org/10.1038/ni.3796.

Liu, S., Shao, S., Huang, Z., Xue, P., Yan, S., Cao, M., & Zeng, X. (2026). A multifunctional manganese-based nanozyme platform for synergistic hypoxia alleviation and cholesterol depletion to potentiate STING-mediated cancer immunotherapy. *Biomaterials, 327*, 123760. https://doi.org/10.1016/j.biomaterials.2025.123760.

Liu, Y., Niu, R., Deng, R., Song, S., Wang, Y., & Zhang, H. (2023). Multi-enzyme Co-expressed dual-atom nanozymes induce cascade immunogenic ferroptosis via activating interferon-γ and targeting arachidonic acid metabolism. *Journal of the American Chemical Society, 145*(16), 8965–8978. https://doi.org/10.1021/jacs.2c13689.

Lu, Y., Sun, Q., Guan, Q., Zhang, Z., He, Q., He, J., Ji, Z., Tian, W., Xu, X., Liu, Y., Yin, Y., Zheng, C., Lian, S., Xu, B., Wang, P., Jiang, R., & Sun, B. (2023). The XOR-IDH3α axis controls macrophage polarization in hepatocellular carcinoma. *Journal of Hepatology, 79*(5), 1172–1184. https://doi.org/10.1016/j.jhep.2023.06.022, http://www.sciencedirect.com/science/journal/01688278.

Lv, H., Han, X., Yang, Y., Shen, J., Yin, Y., & Liu, Y. (2025). Glutamine: A new strategy for targeted metabolic therapy in the tumor microenvironment. *Cell Death Discovery, 11*(1). https://doi.org/10.1038/s41420-025-02767-4, https://www.nature.com/cddiscovery/.

Ma, J., Guo, D., Ji, X., Zhou, Y., Liu, C., Li, Q., Zhang, J., Fan, C., & Song, H. (2023). Composite hydrogel for spatiotemporal lipid intervention of tumor milieu. *Advanced Materials, 35*(14). https://doi.org/10.1002/adma.202211579, http://onlinelibrary.wiley.com/journal/10.1002/(ISSN)1521-4095.

Ma, M., Zhang, Y., Pu, K., & Tang, W. (2025). Nanomaterial-enabled metabolic reprogramming strategies for boosting antitumor immunity. *Chemical Society Reviews, 54*(2), 653–714. https://doi.org/10.1039/D4CS00679H.

Ma, Y., Hu, Y., Liu, H., Li, X., Li, Y., Zhao, Y., Zhang, Q., Zhang, Z., Leng, Q., Luo, L., Li, L., Dai, Y., Chen, G., Zhang, J., & Li, Z. (2024). High-lactate-metabolizing photosynthetic bacteria reprogram tumor immune microenvironment. *Advanced Materials, 36*(36). https://doi.org/10.1002/adma.202405930.

Madsen, H. B., Peeters, M. J., Straten, Pt, & Desler, C. (2023). Nucleotide metabolism in the regulation of tumor microenvironment and immune cell function. *Current Opinion in Biotechnology, 84*. https://doi.org/10.1016/j.copbio.2023.103008, http://www.elsevier.com/locate/copbio.

Malanchi, I., Santamaria-Martínez, A., Susanto, E., Peng, H., Lehr, H. A., Delaloye, J. F., & Huelsken, J. (2012). Interactions between cancer stem cells and their niche govern metastatic colonization. *Nature, 481*(7379), 85–91. https://doi.org/10.1038/nature10694.

Martin, J. D., Cabral, H., Stylianopoulos, T., & Jain, R. K. (2020). Improving cancer immunotherapy using nanomedicines: Progress, opportunities and challenges. *Nature Reviews Clinical Oncology, 17*(4), 251–266. https://doi.org/10.1038/s41571-019-0308-z, http://www.nature.com/nrclinonc/archive/index.html.

Mehta, A., Ratre, Y. K., Soni, V. K., Shukla, D., Sonkar, S. C., Kumar, A., & Vishvakarma, N. K. (2023). Orchestral role of lipid metabolic reprogramming in T-cell malignancy. *Frontiers in Oncology, 13*. https://doi.org/10.3389/fonc.2023.1122789, http://www.frontiersin.org/Oncology/about.

Meng, D., Pan, H., He, W., Jiang, X., Liang, Z., Zhang, X., Xu, X., Wang, Z., Zheng, J., Gong, P., Li, W., & Cai, L. (2022). In situ activated NK cell as bio-orthogonal targeted live-cell nanocarrier augmented solid tumor immunotherapy. *Advanced Functional Materials, 32*(29). https://doi.org/10.1002/adfm.202202603.

Miao, L., Lu, C., Zhang, B., Li, H., Zhao, X., Chen, H., Liu, Y., & Cui, X. (2024). Advances in metabolic reprogramming of NK cells in the tumor microenvironment on the impact of NK therapy. *Journal of Translational Medicine, 22*(1). https://doi.org/10.1186/s12967-024-05033-w.

Milella, M., Rutigliano, M., Pandolfo, S. D., Aveta, A., Crocetto, F., Ferro, M., d'Amati, A., Ditonno, P., Lucarelli, G., & Lasorsa, F. (2025). The metabolic landscape of cancer stem cells: Insights and implications for therapy. *Cells, 14*(10), 717. https://doi.org/10.3390/cells14100717.

Mu, Y., Zhang, Z., Zhou, H., Ma, L., & Wang, D. A. (2024). Applications of nanotechnology in remodeling the tumour microenvironment for glioblastoma treatment. *Biomaterials Science, 12*(16), 4045–4064. https://doi.org/10.1039/d4bm00665h, http://pubs.rsc.org/en/journals/journal/bm.

Mullen, P. J., Yu, R., Longo, J., Archer, M. C., & Penn, L. Z. (2016). The interplay between cell signalling and the mevalonate pathway in cancer. *Nature Reviews. Cancer, 16*(11), 718–731. https://doi.org/10.1038/nrc.2016.76, http://www.nature.com/cancer/.

Myers, J. A., & Miller, J. S. (2021). Exploring the NK cell platform for cancer immunotherapy. *Nature Reviews Clinical Oncology, 18*(2), 85–100. https://doi.org/10.1038/s41571-020-0426-7.

Nel, A. E., Mei, K. C., Liao, Y. P., & Liu, X. (2022). Multifunctional lipid bilayer nanocarriers for cancer immunotherapy in heterogeneous tumor microenvironments, combining immunogenic cell death stimuli with immune modulatory drugs. *ACS Nano, 16*(4), 5184–5232. https://doi.org/10.1021/acsnano.2c01252, http://pubs.acs.org/journal/ancac3.

Nguyen, T. T., Shin, D. H., Jiang, H., Wainwright, D. A., Sohoni, S., Gupta, S., Ossimetha, A., Lang, F., Alonso, M., Gomez-Manzano, C., & Fueyo, J. (2021). Abstract 1785: Inhibition of the IDO-Kyn-AhR cascade optimizes virotherapy in glioblastoma and depends on CD4 T-cell activation. *Cancer Research, 81*(13_Supplement), 1785. https://doi.org/10.1158/1538-7445.am2021-1785 1785.

Ngwa, V. M., Edwards, D. N., Philip, M., & Chen, J. (2019). Microenvironmental metabolism regulates antitumor immunity. *Cancer Research, 79*(16), 4003–4008. https://doi.org/10.1158/0008-5472.CAN-19-0617, https://cancerres.aacrjournals.org/content/79/16/4003.full-text.pdf.

O'neill, L.a J., & Pearce, E. J. (2015). Immunometabolism governs dendritic cell and macrophage function. *The Journal of Experimental Medicine, 213*(1), 15–23. https://doi.org/10.1084/jem.20151570.

Oweira, H., Lahdou, I., Mehrle, S., Khajeh, E., Nikbakhsh, R., Ghamarnejad, O., Terness, P., Reißfelder, C., Sadeghi, M., & Ramouz, A. (2022). Kynurenine is the main metabolite of tryptophan degradation by tryptophan 2,3-dioxygenase in HepaRG Tumor Cells. *Journal of Clinical Medicine, 11*(16), 4794. https://doi.org/10.3390/jcm11164794.

Pacold, M. E., Brimacombe, K. R., Chan, S. H., Rohde, J. M., Lewis, C. A., Swier, L. J. Y. M., Possemato, R., Chen, W. W., Sullivan, L. B., Fiske, B. P., Cho, S., Freinkman, E., Birsoy, K., Abu-Remaileh, M., Shaul, Y. D., Liu, C. M., Zhou, M., Koh, M. J., Chung, H., ... Sabatini, D. M. (2016). A PHGDH inhibitor reveals coordination of serine synthesis and one-carbon unit fate. *Nature Chemical Biology, 12*(6), 452–458. https://doi.org/10.1038/nchembio.2070, http://www.nature.com/nchembio.

Pan, Y., Zhou, S., Liu, C., Ma, X., Xing, J., Parshad, B., Li, W., Wu, A., & Haag, R. (2022). Dendritic polyglycerol-conjugated gold nanostars for metabolism inhibition and targeted photothermal therapy in breast cancer stem cells. *Advanced Healthcare Materials, 11*(8). https://doi.org/10.1002/adhm.202102272.

Patterson, C., Hazime, K. S., Zelenay, S., & Davis, D. M. (2024). Prostaglandin E_2 impacts multiple stages of the natural killer cell antitumor immune response. *European Journal of Immunology, 54*(2). https://doi.org/10.1002/eji.202350635, http://onlinelibrary.wiley.com/journal/10.1002/(ISSN)1521-4141.

Peng, N., Wang, Y., Jia, P., Li, J., Song, C., Lin, J. M., & Wang, Y. (2025). Intracellular glutathione cleaved long-targeting chains of cancer cells and macrophages to exposedly activate mitochondria delivery of liposomes for enhancing antitumor efficacy by metabolic reprogramming. *ACS Applied Materials & Interfaces, 17*(35), 49798–49815. https://doi.org/10.1021/acsami.5c09138.

Peng, X., He, Y., Huang, J., Tao, Y., & Liu, S. (2021). Metabolism of dendritic cells in tumor microenvironment: For immunotherapy. *Frontiers in Immunology, 12*. https://doi.org/10.3389/fimmu.2021.613492.

Pérez-Herrero, E., & Fernández-Medarde, A. (2021). The reversed intra- and extracellular pH in tumors as a unified strategy to chemotherapeutic delivery using targeted nanocarriers. *Acta Pharmaceutica Sinica B, 11*(8), 2243–2264. https://doi.org/10.1016/j.apsb.2021.01.012.

Qi, F., Guo, Y., Xu, Y., Liu, Y., Hu, P., & Shi, J. (2025). Calcium ion nanomodulators induce pyroptosis for tumor immunotherapy. *Nanoscale, 17*(44), 25516–25525. https://doi.org/10.1039/d5nr01897h.

Qi, H., Wang, Y., Yuan, X., Li, P., & Yang, L. (2020). Selective extracellular arginine deprivation by a single injection of cellular non-uptake arginine deiminase nanocapsules for sustained tumor inhibition. *Nanoscale, 12*(47), 24030–24043. https://doi.org/10.1039/d0nr06823c.

Qiao, G., Li, S., Pan, X., Xie, P., Peng, R., Huang, X., He, M., Jiang, J., & Chu, X. (2024). Surgical tumor–derived nanoplatform targets tumor-associated macrophage for personalized postsurgical cancer immunotherapy. *Science Advances, 10*(13). https://doi.org/10.1126/sciadv.adk7955.

Qin, Y.-T., Liu, X.-H., An, J.-X., Liang, J.-L., Li, C.-X., Jin, X.-K., Ji, P., & Zhang, X.-Z. (2023). Dendritic cell-based in situ nanovaccine for reprogramming lipid metabolism to boost tumor immunotherapy. *ACS Nano, 17*(24), 24947–24960. https://doi.org/10.1021/acsnano.3c06784.

Qiu, X., Jiang, S., Xiao, Y., He, Y., Ren, T., Jiang, L., Liu, R., & Chen, Q. (2021). SOX2-dependent expression of dihydroorotate dehydrogenase regulates oral squamous cell carcinoma cell proliferation. *International Journal of Oral Science, 13*(1). https://doi.org/10.1038/s41368-020-00109-x.

Raghavan, S., Mehta, P., Xie, Y., Lei, Y. L., & Mehta, G. (2019). Ovarian cancer stem cells and macrophages reciprocally interact through the WNT pathway to promote pro-tumoral and malignant phenotypes in 3D engineered microenvironments. *Journal for ImmunoTherapy of Cancer, 7*(1). https://doi.org/10.1186/s40425-019-0666-1, http://www.immunotherapyofcancer.org/.

Ravi Kiran, A. V. V. V., Kusuma Kumari, G., Krishnamurthy, P. T., & Khaydarov, R. R. (2021). Tumor microenvironment and nanotherapeutics: Intruding the tumor fort. *Biomaterials Science, 9*(23), 7667–7704. https://doi.org/10.1039/d1bm01127h, http://pubs.rsc.org/en/journals/journal/bm.

Raza, A., Rossi, G. R., Janjua, T. I., Souza-Fonseca-Guimaraes, F., & Popat, A. (2023). Nanobiomaterials to modulate natural killer cell responses for effective cancer immunotherapy. *Trends in Biotechnology, 41*(1), 77–92. https://doi.org/10.1016/j.tibtech.2022.06.011, www.elsevier.com/locate/tibtech.

Ringel, A. E., Drijvers, J. M., Baker, G. J., Catozzi, A., García-Cañaveras, J. C., Gassaway, B. M., Miller, B. C., Juneja, V. R., Nguyen, T. H., Joshi, S., Yao, C. H., Yoon, H., Sage, P. T., LaFleur, M. W., Trombley, J. D., Jacobson, C. A., Maliga, Z., Gygi, S. P., Sorger, P. K., ... Haigis, M. C. (2020). Obesity shapes metabolism in the tumor microenvironment to suppress anti-tumor immunity. *Cell, 183*(7), 1848. https://doi.org/10.1016/j.cell.2020.11.009, https://www.sciencedirect.com/journal/cell.

Sabatino, M. E., Grondona, E., Sosa, Ld. V., Mongi Bragato, B., Carreño, L., Juarez, V., da Silva, R. A., Remor, A., de Bortoli, L., de Paula Martins, R., Pérez, P. A., Petiti, J. P., Gutiérrez, S., Torres, A. I., Latini, A., & De Paul, A. L. (2018). Oxidative stress and mitochondrial adaptive shift during pituitary tumoral growth. *Free Radical Biology and Medicine, 120*, 41–55. https://doi.org/10.1016/j.freeradbiomed.2018.03.019, www.elsevier.com/locate/freeradbiomed.

Saha, S., Ghosh, M., Li, J., Wen, A., Galluzzi, L., Martinez, L. A., & Montrose, D. C. (2024). Serine depletion promotes antitumor immunity by activating mitochondrial DNA-mediated cGAS-STING signaling. *Cancer Research, 84*(16), 2645–2659. https://doi.org/10.1158/0008-5472.CAN-23-1788, https://aacrjournals.org/cancerres/article/84/16/2645/746874/Serine-Depletion-Promotes-Antitumor-Immunity-by.

Schild, T., Wallisch, P., Zhao, Y., Wang, Y. T., Haughton, L., Chirayil, R., Pierpont, K., Chen, K., Nunes-Violante, S., Cross, J., de Stanchina, E., Thompson, C. B., Scheinberg, D. A., Perry, J. S. A., & Keshari, K. R. (2025). Metabolic engineering to facilitate anti-tumor immunity. *Cancer Cell, 43*(3), 552. https://doi.org/10.1016/j.ccell.2025.02.004, https://www.sciencedirect.com/science/journal/15356108.

Sheng, Y., Qiao, C., Zhang, Z., Shi, X., Yang, L., Xi, R., Yu, J., Liu, W., Zhang, G., & Wang, F. (2025). Calcium channel blocker lacidipine promotes antitumor immunity by reprogramming tryptophan metabolism. *Advanced Science, 12*(3). https://doi.org/10.1002/advs.202409310.

Shi, D. D., Savani, M. R., Abdullah, K. G., & McBrayer, S. K. (2023). Emerging roles of nucleotide metabolism in cancer. *Trends in Cancer, 9*(8), 624–635. https://doi.org/10.1016/j.trecan.2023.04.008, http://www.cell.com/trends/cancer/home.

Shi, Q., Shen, Q., Liu, Y., Shi, Y., Huang, W., Wang, X., Li, Z., Chai, Y., Wang, H., Hu, X., Li, N., Zhang, Q., & Cao, X. (2022). Increased glucose metabolism in TAMs fuels O-GlcNAcylation of lysosomal Cathepsin B to promote cancer metastasis and chemoresistance. *Cancer Cell, 40*(10), 1207. https://doi.org/10.1016/j.ccell.2022.08.012.

Shin, E., & Koo, J. S. (2021). Glucose metabolism and glucose transporters in breast cancer. *Frontiers in Cell and Developmental Biology, 9*, 728759. https://doi.org/10.3389/fcell.2021.728759.

Shunxi, W., Xiaoxue, Y., Guanbin, S., Li, Y., Junyu, J., & Wanqian, L. (2023). Serine metabolic reprogramming in tumorigenesis, tumor immunity, and clinical treatment. *Advances in Nutrition, 14*(5), 1050–1066. https://doi.org/10.1016/j.advnut.2023.05.007.

Song, K., Ming, J., Tao, B., Zhao, F., Huang, S., Wu, W., Jiang, C., & Li, X. (2025). Emerging glucose oxidase-delivering nanomedicines for enhanced tumor therapy. *Journal of Controlled Release, 381*, 113580. https://doi.org/10.1016/j.jconrel.2025.02.076.

Su, B., Chen, Q., Li, X., Fang, M., Wang, Y., Song, H., You, H., Zhou, Z., Wu, Y., Zhao, Z., Chen, Y., Fan, H., Li, C., Jiang, C., & Sun, T. (2025). A methionine allocation nanoregulator for the suppression of cancer stem cells and support to the immune cells by epigenetic regulation. *Advanced Science, 12*(15). https://doi.org/10.1002/advs.202415207.

Su, P., Wang, Q., Bi, E., Ma, X., Liu, L., Yang, M., Qian, J., & Yi, Q. (2020). Enhanced lipid accumulation and metabolism are required for the differentiation and activation of tumor-associated macrophages. *Cancer Research, 80*(7), 1438–1450. https://doi.org/10.1158/0008-5472.can-19-2994.

Sun, L., Gao, W., Liu, J., Wang, J., Li, L., Yu, H., & Xu, Z. P. (2022). O2-supplying nanozymes alleviate hypoxia and deplete lactate to eliminate tumors and activate antitumor immunity. *ACS Applied Materials and Interfaces, 14*(51), 56644–56657. https://doi.org/10.1021/acsami.2c18960, http://pubs.acs.org/journal/aamick.

Sun, M., Yang, M., Li, S., Wang, C., Zhang, F., Xu, B., Zhang, Y., Sun, X., Yuan, Q., & Liu, H. (2023). Photothermal lysis of engineered bacteria to modulate amino acid metabolism against tumors. *Advanced Functional Materials, 33*(13). https://doi.org/10.1002/adfm.202212226.

Tadros, S., Shukla, S. K., King, R. J., Gunda, V., Vernucci, E., Abrego, J., Chaika, N. V., Yu, F., Lazenby, A. J., Berim, L., Grem, J., Sasson, A. R., & Singh, P. K. (2017). De Novo lipid synthesis facilitates gemcitabine resistance through endoplasmic reticulum stress in pancreatic cancer. *Cancer Research, 77*(20), 5503–5517. https://doi.org/10.1158/0008-5472.CAN-16-3062, http://cancerres.aacrjournals.org/content/77/20/5503.full-text.pdf.

Tang, M., Ren, X., Fu, C., Ding, M., & Meng, X. (2021). Regulating glucose metabolism using nanomedicines for cancer therapy. *Journal of Materials Chemistry B, 9*(29), 5749–5764. https://doi.org/10.1039/d1tb00218j.

Thomas, T. M., & Yu, J. S. (2017). Metabolic regulation of glioma stem-like cells in the tumor micro-environment. *Cancer Letters, 408*, 174–181. https://doi.org/10.1016/j.canlet.2017.07.014.

Tu, B., Gao, Y., Sun, F., Shi, M., & Huang, Y. (2022). Lipid metabolism regulation based on nanotechnology for enhancement of tumor immunity. *Frontiers in Pharmacology, 13*. https://doi.org/10.3389/fphar.2022.840440.

Valcarcel-Jimenez, L., Gaude, E., Torrano, V., Frezza, C., & Carracedo, A. (2017). Mitochondrial metabolism: Yin and Yang for tumor progression. *Trends in Endocrinology & Metabolism, 28*(10), 748–757. https://doi.org/10.1016/j.tem.2017.06.004.

Vander Heiden, M. G. (2011). Targeting cancer metabolism: A therapeutic window opens. *Nature Reviews. Drug Discovery, 10*(9), 671–684. https://doi.org/10.1038/nrd3504.

Viel, S., Vivier, E., Walzer, T., & Marçais, A. (2025). Targeting metabolic dysfunction of CD8 T cells and natural killer cells in cancer. *Nature Reviews. Drug Discovery, 24*(3), 190–208. https://doi.org/10.1038/s41573-024-01098-w.

Vitale, I., Manic, G., Coussens, L. M., Kroemer, G., & Galluzzi, L. (2019). Macrophages and metabolism in the tumor microenvironment. *Cell Metabolism, 30*(1), 36–50. https://doi.org/10.1016/j.cmet.2019.06.001, http://www.cellmetabolism.org/.

Wan, M., Ding, Y., Li, Z., Wang, X., & Xu, M. (2022). Metabolic manipulation of the tumour immune microenvironment. *Immunology, 165*(3), 290–300. https://doi.org/10.1111/imm.13444.

Wang, N., Lu, S., Cao, Z., Li, H., Xu, J., Zhou, Q., Yin, H., Qian, Q., Zhang, X., Tao, M., Jiang, Q., Zhou, P., Zheng, L., Han, L., Li, H., Yin, L., Gu, Y., Dou, X., Sun, H., ... Liu, J. (2025). Pyruvate metabolism enzyme DLAT promotes tumorigenesis by suppressing leucine catabolism. *Cell Metabolism, 37*(6), 1381–1399. https://doi.org/10.1016/j.cmet.2025.02.008.

Wang, R., Dillon, C. P., Shi, L. Z., Milasta, S., Carter, R., Finkelstein, D., McCormick, L. L., Fitzgerald, P., Chi, H., Munger, J., & Green, D. R. (2011). The transcription factor myc controls metabolic reprogramming upon T lymphocyte activation. *Immunity, 35*(6), 871–882. https://doi.org/10.1016/j.immuni.2011.09.021.

Wang, W., Guo, Y., Yang, Z., Su, G., & Sun, Z. (2023). Sniping cancer stem cells with nanomaterials. *ACS Nano, 17*(23), 23262–23298. https://doi.org/10.1021/acsnano.3c07828.

Wang, Z., Wang, Q., Cao, H., Wang, Z., Wang, D., Liu, J., Gao, T., Ren, C., & Liu, J. (2024). Mitochondrial localized in situ self-assembly reprogramming tumor immune and metabolic microenvironment for enhanced cancer therapy. *Adv. Mater. 36*(15), 2311043. https://doi.org/10.1002/adma.202311043.

Watson, M. L. J., Vignali, P. D. A., Mullett, S. J., Overacre-Delgoffe, A. E., Peralta, R. M., Grebinoski, S., Menk, A. V., Rittenhouse, N. L., DePeaux, K., Whetstone, R. D., Vignali, D. A. A., Hand, T. W., Poholek, A. C., Morrison, B. M., Rothstein, J. D., Wendell, S. G., & Delgoffe, G. M. (2021). Metabolic support of tumour-infiltrating regulatory T cells by lactic acid. *Nature, 591*(7851), 645–651. https://doi.org/10.1038/s41586-020-03045-2, http://www.nature.com/nature/index.html.

Wilfahrt, D., & Delgoffe, G. M. (2024). Metabolic waypoints during T cell differentiation. *Nature Immunology, 25*(2), 206–217. https://doi.org/10.1038/s41590-023-01733-5.

Wu, C., Xu, T., Zhang, H., Hu, Y., Jiao, J., Qiu, K., Gu, J., Li, W., & Sun, L. (2025). Hypoxia and immunometabolism in the tumor microenvironment: insights into mechanisms and therapeutic potential. *Cancer Letters, 631*, 217913. https://doi.org/10.1016/j.canlet.2025.217913.

Wu, J., Bai, X., Yan, L., Baimanov, D., Cong, Y., Quan, P., Cai, R., Guan, Y., Bu, W., Lin, B., Wang, J., Yu, S., Li, S., Chong, Y., Li, Y., Hu, G., Zhao, Y., Chen, C., & Wang, L. (2024). Selective regulation of macrophage lipid metabolism via nanomaterials' surface chemistry. *Nature Communications, 15*(1), 8349. https://doi.org/10.1038/s41467-024-52609-7.

Wu, S., Xu, L., He, C., Wang, P., Qin, J., Guo, F., & Wang, Y. (2023). Lactate efflux inhibition by syrosingopine/LOD co-loaded nanozyme for synergetic self-replenishing catalytic cancer therapy and immune microenvironment remodeling. *Advanced Science, 10*(26). https://doi.org/10.1002/advs.202300686.

Xia, C., Li, M., Ran, G., Wang, X., Lu, Z., Li, T., Tang, X., Zhang, Z., & He, Q. (2021). Redox-responsive nanoassembly restrained myeloid-derived suppressor cells recruitment through autophagy-involved lactate dehydrogenase A silencing for enhanced cancer immunochemotherapy. *Journal of Controlled Release, 335*, 557–574. https://doi.org/10.1016/j.jconrel.2021.05.034.

Xie, T.-Q., Yan, X., Qin, Y.-T., Zhang, C., Jin, X.-K., Li, Q.-R., Rao, Z.-Y., Zhou, H., Chen, W.-H., & Zhang, X.-Z. (2024). Lactate/cysteine dual-consuming probiotic–nanomedicine biohybrid system for enhanced cancer chemo-immunotherapy. *Nano Letters, 24*(50), 16132–16142. https://doi.org/10.1021/acs.nanolett.4c04938.

Xie, W., Deng, W.-W., Zan, M., Rao, L., Yu, G.-T., Zhu, D.-M., Wu, W.-T., Chen, B., Ji, L.-W., Chen, L., Liu, K., Guo S.-S., Huang, H.-M., Zhang, W.-F., Zhao, X., Yuan, Y., Dong, W., Sun, Z.-J., & Liu, W. (2019). Cancer cell membrane camouflaged nanoparticles to realize starvation therapy together with checkpoint blockades for enhancing cancer therapy. *ACS Nano, 13*(3), 2849–2857. https://doi.org/10.1021/acsnano.8b03788.

Xia, Y., Xie, Y., Yu, Z., Xiao, H., Jiang, G., Zhou, X., Yang, Y., Li, X., Zhao, M., Li, L., Zheng, M., Han, S., Zong, Z., Meng, X., Deng, H., Ye, H., Fa, Y., Wu, H., Oldfield, E., ... Zhang, Y. (2018). The mevalonate pathway is a druggable target for vaccine adjuvant discovery. *Cell, 175*(4), 1059. https://doi.org/10.1016/j.cell.2018.08.070.

Xiong, B., Yu, J., Wen, C., Li, S., Zhang, S., Fang, Y., Cao, Y., Guan, X., Shen, Y., Zhu, M., Li, X., Zhu, Y., Guo, L., Xu, H., & Yin, H. (2025). Antisense oligonucleotide-loaded nanozyme reverses tumor immune suppression through sonogenetic metabolic therapy. *Journal of Controlled Release, 387*, 114236. https://doi.org/10.1016/j.jconrel.2025.114236.

Xu, C., Ji, X., Zhou, Y., Cheng, Y., Guo, D., Li, Q., Chen, N., Fan, C., & Song, H. (2023). Slimming and reinvigorating tumor-associated dendritic cells with hierarchical lipid rewiring nanoparticles. *Advanced Materials, 35*(30). https://doi.org/10.1002/adma.202211415.

Xu, L., Peng, M., Gao, T., Wang, D., Lian, X., Sun, H., Shi, J., Wang, Y., & Wang, P. (2024). Nanoenabled intracellular metal ion homeostasis regulation for tumor therapy. *Advancement of Science, 11*(7), 2306203. https://doi.org/10.1002/advs.202306203.

Xu, Y., Li, S., Wu, J., Xu, S., Shen, M., Wang, C., Lundqvist, A., Yu, J., Xu, Z., Shi, Y., Liu, N., Yang, Y., Zhao, J., Yang, Y., Wang, P., Yi, P., Cheng, J., Sun, J., Li, M., ... Wang, K. (2025). Targeting cystine metabolism in the lung cancer environment enhances the efficacy of immune checkpoint inhibition. *Advancement of Science, 12*(35), e13084. https://doi.org/10.1002/advs.202413084.

Yan, J., Li, W., Tian, H., Li, B., Yu, X., Wang, G., Sang, W., & Dai, Y. (2023). Metal-phenolic nanomedicines regulate t-cell antitumor function for sono-metabolic cancer therapy. *ACS Nano, 17*(15), 14667–14677. https://doi.org/10.1021/acsnano.3c02428.

Yan, Y., Huang, L., Liu, Y., Yi, M., Chu, Q., Jiao, D., & Wu, K. (2022). Metabolic profiles of regulatory T cells and their adaptations to the tumor microenvironment: Implications for antitumor immunity. *Journal of Hematology & Oncology, 15*(1). https://doi.org/10.1186/s13045-022-01322-3.

Yang, J., & Zhang, C. (2020). Regulation of cancer-immunity cycle and tumor microenvironment by nanobiomaterials to enhance tumor immunotherapy. *WIREs Nanomed. Nanobi. 12*(4), e1612. https://doi.org/10.1002/wnan.1612.

Yang, L., Xue, R., Yang, C., Lv, Y., Li, S., Xiang, W., Guo, X., & Zhou, J. (2025). Endoplasmic reticulum stress on glioblastoma: Tumor growth promotion and immunosuppression. *International Immunopharmacology, 157*, 114806. https://doi.org/10.1016/j.intimp.2025.114806.

Yao, X., Yang, H., Guo, S., Liu, Y., Zhang, Q., Zhou, Z., Li, M., & Luo, Z. (2025). Radiation-triggerable bioreactors enable bioenergetic reprograming of cancer stem cell plasticity via targeted arginine metabolism disruption for augmented radio-immunotherapy. *Biomaterials, 322*, 123391. https://doi.org/10.1016/j.biomaterials.2025.123391.

Yin, X., Zeng, W., Wu, B., Wang, L., Wang, Z., Tian, H., Wang, L., Jiang, Y., Clay, R., Wei, X., Qin, Y., Zhang, F., Zhang, C., Jin, L., & Liang, Wei (2020). PPARα inhibition overcomes tumor-derived exosomal lipid-induced dendritic cell dysfunction. *Cell Reports, 33*(3), 108278. https://doi.org/10.1016/j.celrep.2020.108278.

Yin, Z., Bai, L., Li, W., Zeng, T., Tian, H., & Cui, J. (2019). Targeting T cell metabolism in the tumor microenvironment: An anti-cancer therapeutic strategy. *Journal of Experimental & Clinical Cancer Research: CR, 38*(1), 403. https://doi.org/10.1186/s13046-019-1409-3.

Yoo, H. C., Park, S. J., Nam, M., Kang, J., Kim, K., Yeo, J. H., Kim, J. K., Heo, Y., Lee, H. S., Lee, M. Y., Lee, C. W., Kang, J. S., Kim, Y. H., Lee, J., Choi, J., Hwang, G. S., Bang, S., & Han, J. M. (2020). A Variant of SLC1A5 Is a mitochondrial glutamine transporter for metabolic reprogramming in cancer cells. *Cell Metabolism, 31*(2), 267. https://doi.org/10.1016/j.cmet.2019.11.020, http://www.cellmetabolism.org/.

Yu, M., Guo, G., Huang, L., Deng, L., Chang, C. S., Achyut, B. R., Canning, M., Xu, N., Arbab, A. S., Bollag, R. J., Rodriguez, P. C., Mellor, A. L., Shi, H., Munn, D. H., & Cui, Y. (2020). CD73 on cancer-associated fibroblasts enhanced by the A2B-mediated feedforward circuit enforces an immune checkpoint. *Nature Communications, 11*(1). https://doi.org/10.1038/s41467-019-14060-x, http://www.nature.com/ncomms/index.html.

Yu, W., Lei, Q., Yang, L., Qin, G., Liu, S., Wang, D., Ping, Y., & Zhang, Y. (2021). Contradictory roles of lipid metabolism in immune response within the tumor microenvironment. *Journal of Hematology & Oncology, 14*(1). https://doi.org/10.1186/s13045-021-01200-4.

Zdioruk, M., Jimenez-Macias, J. L., Nowicki, M. O., Manz, K. E., Pennell, K. D., Koch, M. S., Finkelberg, T., Wu, B., Boucher, P., Takeda, Y., Li, W., Piranlioglu, R., Ling, A. L., Chiocca, E. A., & Lawler, S. E. (2023). PPRX-1701, a nanoparticle formulation of 6′-bromoindirubin acetoxime, improves delivery and shows efficacy in preclinical GBM models. *Cell Reports Medicine, 4*(5). https://doi.org/10.1016/j.xcrm.2023.101019, www.cell.com/cell-reports-medicine.

Zhang, B., Fan, R., Hai, Y., Chen, Y., Lu, X., Wang, W., Dou, J., Yan, J., Su, C., Chen, Y., Yang, L., Zhao, M., Liang, L., & Wei, G. (2025). Immunometabolic rewiring of dendritic cells to overcome glutamine-driven immune suppression in colorectal cancer. *Advancement of Science*e13986. https://doi.org/10.1002/advs.202513986.

Zhang, M., Liu, Q., Zhang, M., Cao, C., Liu, X., Zhang, M., Li, G., Xu, C., & Zhang, X. (2020). Enhanced antitumor effects of follicle-stimulating hormone receptor-mediated hexokinase-2 depletion on ovarian cancer mediated by a shift in glucose metabolism. *Journal of Nanobiotechnology, 18*(1). https://doi.org/10.1186/s12951-020-00720-4.

Zhang, Q., Wang, X., Zhao, Y., Cheng, Z., Fang, D., Liu, Y., Tian, G., Li, M., & Luo, Z. (2023). Nanointegrative in situ reprogramming of tumor-intrinsic lipid droplet biogenesis for low-dose radiation-activated ferroptosis immunotherapy. *ACS Nano, 17*(24), 25419–25438. https://doi.org/10.1021/acsnano.3c08907.

Zhang, S., Zhang, Y., Feng, Y., Wu, J., Hu, Y., Lin, L., Xu, C., Chen, J., Tang, Z., Tian, H., & Chen, X. (2022). Biomineralized two-enzyme nanoparticles regulate tumor glycometabolism inducing tumor cell pyroptosis and robust antitumor immunotherapy. *Advanced Materials, 34*(50). https://doi.org/10.1002/adma.202206851, http://onlinelibrary.wiley.com/journal/10.1002/(ISSN)1521-4095.

Zhao, S., Hou, J., Deng, L., Qi, Z., Tao, N., Ruan, W., Zheng, J., Wang, W., Xu, Q., Saiding, Q., Kong, N., Liu, Y.-N., & Tao, W. (2025). Lactate-modulating nanozyme-mediated mitochondrial respiration block for tumor immunosuppression remodeling. *Angewandte Chemie International Edition, 64*(17). https://doi.org/10.1002/anie.202422203.

Zhao, S., Li, H., Liu, R., Tao, N., Deng, L., Xu, Q., Hou, J., Sheng, J., Zheng, J., Wang, L., Chen, W., Guo, S., & Liu, Y.-N. (2023). Nitrogen-centered lactate oxidase nanozyme for tumor lactate modulation and microenvironment remodeling. *Journal of the American Chemical Society, 145*(18), 10322–10332. https://doi.org/10.1021/jacs.3c02005.

Zheng, J., Meng, W., Cui, Z., Tian, J., & Zhang, W. (2024). A dual-enzyme-like photosensitive nanozyme for remodeling the tumor immunosuppressive microenvironment to enhance immunotherapy. *Biomaterials, 311*, 122660. https://doi.org/10.1016/j.biomaterials.2024.122660.

Zhou, X., Deng, R., Liao, Z., Huang, X., Huang, J., Yang, H., Leong, K. W., & Zhong, Y. (2025). Integrating metabolic modulation and nanomedicine for cancer immunotherapy. *Advanced Science, 12*(40). https://doi.org/10.1002/advs.202510004, http://onlinelibrary.wiley.com/journal/10.1002/(ISSN)2198-3844.

Zhou, X., Tian, C., Cao, Y., Zhao, M., & Wang, K. (2023). The role of serine metabolism in lung cancer: From oncogenesis to tumor treatment. *Frontiers in Genetics, 13*. https://doi.org/10.3389/fgene.2022.1084609.

Zhou, Z., Li, C., Li, C., Zhou, L., Tan, S., Hou, W., Xie, C., Wang, L., Shen, J., & Xiong, W. (2024). Mitochondria-targeted nanoadjuvants induced Multi-functional immune-microenvironment remodeling to sensitize tumor radio-immunotherapy. *Advancement of Science, 11*(26), 2400297. https://doi.org/10.1002/advs.202400297.

Zhu, Y., Li, W., Zhang, Y., Li, J., Liang, L., Zhang, X., Chen, N., Sun, Y., Chen, W., Tai, R., Fan, C., & Huang, Q. (2012). Excessive sodium ions delivered into cells by nanodiamonds: Implications for tumor therapy. *Small (Weinheim an der Bergstrasse, Germany), 8*(11), 1771–1779. https://doi.org/10.1002/smll.201102539.

Zhu, Z., Wang, H., Liu, M., Ji, Y., Song, A., Ren, J., & Qu, X. (2025). A sodium iron phosphate nanocatalyst-regulated high-mobility ion reservoir enables tumor-selective immunotherapy. *Journal of the American Chemical Society, 147*(42), 38958–38972. https://doi.org/10.1021/jacs.5c16505.

Zi, Y., Yang, K., He, J., Wu, Z., Liu, J., & Zhang, W. (2022). Strategies to enhance drug delivery to solid tumors by harnessing the EPR effects and alternative targeting mechanisms. *Advanced Drug Delivery Reviews, 188*, 114449. https://doi.org/10.1016/j.addr.2022.114449.

Zou, W., Han, Z., Wang, Z., & Liu, Q. (2025). Targeting glutamine metabolism as a potential target for cancer treatment. *Journal of Experimental & Clinical Cancer Research, 44*(1). https://doi.org/10.1186/s13046-025-03430-7.

Zou, Y., Jin, B., Li, H., Wu, X., Liu, Y., Zhao, H., Zhong, D., Wang, L., Chen, W., Wen, M., & Liu, Y.-N. (2022). Cold nanozyme for precise enzymatic antitumor immunity. *ACS Nano, 16*(12), 21491–21504. https://doi.org/10.1021/acsnano.2c10057.

SECTION IV

Biomarkers and personalized medicine

CHAPTER

7

Biomarker discovery and validation in inflammatory cancer research

Xiangfeng Guan

Department of Cardiology, The Affiliated Hospital of Southwest Medical University, Luzhou, Sichuan, P.R. China

7.1 Introduction

Cancer remains a leading cause of morbidity and mortality worldwide. While genetic mutations have traditionally been viewed as the primary drivers of tumorigenesis, growing evidence now supports the pivotal roles of chronic inflammation, metabolic dysregulation, and immune dysfunction in cancer initiation, progression, and therapeutic resistance (Bharadwaj et al., 2020; de Visser & Joyce, 2023; Hu et al., 2024). Central to this interplay is the tumor microenvironment (TME)—a dynamic, immunometabolically active compartment composed of malignant cells, immune infiltrates, fibroblasts, endothelial cells, and extracellular matrix (ECM). These components do not merely coexist but engage in bidirectional interactions that collectively shape tumor behavior.

At the core of this interaction lies the emerging field of immunometabolism, which explores how metabolic programming regulates immune cell fate and function. Unlike homeostatic tissues, the TME presents a metabolically hostile milieu—characterized by hypoxia, nutrient depletion (e.g., glucose, arginine, tryptophan), oxidative stress, acidosis, and the accumulation of immunosuppressive metabolites such as lactate, kynurenine, and adenosine (Hu et al., 2025; Jennings et al., 2021; Watson & Delgoffe, 2022). These conditions impair effector immune cells while favoring the expansion of immunosuppressive populations such as regulatory T cells (Tregs), myeloid-derived suppressor cells (MDSCs), and tumor-associated macrophages (TAMs) (Kaymak et al., 2021; Poznanski et al., 2021; Shi et al., 2020).

Importantly, immune cell subsets exhibit distinct metabolic preferences. Cytotoxic T lymphocytes (CTLs) and natural killer (NK) cells depend on aerobic glycolysis for rapid proliferation and cytokine production, whereas Tregs and MDSCs preferentially utilize fatty acid oxidation (FAO) and oxidative phosphorylation (OXPHOS), enabling their survival in nutrient-depleted environments (Geltink et al., 2018). This metabolic asymmetry contributes to immune evasion strategies exploited by tumors.

Inflammation in Tumorigenesis and Cancer Treatment
DOI: https://doi.org/10.1016/B978-0-443-36649-9.00002-5

Chronic inflammation—a hallmark of many cancers—further exacerbates immunometabolic dysfunction. Proinflammatory cytokines such as TNF-α, IL-6, and IL-1β, along with lipid-derived eicosanoids, activate nutrient-sensing pathways including mTOR (mechanistic target of rapamycin), HIF-1α (hypoxia-inducible factor 1α), and AMPK (AMP-activated protein kinase), altering immune cell metabolism and tumor–immune interactions (Traba et al., 2021; Yan et al., 2022). Tumor cells often hijack these inflammatory signals to reprogram metabolic networks in their favor. For example, the IDO1–kynurenine–aryl hydrocarbon receptor (AhR) axis not only depletes tryptophan but generates immunosuppressive ligands that suppress T cell activation. Similarly, arginase-mediated arginine depletion, adenosine accumulation via CD39/CD73, and glutaminolysis represent key metabolic checkpoints that impair immune surveillance (Azizi et al., 2018; Braun & Weichhart, 2021; Cui et al., 2023).

These mechanisms are particularly prominent in inflammation-associated malignancies such as hepatocellular carcinoma (HCC), colorectal cancer (CRC), pancreatic ductal adenocarcinoma (PDAC), and gastric cancer, which frequently arise in the context of chronic infection or tissue damage, including HBV/HCV infection, inflammatory bowel disease, chronic pancreatitis, and Helicobacter pylori–induced gastritis. In such settings, persistent inflammation reprograms immune cells—particularly macrophages and dendritic cells (DCs)—toward metabolically suppressed, tolerogenic phenotypes (Binnewies et al., 2018; G. Biswas & Mantovani, 2010; Wang et al., 2023). For instance, IL-6–driven STAT3 activation in CRC promotes tumor proliferation while skewing macrophages toward M2-like polarization, thereby facilitating angiogenesis and matrix remodeling (Erez et al., 2010). In HCC, chronic inflammation driven by HCV shapes Kupffer cell metabolism by enhancing oxidative stress responses and impairing glycolytic capacity, fostering immune evasion and tumor growth (Wen et al., 2025).

These insights have catalyzed the development of metabolic therapies targeting TME vulnerabilities. Approaches include inhibition of tumor glycolysis (e.g., GLUT1 antagonists), restoration of T cell mitochondrial function (e.g., PGC-1α activators), blockade of lactate signaling (e.g., MCT1/4 inhibitors), and combination regimens pairing immune checkpoint inhibitors (ICIs) with metabolic modulators such as IDO1 inhibitors or adenosine receptor antagonists (Kalluri, 2016; Llibre et al., 2025; Hao et al., 2024). Early clinical trials report encouraging results in selected patient populations, showing improved immune activation and tumor control.

In summary, immunometabolic dysregulation is a central feature of tumor progression, influencing immune cell differentiation, inflammatory tone, and treatment outcomes. Recognizing immune metabolism as a programmable and therapeutically actionable axis presents an opportunity to enhance antitumor immunity, particularly in cancers characterized by chronic inflammation or resistance to immunotherapy.

This chapter provides a comprehensive overview of immunometabolism within the inflammatory TME. It examines the metabolic plasticity of key immune populations, the tumor–immune metabolic crosstalk, and the role of inflammatory mediators in shaping immunometabolic reprogramming. Emphasis is placed on therapeutically actionable pathways, the potential for personalized metabolic interventions, and translational challenges in clinical implementation.

7.2 Overview of the tumor microenvironment

Overview of the TME has emerged as a pivotal determinant of cancer progression, immune evasion, and treatment response. Far from being a passive scaffold, the TME constitutes a metabolically, immunologically, and structurally dynamic ecosystem composed of neoplastic cells, stromal fibroblasts, vascular and lymphatic networks, immune infiltrates, and a constantly remodeling ECM (Binnewies et al., 2018; G. Biswas & Mantovani, 2010; Wang et al., 2023). Both intrinsic oncogenic signaling and extrinsic inflammatory cues shape the TME, orchestrating processes that promote immune suppression, angiogenesis, epithelial–mesenchymal transition, and resistance to therapy.

7.2.1 Structural and cellular complexity

A defining feature of the TME is its immunological heterogeneity, characterized by a dynamic equilibrium between pro- and antitumor immune subsets. Cytotoxic $CD8^+$ T cells and NK cells mediate antitumor immunity, whereas Tregs, TAMs, MDSCs, and tolerogenic DCs contribute to immunosuppression (Biswas & Mantovani, 2010; Erez et al., 2010). TAMs, in particular, exist along a functional spectrum ranging from M1-like (proinflammatory, antitumor) to M2-like (antiinflammatory, tumor-promoting) phenotypes. The polarization of macrophages is influenced by cytokines such as IL-4, IL-13, and CSF1, as well as metabolic signals including lactate and adenosine (Hao et al., 2024; Llibre et al., 2025).

In parallel, cancer-associated fibroblasts (CAFs) impede immune infiltration through secretion of TGF-β and ECM components, and by producing chemokines such as CXCL12 and CCL5, which establish immune-excluded niches within tumors (Erez et al., 2010; Kalluri, 2016).

7.2.2 Metabolic constraints and immune dysfunction

The metabolic landscape of the TME is shaped by high proliferative demand, hypoxia, and insufficient vascularization. Tumor cells undergo metabolic reprogramming—shifting toward aerobic glycolysis and enhanced lipid biosynthesis—which depletes essential nutrients like glucose, glutamine, and arginine (Cruz-Bermúdez et al., 2021; Kelly & O'Neill, 2015). This nutrient competition impairs effector immune cells, especially T and NK cells, which depend on these substrates for activation and cytokine production.

In addition, metabolic byproducts such as lactate, reactive oxygen species (ROS), kynurenine, and adenosine directly inhibit immune cell function. Extracellular lactate suppresses cytotoxicity in $CD8^+$ T cells and NK cells while promoting the differentiation of immunosuppressive macrophages and Tregs (Chen et al., 2025; Hao et al., 2024; Llibre et al., 2025). Kynurenine, a product of IDO1/TDO2-mediated tryptophan catabolism, activates the AhR, inducing T cell exhaustion and functional anergy (Y. Wang et al., 2023).

7.2.3 Inflammation as a metabolic driver

The interplay between inflammation and metabolism within the TME is reciprocal. Chronic inflammation—arising from oncogenic stress, infection, therapeutic injury, or persistent tissue damage—drives sustained cytokine production (e.g., IL-1β, IL-6, TNF-α) and activation of transcriptional programs such as NF-κB, STAT3, and HIF-1α. These factors enhance glycolysis and biosynthetic pathways in both tumor and immune cells (Biswas & Mantovani, 2010; Fan et al., 2013).

Tumor-infiltrating macrophages and neutrophils act as both sources and targets of metabolic inflammation. For example, oxidized lipids in the TME activate TLR4 on macrophages, promoting M2-like polarization, while IL-6–STAT3 signaling induces glycolysis and lipid droplet formation in cancer and myeloid cells alike (Kelly & O'Neill, 2015; Yan et al., 2022). These positive feedback loops reinforce fibrosis, neovascularization, and immunosuppression.

7.2.4 Spatial and temporal heterogeneity of immunometabolism

The metabolic architecture of the TME exhibits profound spatial and temporal heterogeneity. Hypoxic gradients create metabolic zonation, with central tumor regions accumulating lactate and ROS, while better-perfused peripheral zones sustain oxidative metabolism and immune infiltration. Temporally, the composition of the TME evolves through tumor progression, metastasis, and treatment exposure. Immune profiling has revealed that metabolically "cold" tumors—characterized by low T cell infiltration and high CAF/MDSC content—respond poorly to immunotherapy, whereas "hot" tumors with enriched effector cells exhibit better clinical outcomes (Z. Hsieh et al., 2022; Liu, Zhang, Zhang, et al., 2024).

Technological advances such as spatial transcriptomics, metabolomic imaging, and intravital microscopy have enabled real-time visualization of immunometabolic remodeling, emphasizing the importance of temporally and spatially resolved therapeutic strategies (Z. Hsieh et al., 2022; Liu, Zhang, Zhang, et al., 2024).

7.2.5 Translational implications and therapeutic targeting

The metabolic dysregulation of the TME offers multiple opportunities for therapeutic intervention. Promising approaches include: IDO1 inhibitors to prevent tryptophan depletion and T cell suppression; CD73 and A2A receptor antagonists to inhibit adenosine signaling; MCT1/4 inhibitors to reduce lactate efflux; arginase inhibitors to restore arginine availability; glutaminase inhibitors targeting glutaminolysis in immunosuppressive cells (Cruz-Bermúdez et al., 2021; Y. Vezina et al., 2021; Wang et al., 2023).

Furthermore, metabolic adjuvants such as metformin (an AMPK activator) and 2-deoxyglucose (2-DG, a glycolytic inhibitor) are under investigation in combination with ICIs and CAR-T cell therapies, aiming to overcome metabolic barriers to immune activation (Cruz-Bermúdez et al., 2021; Wang et al., 2023).

Reprogramming the TME from a metabolically suppressive to an immunologically supportive state represents a compelling avenue for enhancing cancer immunotherapy. As the field evolves, rational combination therapies that integrate metabolic and immunologic modulation hold promise for improving patient outcomes across diverse tumor types.

7.3 Immunometabolism: concept and regulatory axes

Immunometabolism: concept and regulatory axes: Immunometabolism is a field that investigates how metabolic pathways govern immune cell function, particularly within pathological environments such as cancer. In contrast to earlier paradigms that viewed metabolism as a downstream consequence of immune activation, current understanding emphasizes that metabolic reprogramming acts as an instructive signal—shaping immune cell fate, functional plasticity, and effector capacity. In the TME, where oxygen, nutrient availability, and cytokine levels fluctuate dramatically, immune cells adapt distinct metabolic profiles that determine whether they mount an effective response, enter tolerance, or contribute to tumor progression (Kornberg, 2020; Ma et al., 2024; Rao et al., 2021).

7.3.1 Core metabolic programs and immune cell fate

Distinct immune subsets utilize specialized metabolic pathways tailored to their functional roles. For instance, Effector T (Teff) cells, including Th1 and $CD8^+$ cytotoxic lymphocytes, depend heavily on aerobic glycolysis (the Warburg effect), even under normoxic conditions. This facilitates rapid ATP generation and the synthesis of nucleotides, amino acids, and lipids required for clonal expansion and cytokine secretion. In contrast, Tregs and memory T cells rely on FAO and OXPHOS to maintain long-term survival and suppressive or surveillance functions in nutrient-deprived environments (Ma et al., 2024; Rao et al., 2021). Macrophages exhibit metabolic polarization: M1-like (classically activated) macrophages utilize glycolysis to support proinflammatory functions and generate reactive oxygen and nitrogen species for antimicrobial and antitumor activity; M2-like (alternatively activated) macrophages favor FAO and mitochondrial respiration to support tissue remodeling and immunosuppression (Yi et al., 2023). Similarly, DCs shift toward glycolysis during activation to facilitate antigen presentation, while tolerogenic DCs maintain OXPHOS and lipid metabolism patterns comparable to Tregs. These metabolic profiles are not static but respond dynamically to the local environmental context of the TME.

7.3.2 Key regulatory axes of immunometabolism

Several intracellular signaling networks regulate metabolic programming in immune cells by integrating nutrient availability and inflammatory cues: mTOR: mTORC1 and mTORC2 respond to amino acids, glucose, and cytokines to promote anabolic metabolism. In immune cells, mTORC1 activation is essential for Teff cell growth, glycolytic flux, and proinflammatory cytokine production. However, persistent mTOR activation in tumors may drive T cell senescence and reduce CAR-T cell persistence (Chi, 2012; Ma et al., 2024). AMPK: A cellular energy sensor activated under metabolic stress, AMPK promotes catabolic processes such as FAO, autophagy, and mitochondrial maintenance. AMPK activation enhances the longevity and function of Tregs and memory T cells, and is being explored as a target of metabolic adjuvants like metformin (Zeng & Chi, 2017). HIF-1α: Stabilized under low oxygen, HIF-1α promotes glycolytic gene expression and suppresses mitochondrial respiration. While it enhances acute Teff activation, chronic HIF-1α signaling contributes to M2 macrophage skewing and T cell exhaustion in hypoxic tumors (Kumagai et al., 2022; Phan & Goldrath, 2015). c-Myc: A key transcription factor for glucose and glutamine metabolism in proliferating immune cells. While c-Myc is necessary for Teff activation, its sustained expression in the TME may drive metabolic exhaustion and immune dysfunction (Wang et al., 2011). PGC-1α (peroxisome proliferator-activated receptor gamma coactivator 1α): A central regulator of mitochondrial biogenesis, PGC-1α promotes OXPHOS and supports the survival and persistence of memory and resilient Teff cells. Its suppression in the TME is associated with mitochondrial fragmentation and T cell senescence (Dumauthioz et al., 2021). SREBP, LXR, and PPARs: These nuclear receptors regulate lipid metabolism. In the TME: SREBP promotes lipogenesis and MDSC expansion; PPARγ facilitates TAM immunosuppressive polarization; LXR agonists are under investigation for reprogramming myeloid cells toward proinflammatory phenotypes (Tang et al., 2024). Collectively, these pathways function as metabolic switches that can be pharmacologically manipulated to enhance immune competence or dampen tumor-promoting inflammation.

7.3.3 Crosstalk with inflammatory signaling

Immunometabolism is deeply intertwined with inflammatory signaling cascades. In the TME: Proinflammatory cytokines such as IL-6, IL-1β, and TNF-α drive glycolytic reprogramming through transcriptional regulators including NF-κB, STAT3, and HIF-1α, fostering anabolic metabolism and immune polarization (Taniguchi & Karin, 2018). Conversely, antiinflammatory cytokines like IL-10 and TGF-β support OXPHOS and lipid storage in Tregs and M2 macrophages, reinforcing a tolerogenic milieu (O'Neill & Pearce, 2016). Tumor-derived factors such as VEGF, adenosine, lactate, and oxidized lipids further drive immune metabolic suppression. For example, adenosine accumulation via CD39/CD73 inhibits Teff proliferation and enhances MDSC-mediated suppression (Xia et al., 2023). Moreover, tumor-secreted exosomes carrying lipids, metabolites, and microRNAs have been shown to reprogram T cell metabolism and dampen antigen-presenting cell (APC) function, further contributing to immune evasion (Park et al., 2022).

7.3.4 Therapeutic targeting of metabolic checkpoints

Given the pivotal role of metabolism in immune regulation, targeting metabolic checkpoints offers a novel avenue for cancer immunotherapy. Strategies under active investigation include: mTOR inhibitors (e.g., rapamycin, everolimus): Support memory T cell development and mitigate exhaustion, though careful titration is required to avoid general immunosuppression (Chi, 2012). AMPK activators (e.g., metformin, AICAR): Improve T cell metabolic resilience and mitigate inflammatory signaling within the TME (Zeng & Chi, 2017). HIF-1α inhibitors: Aim to reverse hypoxia-induced dysfunction, enhance Teff infiltration, and synergize with adoptive cell therapies (Phan & Goldrath, 2015). PGC-1α agonists: Investigational agents that seek to restore mitochondrial function and improve Teff persistence under metabolic stress (Dumauthioz et al., 2021). Dual immunometabolic blockade: Combinatorial regimens involving IDO1 inhibitors, glutaminase antagonists, and CD73 inhibitors are being tested alongside ICIs to reverse immune suppression at both metabolic and signaling levels (Park et al., 2022; Xia et al., 2023). These approaches reflect a growing understanding that effective cancer immunotherapy must not only target immune checkpoints but also reprogram the metabolic foundations upon which immune cells operate.

7.4 Key immune cells and their metabolic reprogramming in the tumor microenvironment

Immunometabolic reprogramming is a fundamental determinant of how immune cells function—or fail to function—within the TME. The metabolic phenotype of each immune cell subset governs not only its survival and activation status, but also its differentiation and immunological role. Tumor-induced metabolic stressors—including hypoxia, acidosis, nutrient deprivation, and chronic inflammation—reconfigure immune cell function toward exhausted, suppressive, or tolerogenic phenotypes. Deciphering the immunometabolic features of major immune populations within the TME provides key insights into mechanisms of immune evasion and therapeutic resistance, and opens opportunities for targeted intervention.

7.4.1 Tumor-associated macrophages

TAMs are among the most abundant immune cells in solid tumors and exhibit remarkable metabolic and functional plasticity. They polarize along an M1–M2 spectrum depending on local stimuli: M1-like macrophages possess proinflammatory and cytotoxic properties, producing nitric oxide (NO) via inducible nitric oxide synthase (iNOS) and relying on glycolysis to sustain antimicrobial and antitumor activities. Conversely, M2-like TAMs adopt an oxidative metabolic profile dominated by FAO and mitochondrial respiration, which supports protumorigenic functions including angiogenesis, matrix remodeling, and immunosuppression (Colegio et al., 2014; Mantovani et al., 2004). Within the TME, signals such as IL-4, IL-10, TGF-β, lactic acid, and hypoxia promote M2 polarization. Lactic acid enhances arginase-1 expression through HIF-1α and GPR132 activation, leading to T cell suppression. Concurrently, lipid accumulation in TAMs activates PPARγ and SREBP transcriptional programs, reinforcing an immunosuppressive phenotype (Gu et al., 2025). Therapeutically, reprogramming TAMs toward an M1-like phenotype—or depleting M2-like TAMs—is a promising strategy. Agents such as CSF1R inhibitors, PI3Kγ inhibitors, and TLR agonists are currently under clinical investigation.

7.4.2 T cells: effector, exhausted, and regulatory

T cells play a pivotal role in antitumor immunity, but their metabolic competence is often compromised in the TME. Effector $CD8^+$ T cells and Th1 cells require aerobic glycolysis to support clonal expansion, cytokine production (e.g., IFN-γ, TNF-α), and cytotoxic activity. However, intense nutrient competition with tumor cells limits glucose availability, impairing T cell function. Tumor-derived immunosuppressive metabolites—such as adenosine, ROS, and kynurenine—further inhibit T cell receptor (TCR) signaling and proliferation (Chang et al., 2015). Exhausted T cells, characterized by sustained expression of inhibitory receptors such as PD-1, LAG-3, and TIM-3, exhibit a metabolically dysfunctional phenotype: Mitochondrial depolarization and ROS leakage; Suppressed PGC-1α expression, reducing mitochondrial biogenesis and respiration; Heightened reliance on glycolysis, which fails to meet energetic demands in a nutrient-deprived TME (Ikeda et al., 2025). Tregs, by contrast, are metabolically adapted to the TME: They preferentially utilize FAO and OXPHOS, ensuring survival under glucose-limited and hypoxic conditions; express high levels of CD36 and related lipid uptake proteins, enabling persistence in lipid-rich, immunosuppressive niches; Suppress Teff function through IL-10, TGF-β, and metabolic competition (Berod et al., 2014). Therapeutic strategies that restore mitochondrial fitness in Teff cells (e.g., via PGC-1α agonists) or block immunosuppressive signals (e.g., adenosine–A2A antagonists) are being developed to reverse exhaustion and enhance the efficacy of checkpoint inhibitors.

7.4.3 Dendritic cells

DCs are central to initiating adaptive antitumor responses through antigen presentation and T cell priming. Their metabolic programming is tightly coupled to their maturation status. Upon activation, DCs switch to glycolysis, which supports cytokine production (e.g., IL-12, IFN-β), antigen processing, and costimulation (Cubillos-Ruiz et al., 2015). However, in the TME, DC function is impaired by lipid accumulation—particularly oxidized lipids—which induces endoplasmic reticulum (ER) stress and activation of XBP1. This results in downregulation of MHC class I/II molecules and a tolerogenic phenotype that fails to activate Teff cells (Herber et al., 2010). Additional tumor-derived factors such as VEGF, prostaglandins, and lactic acid further suppress DC maturation and migration. Restoring DC function by targeting lipid metabolism (e.g., inhibition of FATP2 or SCD1) or alleviating ER stress (e.g., XBP1 silencing) has shown potential to improve the performance of DC vaccines and combination immunotherapies (Moreews & Karlsson, 2025).

7.4.4 Myeloid-derived suppressor cells

MDSCs are a heterogeneous group of immature myeloid cells that expand during cancer and play a central role in immune evasion by inhibiting T cell responses, promoting angiogenesis, and facilitating matrix remodeling. Metabolically, MDSCs are characterized by: High arginase-1 (ARG1) and iNOS expression, depleting extracellular arginine and generating ROS/NO, thereby impairing T cell proliferation and activation; A dependence on FAO, glutaminolysis, and cholesterol metabolism, supporting their expansion and suppressive activity (Goldmann & Medina, 2024); Upregulation of lipid metabolism pathways (e.g., CD36, FABP4, LXR), promoting lipid uptake and storage, which correlates with enhanced immunosuppression. Pharmacological inhibition of MDSC metabolism using agents such as FAO inhibitors (e.g., etomoxir), glutaminase inhibitors, or statins has demonstrated efficacy in preclinical models, particularly when combined with immune checkpoint blockade or cancer vaccines (Gabrilovich & Nagaraj, 2009; Li et al., 2021; H.R. Jin, Wang, et al., 2023).

7.4.4.1 Therapeutic outlook

Targeting the metabolic vulnerabilities of immune cell populations within the TME represents a promising direction for next-generation immunotherapy. Strategies that restore metabolic fitness in effector immune cells or disrupt the metabolic support of suppressive populations may enable the conversion of immunologically "cold" tumors into "hot" and responsive ones. Personalized metabolic reprogramming, in combination with existing immunotherapies, offers the potential to enhance clinical outcomes across diverse cancer types.

7.5 Metabolic crosstalk between tumor and immune cells in the tumor microenvironment

Immunometabolic reprogramming fundamentally determines how immune cells function in the TME. The metabolic phenotype of each immune subset governs not only survival and activation, but also polarization toward effector or suppressive roles. Tumor-induced metabolic constraints—including hypoxia, acidosis, nutrient depletion, and inflammatory cytokines—drive immune cells toward dysfunctional, exhausted, or tolerogenic states. Dissecting the immunometabolic interactions between tumor and immune compartments is critical to understanding immune escape and informing therapeutic strategies.

7.5.1 Nutrient competition: a central driver of immunosuppression

One of the most fundamental metabolic interactions in the TME is nutrient competition. Tumor cells, through aerobic glycolysis (Warburg effect) and glutaminolysis, consume disproportionate amounts of key nutrients such as glucose, glutamine, arginine, and tryptophan: Glucose depletion deprives $CD8^{+}$ T cells and NK cells of metabolic fuel, suppressing mTORC1 signaling, limiting glycolysis, and curtailing cytokine production (e.g., IFN-γ) and cytolytic function (Chang et al., 2015). Glutamine consumption by tumor cells limits availability for immune cells, suppressing T cell proliferation and impairing DC activation. Tumor-targeted inhibition of glutamine uptake can restore antigen presentation and T cell effector functions (Leone et al., 2019). Arginine deprivation, mediated by tumor cells and MDSCs via arginase-1, leads to cell cycle arrest in T cells, increased oxidative stress, and activation of GCN2 kinase, which inhibits protein translation and T cell function under amino acid scarcity (Niu et al., 2022). Tryptophan catabolism, driven by upregulation of IDO1 and TDO2 in tumor and tolerogenic APCs, depletes tryptophan while generating kynurenine, a suppressive metabolite that engages the AhR in T cells, promoting $Foxp3^{+}$ Treg differentiation (Campesato et al., 2020). These nutrient-driven interactions vary according to local perfusion, vascular density, and metabolic zonation. Spatial metabolomic analyses demonstrate that perivascular regions retain relatively higher nutrient and oxygen levels, while hypoxic cores are severely nutrient-depleted, correlating with impaired immune infiltration and function (Karamitopoulou et al., 2024).

7.5.2 Immunomodulatory metabolites: suppression through secretion

Beyond substrate competition, tumors actively secrete metabolites that alter immune cell fate and suppress antitumor immunity: Lactate, a byproduct of glycolysis exported via MCT1/4, accumulates in the extracellular space and: Acidifies the microenvironment, disrupting TCR signaling; Inhibits maturation of DCs and CTLs; Promotes M2 macrophage polarization through HIF-1α and GPR81 activation (Chen et al., 2025; Llibre et al., 2025). Kynurenine, produced via IDO1/TDO2, binds AhR in T cells and DCs, leading to expansion of $Foxp3^{+}$ Tregs; suppression of Th17 differentiation; impaired antigen presentation and Teff cell activity (Campesato et al., 2020). Adenosine, formed through CD39/CD73-mediated ATP hydrolysis, binds A2A/A2B receptors on T cells and NK cells to inhibit cytokine production; suppress proliferation; promote T cell exhaustion and immune tolerance

(Saigí et al., 2023; Xia et al., 2023). ROS and lipid peroxides, generated by tumor metabolism and TAMs, disrupt TCR signaling and reprogram DCs and MDSCs into tolerogenic or dysfunctional states (Di Conza et al., 2021).

7.5.3 Immune feedback on tumor metabolism

Immune cells reciprocally influence tumor metabolism through cytokines and stress responses: IFN-γ released by Teff cells and NK cells induces PD-L1 expression and autophagy in tumor cells, while shifting their metabolism toward FAO to enhance stress tolerance (Chang et al., 2015). Macrophage-derived VEGF and matrix metalloproteinases reshape vasculature and ECM, indirectly influencing oxygen and nutrient gradients that promote tumor progression (Wang et al., 2024). TNF-α and FasL produced by T cells can impair tumor mitochondrial integrity, yet chronic exposure under metabolic stress may paradoxically promote immune editing and selection of resistant tumor clones (Deng et al., 2018).

7.5.4 Spatial and temporal organization of metabolic crosstalk

Tumor–immune metabolic interactions are highly heterogeneous in both space and time: Tumor cores are typified by profound hypoxia, elevated lactate and kynurenine levels, and accumulation of Tregs, MDSCs, and exhausted T cells (Karamitopoulou et al., 2024). Invasive fronts often contain more metabolically active immune populations (e.g., Th1 cells, NK cells, M1-like TAMs), supported by proximity to blood vessels and greater nutrient access (Wang et al., 2024). Temporal adaptation occurs during immunotherapy. For instance, anti-PD-1 treatment can lead to upregulation of CD73, increasing adenosine production and driving adaptive resistance (Saigí et al., 2023). Understanding the dynamic and regional organization of immunometabolism is essential for designing rational interventions, such as hypoxia-activated prodrugs, zone-targeted metabolic inhibitors, or time-coordinated immunometabolic combination therapies.

7.5.5 Therapeutic implications and strategies

Targeting metabolic crosstalk between tumors and immune cells represents a compelling therapeutic strategy. Notable approaches include: IDO1 inhibitors (e.g., epacadostat), which aim to block kynurenine production and restore T cell activation. However, monotherapy trials have yielded mixed results, emphasizing the need for combinatorial regimens (Campesato et al., 2020). CD73 and A2A receptor antagonists (e.g., CPI-006, ciforadenant) lift adenosine-mediated immunosuppression and augment responses to checkpoint inhibitors (Saigí et al., 2023; Xia et al., 2023). MCT1/4 inhibitors reduce lactate export and extracellular acidification, reprogramming TAMs toward proinflammatory phenotypes (Chen et al., 2025). Arginase inhibitors (e.g., INCB001158) restore arginine levels and enhance T cell proliferation and effector function (Niu et al., 2022). Dual-targeting strategies, combining metabolic blockade (e.g., glutaminase inhibitors, metformin) with ICIs or CAR-T therapy, aim to overcome resistance by reshaping the immunosuppressive TME (Leone et al., 2019).

Metabolic crosstalk between tumor and immune cells is a core determinant of immune competence within the TME. By decoding and therapeutically targeting these intercellular exchanges, it is possible to transform immunologically "cold" tumors into "hot," immune-permissive microenvironments. This paradigm shift holds the potential to broaden the efficacy and durability of cancer immunotherapies.

7.6 Critical metabolic pathways involved in immunoregulation

Immune cells exhibit remarkable metabolic plasticity, engaging distinct bioenergetic and biosynthetic pathways to fulfill effector, regulatory, or memory functions. These pathways not only sustain cellular viability but also instruct immune cell fate, cytokine production, and responsiveness to environmental stimuli. In cancer, the metabolic landscape of the TME is profoundly altered, exerting selective pressure that often skews immune cells toward dysfunctional or suppressive phenotypes. This section delineates five critical immunometabolic pathways and their therapeutic relevance (Fig. 7.1).

The central tumor cell creates a hostile metabolic milieu—consuming glucose and glutamine, and secreting high levels of lactate and kynurenine—that drives nutrient competition and metabolite-mediated suppression of surrounding immune effectors. Five key pathways are engaged by different immune subsets: Glycolysis in $CD8^+$ T cells (left) and DCs supports rapid effector functions but is impaired by glucose depletion and lactate accumulation. Glutaminolysis in DCs fuels antigen presentation and cytokine production but is outcompeted by tumor glutamine uptake via GLS1. OXPHOS/FAO in Tregs (top right) underpins regulatory survival in low-nutrient niches. Lipid metabolism in MDSCs (bottom right) drives immunosuppression through CD36-mediated lipid uptake and SREBP/PPAR signaling. Amino acid metabolism in macrophages (bottom center) governs nitric oxide production and TCR ζ-chain expression. On the right, therapeutic inhibitors (GLS1, LDHA, IDO1) are shown intercepting these pathways to restore immune competence. The lower panel contrasts immune (left) versus inhibitor-driven (right) strategies, highlighting metabolic checkpoints as actionable targets to reinvigorate antitumor immunity.

7.6.1 Glycolysis: a double-edged sword for effector function

Aerobic glycolysis (Warburg metabolism) is the dominant pathway in activated $CD8^+$ T cells, Th1 cells, NK cells, and mature DCs, supporting rapid ATP generation and supplying intermediates for nucleotide, amino acid, and lipid biosynthesis via the pentose phosphate pathway (Shyer et al., 2020).

However, within the TME, glycolytic flux is constrained by: Glucose depletion and lactate accumulation; Inhibition of hexokinase 2 (HK2) and phosphofructokinase; Increased LDHA activity in tumor cells, diverting pyruvate from mitochondria; Suppressed mTORC1 activation due to nutrient stress. Furthermore, lactate serves as an immunosuppressive metabolite, impairing T cell proliferation, cytokine production (e.g., IFN-γ, IL-2), and enhancing Treg stability. Inhibiting lactate efflux via MCT1/MCT4 or targeting LDHA is under investigation as a means of restoring effector immune function (Brand et al., 2016).

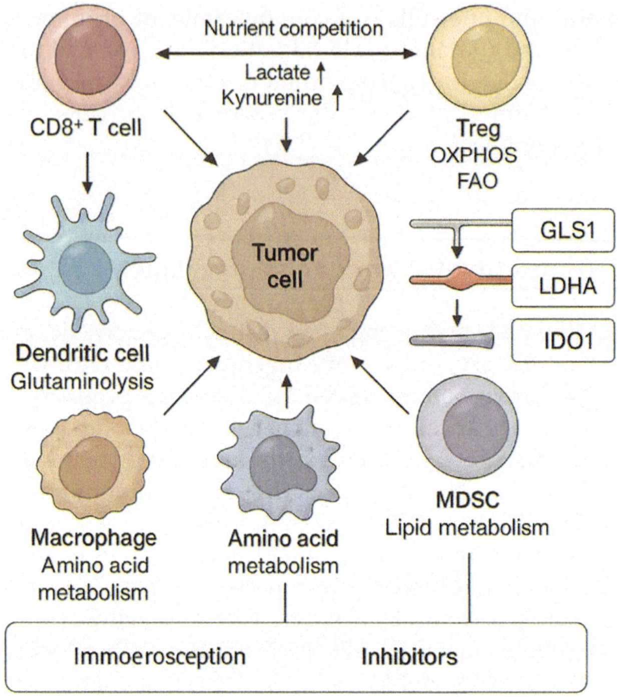

FIGURE 7.1 Critical metabolic pathways involved in immunoregulation within the tumor microenvironment. *FAO*, Fatty acid oxidation; *MDSC*, myeloid-derived suppressor cell; *OXPHOS*, oxidative phosphorylation; *Tregs*, regulatory T cells.

7.6.2 Oxidative phosphorylation and fatty acid oxidation

OXPHOS underlies the long-term persistence of $CD8^+$ memory T cells and Tregs, providing sustained energy production and supporting quiescent or regulatory phenotypes. These cells preferentially utilize FAO, which is regulated by AMPK signaling and PGC-1α–mediated mitochondrial biogenesis (Pearce et al., 2009).

Yet, within the TME, sustained OXPHOS may lead to excessive mitochondrial ROS generation, damaging mtDNA and membranes; loss of mitochondrial mass and membrane potential, promoting exhaustion; engagement of exhaustion-related pathways (e.g., PD-1, TOX, NR4A). Therapeutic restoration of mitochondrial integrity through PGC-1α agonists, ROS scavengers, or FAO-promoting agents has shown potential to rejuvenate T cell function, especially in CAR-T contexts (Ikeda et al., 2025).

7.6.3 Glutaminolysis: tumor–immune competition for a central metabolite

Glutamine is vital for: Nucleotide biosynthesis via glutamate and α-ketoglutarate; TCA cycle anaplerosis; Glutathione production for redox control; Activation of mTORC1 in proliferative immune subsets. Tumor cells often upregulate GLS1 (glutaminase 1), enhancing glutaminolysis and outcompeting immune cells. Additionally, MDSCs and M2 macrophages exploit glutamine metabolism to maintain suppressive phenotypes. Inhibition of GLS1 (e.g., with CB-839) has been shown to reduce MDSC viability; suppress tumor growth; enhance T cell function in glutamine-limited settings (Leone et al., 2019). Combining GLS1 inhibition with immune checkpoint blockade has yielded synergistic effects in preclinical studies.

7.6.4 Lipid metabolism: fuel for immunosuppression or inflammation

Lipid metabolism exerts divergent effects on immune responses: Teff cells depend on de novo lipogenesis (via ACC, SREBP1) for membrane synthesis and cytokine secretion. Tregs, MDSCs, and M2-like macrophages preferentially utilize FAO and lipid uptake to sustain suppressive function. In the TME, abnormal lipid accumulation contributes to ER stress and XBP1 activation in DCs, impairing antigen presentation; CD36-mediated uptake of oxidized lipids, promoting Treg stability; lipid droplet formation in MDSCs, associated with increased ROS and immunosuppression (Saravia & Chi, 2025; Veglia et al., 2017; Xu et al., 2021). Potential interventions include CD36 inhibition, ACC blockade, and modulation of LXR/PPAR signaling to reprogram immune cells toward inflammatory phenotypes.

7.6.5 Amino acid metabolism: gatekeeper of T cell function

Several amino acids critically regulate immune responses within the TME: Arginine: Depleted by arginase-1 in TAMs and MDSCs, arginine deficiency disrupts T cell proliferation, downregulates TCR ζ-chain, and induces mitochondrial dysfunction. Arginine supplementation or arginase inhibitors (e.g., INCB001158) can restore T cell activity (Feng et al., 2025; Taheri et al., 2001). Tryptophan: Catabolized by IDO1/TDO2 into kynurenine, which activates AhR, fostering Treg induction and T cell anergy. IDO1 inhibitors are being tested alongside ICIs. Cysteine: Required for glutathione synthesis. Tumor cells limit cysteine availability by competing for xCT (SLC7A11)-mediated uptake. Inhibiting tumor xCT may improve T cell antioxidant capacity and function (Linher-Melville et al., 2015). Methionine: Essential for *S*-adenosylmethionine production and histone methylation. Methionine scarcity impairs epigenetic regulation in T cells, reducing IFN-γ production and effector differentiation.

7.6.5.1 Therapeutic outlook

Targeting metabolic pathways in immune cells has moved beyond theoretical interest and into translational application. Metabolism-centered strategies can enhance the fitness of effector lymphocytes; reprogram suppressive myeloid subsets; improve response rates to checkpoint blockade and adoptive cell therapies; selectively impair metabolically addicted tumor cells.

Clinical trials are now testing combination therapies involving metabolic modulators and ICIs, offering a promising route to overcome resistance and expand the efficacy of modern immunotherapy.

7.7 Therapeutic targeting of immunometabolism in cancer

The metabolic reprogramming of tumor and immune cells within the TME is increasingly recognized as a pivotal driver of immune evasion and therapy resistance. Unlike ICIs, which

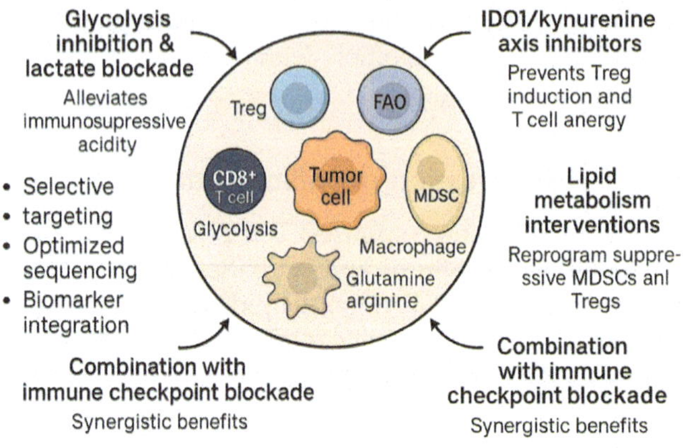

FIGURE 7.2 Therapeutic targeting strategies in cancer immunometabolism. *MDSC*, Myeloid-derived suppressor cell; *Tregs*, regulatory T cells.

release inhibitory immune signals, immunometabolism-based therapies reshape the bioenergetic and biosynthetic context in which immune decisions are executed. These interventions seek to disrupt the tumor's metabolic dominance while restoring immune effector function. This section reviews key therapeutic targets and strategies currently in development or clinical testing (Fig. 7.2).

This schematic illustrates how key metabolic pathways within the TME can be manipulated to restore antitumor immunity. At its core, the TME comprises a tumor cell surrounded by diverse immune subsets—$CD8^+$ T cells (glycolysis-dependent), Tregs (FAO-dependent), MDSCs (lipid-metabolism reliant), macrophages (glutamine/arginine metabolism), and DCs. Arrows denote major intervention points: Glycolysis inhibition and lactate blockade to relieve immunosuppressive acidity; IDO1/kynurenine axis inhibitors to prevent Treg induction and T cell anergy; lipid metabolism interventions (e.g., CD36, SREBP, PPAR modulators) to reprogram suppressive myeloid and regulatory cells; glutamine and arginine metabolism targeting (e.g., GLS1, ARG1 inhibitors) to support Teff cell proliferation and function; combination with immune checkpoint blockade to achieve synergistic enhancement of antitumor responses. The side panel emphasizes the necessity for selective targeting, optimized therapeutic sequencing, and biomarker integration to maximize efficacy and precision in immunometabolic therapy.

7.7.1 Targeting glycolysis and lactate metabolism

Targeting glycolysis and lactate metabolism, tumor cells exhibit heightened glycolysis, leading to glucose depletion; accumulation of lactate; acidification of the TME. These conditions suppress the function of $CD8^+$ T cells, NK cells, and DCs. Pharmacologic agents such as 2-DG inhibit hexokinase, thereby limiting glycolytic flux. MCT1/4 inhibitors (e.g., AZD3965) block lactate efflux from tumor cells, preventing extracellular acidification and alleviating T cell suppression (Beloueche-Babari et al., 2020; Bénéteau et al., 2012; Sharma et al., 2022). Targeting LDHA redirects pyruvate toward mitochondrial metabolism, supporting OXPHOS and improving T cell viability. However, systemic inhibition of glycolysis carries off-target toxicity risks. To overcome this, tumor-selective delivery strategies—such as nanoparticles or hypoxia-activated prodrugs—are under development.

7.7.2 Inhibition of indoleamine 2, 3-dioxygenase 1 and the kynurenine pathway

The tryptophan–IDO1–kynurenine–AhR axis is a well-established mediator of immune tolerance. IDO1 catalyzes tryptophan degradation into kynurenine, which activates AhR in T cells; induces Treg differentiation; suppresses Th1 and CTL responses. Although early clinical trials of epacadostat (e.g., ECHO-301) in combination with PD-1 inhibitors yielded disappointing results (Long et al., 2019), this outcome likely reflects compensatory pathways, including TDO2 and IL4I1 activity (Wu et al., 2023). More recent strategies focus on dual inhibition (e.g., IDO1+TDO2) or direct AhR antagonism (e.g., BAY2416964) (Olafsen et al., 2024). Preclinical studies show that combining IDO1 blockade with STING agonists or radiotherapy enhances DC activation and antigen presentation.

7.7.3 Modulating fatty acid and lipid metabolism

Lipid metabolism sustains immunosuppressive cell populations within the TME: Tregs and MDSCs rely on FAO for persistence; CD36-mediated lipid uptake promotes Treg stability and oxidative stress in DCs; SREBP1 activation drives de novo lipogenesis in tumors and suppressive myeloid cells (Li et al., 2021). Therapeutic interventions include FAO blockade via etomoxir (a CPT1a inhibitor) and modulation of LXR/PPAR pathways to repolarize macrophages toward proinflammatory states (Li et al., 2021). Inhibition of ACC1, a key lipogenic enzyme, has also enhanced DC-mediated T cell priming in preclinical models (Li et al., 2022). Additional strategies involve inhibiting lipid peroxidation in T cells to prevent ferroptosis; enhancing PGC-1α signaling to improve mitochondrial lipid metabolism and T cell fitness.

7.7.4 Targeting arginine and glutamine metabolism

Arginase-1 (ARG1), expressed by MDSCs and TAMs, depletes extracellular arginine, impairing TCR ζ-chain expression; T cell proliferation and cytokine production. CB-1158 (INCB001158), an oral arginase inhibitor, is currently in clinical trials (NCT02903914), with preliminary results indicating increased $CD8^+$ infiltration and IFN-γ production (Steggerda et al., 2017). Similarly, glutaminase (GLS1) inhibitors (e.g., CB-839, telaglenastat) suppress glutamine metabolism in both tumor cells and immunosuppressive myeloid cells. Combined with checkpoint blockade, CB-839 improves T cell metabolic fitness and enhances tumor clearance (Zhu, Zhu and Wu, 2022; J. Jin, Wang, et al., 2023). Other glutamine-targeting strategies include use of glutamine antagonists (e.g., DON derivatives); inhibition of glutamine transporters (e.g., ASCT2/SLC1A5).

7.7.5 Combining metabolic interventions with immune checkpoint blockade

Metabolic modulation can prime the immune microenvironment for enhanced response to ICIs. For instance, AMPK activators (e.g., metformin) alleviate hypoxia, support T cell persistence, and synergize with PD-1 blockade (Scharping et al., 2017); MCT inhibitors combined with anti–PD-1 enhance tumor-infiltrating lymphocyte infiltration and cytotoxicity (Beloueche-Babari et al., 2020); GLS1 inhibition alongside

CTLA-4 blockade fosters epitope spreading and memory T cell development. Representative clinical trials include NCT03422627: CB-839 + nivolumab in renal cell carcinoma; NCT03145064: anti-PD-L1 combined with arginase inhibition; NCT04265534: metformin with anti-PD-1 in non–small cell lung cancer. These approaches reflect a strategic shift—from monotherapy toward TME metabolic conditioning—to enable more durable and comprehensive immunotherapy responses.

7.7.6 Future perspectives and considerations

Despite promising advances, several challenges must be addressed: Cell-type specificity: Many metabolic targets are shared between immune and tumor cells; thus, selective modulation is critical to avoid off-target immunosuppression. Temporal sequencing: Optimal scheduling of metabolic and immune interventions remains poorly defined and may influence therapeutic synergy. Biomarkers of response: Real-time monitoring tools, including metabolic imaging, metabolomics, and single-cell transcriptomics, are essential to identify responsive patients. Looking forward, integration of multiomics, AI-guided metabolic modeling, and spatial metabolic profiling will be pivotal in designing personalized, mechanism-driven metabolic immunotherapies.

7.8 Challenges and future perspectives

Targeting immunometabolism represents a novel and promising frontier in oncology by modulating core metabolic programs that regulate immune function. However, its successful clinical translation is challenged by biochemical redundancy, spatial and temporal heterogeneity, systemic toxicity, and the dynamic nature of immune–tumor metabolic interactions. Addressing these multifaceted barriers is essential to realize the full therapeutic potential of metabolic interventions (Fig. 7.3).

This conceptual schematic illustrates major barriers to translating immunometabolic therapies (arrows pointing into the tumor-immune microenvironment) alongside emerging strategies to overcome them. Metabolic plasticity: Immune and tumor cells compensate for single-pathway inhibition by engaging alternative fuel sources, necessitating multitarget approaches. Systemic toxicity: On-target inhibition in normal tissues (e.g., FAO blockade) underscores the need for tumor-selective delivery and isoform-specific agents. Spatial and temporal heterogeneity: Metabolic zonation within tumors and dynamic shifts during treatment demand precision, guided by spatial multiomics and machine learning. Biomarker gap: The absence of validated metabolic readouts impairs patient stratification and real-time response monitoring. Context- and time-sensitive metabolism: Divergent acute versus chronic metabolic dependencies require adaptable dosing regimens. At the base, future platforms—single-cell metabolic imaging, CRISPR-based metabolic screens, AI-guided modeling, and nonpharmacological interventions (dietary and microbiome modulation)—are proposed to refine immunometabolic therapies into selective, dynamic, and patient-specific cancer treatments.

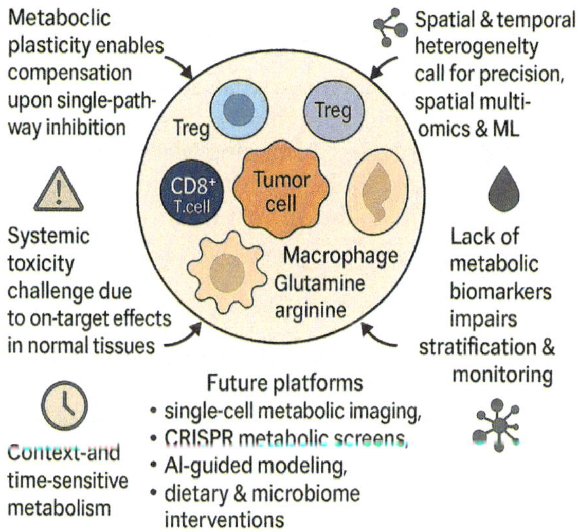

FIGURE 7.3 Challenges and future directions in targeting immunometabolism.

7.8.1 Metabolic redundancy and plasticity

Immune and cancer cells exhibit substantial metabolic plasticity, enabling compensation upon inhibition of a single pathway. For example, glycolysis blockade often induces compensatory upregulation of glutaminolysis or FAO. Tumor cells can adapt to utilize alternative substrates such as acetate, ketone bodies, or branched-chain amino acids under metabolic stress (Tufail et al., 2024). Immunosuppressive populations like Tregs and MDSCs maintain function even when key metabolic axes are disrupted. Overcoming this adaptability requires multipronged strategies, including sequential inhibition (e.g., glutaminase plus CD36 blockade), combination with ICIs, and targeting stress response pathways (e.g., HSP90 or UPR modulators) to prevent compensatory reprogramming.

7.8.2 Systemic toxicity and tissue specificity

Metabolic targets often play essential roles in normal physiology, creating challenges in achieving tumor selectivity. For instance, IDO1 inhibitors may disturb neuroimmune homeostasis via systemic kynurenine depletion; glutaminase inhibition can impact hepatic detoxification and CNS function; and FAO inhibitors such as etomoxir have induced cardiac toxicity in clinical trials (O'Connor et al., 2018). To mitigate systemic side effects, current approaches include TME-activated prodrugs responsive to hypoxia, ROS, or acidic pH; immune cell–targeted nanoparticles for selective drug delivery; and isoform-specific inhibitors (e.g., targeting HK2 in tumors while sparing HK1 in normal tissue). These strategies aim to reprogram immune metabolism with minimal impact on nontarget tissues.

7.8.3 Intratumoral and intertumoral heterogeneity

Metabolic phenotypes vary significantly across and within tumors: Hypoxic cores harbor glycolysis-dependent M2-like TAMs, oxygen-rich peripheries support Teff infiltration and mitochondrial metabolism, desmoplastic tumors (e.g., PDAC) exhibit dense stroma with poor nutrient diffusion, and inflamed tumors (e.g., melanoma) are highly glycolytic and immune-permissive (Shan Liu, Zhang, Zhang, et al., 2024). This spatial and intertumoral diversity limits the effectiveness of one-size-fits-all therapies. Advancing precision immunometabolic strategies requires spatial multiomics platforms (e.g., Imaging Mass Cytometry, MIBI, CODEX), machine learning–guided mapping of metabolic–immune landscapes, and longitudinal metabolomic profiling to guide therapy adjustment in real time.

7.8.4 Lack of reliable metabolic biomarkers

Unlike genomics-driven therapies, immunometabolism lacks well-validated biomarkers for predicting therapeutic response or immune fitness. This impairs: patient stratification, real-time monitoring of treatment efficacy, and assessment of metabolic reprogramming in immune subsets. Emerging candidate tools include radiometabolic PET tracers (e.g., $[^{18}F]$F-Gln, $[^{11}C]$acetate), circulating metabolite ratios (e.g., kynurenine/tryptophan, lactate/pyruvate), SCENITH-based flow cytometric profiling of immune metabolic activity (Argüello et al., 2020), and exosome-derived metabolic cargo for liquid biopsy applications (Huang & Mcconathy, 2013; Seo et al., 2022).

7.8.5 Temporal and contextual complexity

Immune metabolism is context- and time-sensitive, evolving with disease progression, immunotherapy exposure, cytokine milieu, and nutrient flux during cachexia or inflammation. For example, while glycolysis may support acute T cell activation, it promotes exhaustion in chronic settings. Thus, metabolic therapy must be cell-specific, pathway-specific, and time-adapted. Future directions include pulsatile or intermittent dosing regimens to minimize adaptation, dynamic treatment algorithms based on real-time metabolic monitoring, and circadian-informed interventions, given that immune metabolism follows diurnal patterns (Koppula et al., 2021).

7.8.6 Future directions and technological integration

Advancing immunometabolic therapies will require integration of biological insight with cutting-edge technology. Key innovations include: Single-cell metabolic imaging (e.g., FLIM for NADH/FAD, MALDI-MS); CRISPR-based metabolic screens in patient-derived organoids; AI-driven modeling integrating transcriptomics, metabolomics, and immune profiling to predict therapeutic response, resistance, and optimal drug combinations. In parallel, nonpharmacological strategies—such as dietary methionine restriction, ketogenic diets, and microbiome modulation using short-chain fatty acid–producing bacteria—are being investigated for their capacity to reprogram host–tumor metabolism.

The interface of immunity, metabolism, and inflammation presents a powerful therapeutic axis in cancer. While targeting immunometabolism holds transformative potential, clinical translation demands solutions for selectivity, resistance, and personalization. With advances in imaging, single-cell analysis, and computational modeling, immunometabolic therapies may soon evolve from conceptual frameworks to clinical standards—bringing forth a new era in precision oncology.

7.9 Conclusion

The convergence of metabolism, immunity, and cancer biology has fundamentally reshaped our understanding of the TME. Once regarded as a niche topic, immunometabolism has now emerged as a central regulatory axis that orchestrates immune cell differentiation, effector function, exhaustion, and survival within the nutrient-deprived and inflammatory milieu of the TME. Tumor cells do not merely adapt to this metabolic landscape—they actively manipulate it to evade immune surveillance and sustain malignant progression.

Crucially, the metabolic status of immune cells is not simply a reflection of their activation but a determinant of their fate and function. CTLs, DCs, macrophages, and MDSCs adopt distinct metabolic programs that govern their immunological behavior. Aberrant immunometabolism—driven by tumor-derived metabolites, cytokines, and hypoxic stress—contributes to immunosuppression and limits the efficacy of immunotherapies, including immune checkpoint blockade and adoptive cell therapies.

These insights have fostered the development of metabolically guided therapeutic strategies aimed at: Reinvigorating exhausted T cells by promoting mitochondrial biogenesis or restoring nutrient availability; Reprogramming suppressive myeloid populations by targeting FAO, arginine, or glutamine metabolism; Enhancing DC function through modulation of lipid homeostasis or alleviation of ER stress; Normalizing the TME by inhibiting immunoregulatory pathways involving lactate, adenosine, or tryptophan metabolism.

Several small-molecule modulators—such as IDO1 inhibitors, arginase inhibitors, GLS1 antagonists, and MCT blockers—are already undergoing clinical evaluation, frequently in combination with checkpoint inhibitors or cytotoxic therapies. In parallel, the rise of systems immunometabolism—an approach integrating multiomics technologies, spatial biology, and artificial intelligence—is enabling the precise mapping of metabolic vulnerabilities and immune niches within diverse tumor ecosystems. This paves the way for precision immunometabolism: the customization of treatment strategies not only to genetic or immunological profiles, but also to the dynamic metabolic constraints within the TME.

Looking ahead, the incorporation of dietary interventions, microbiome modulation, circadian rhythm alignment, and advanced metabolic imaging will further refine our ability to reprogram immune metabolism in a patient-specific manner. Moreover, inflammation—an established driver of tumorigenesis—intersects with immunometabolism at multiple levels, influencing cytokine networks, oxidative stress responses, energy production, and metabolic checkpoint signaling. Targeting this intersection offers a dual-benefit approach: suppressing tumor-promoting inflammation while simultaneously enhancing antitumor immunity.

In summary, immunometabolism is not merely adjunctive to immunotherapy—it is a fundamental determinant of therapeutic success. Deciphering and therapeutically manipulating the metabolic language of the immune system has the potential to not only enhance existing treatment modalities but also usher in a new era of interventions that are adaptive, durable, and tailored to the metabolic realities of disease. As research in this field accelerates, immunometabolism is poised to become a cornerstone of personalized oncology, shifting the paradigm from reactive treatment to proactive metabolic reprogramming.

References

Argüello, R. J., Combes, A. J., Char, R., Gigan, J. P., Baaziz, A. I., Bousiquot, E., Camosseto, V., Samad, B., Tsui, J., Yan, P., Boissonneau, S., Figarella-Branger, D., Gatti, E., Tabouret, E., Krummel, M. F., & Pierre, P. (2020). SCENITH: A flow cytometry-based method to functionally profile energy metabolism with single-cell resolution. *Cell Metabolism, 32*(6), 1063. https://doi.org/10.1016/j.cmet.2020.11.007, http://www.cellmetabolism.org/.

Azizi, E., Carr, A. J., Plitas, G., Cornish, A. E., Konopacki, C., Prabhakaran, S., Nainys, J., Wu, K., Kiseliovas, V., Setty, M., Choi, K., Fromme, R. M., Dao, P., McKenney, P. T., Wasti, R. C., Kadaveru, K., Mazutis, L., Rudensky, A. Y., & Pe'er, D. (2018). Single-cell map of diverse immune phenotypes in the breast tumor microenvironment. *Cell, 174*(5), 1293. https://doi.org/10.1016/j.cell.2018.05.060, https://www.sciencedirect.com/journal/cell.

Beloueche-Babari, M., Casals Galobart, T., Delgado-Goni, T., Wantuch, S., Parkes, H. G., Tandy, D., Harker, J. A., & Leach, M. O. (2020). Monocarboxylate transporter 1 blockade with AZD3965 inhibits lipid biosynthesis and increases tumour immune cell infiltration. *Journal of Cancer, 122*(6), 895–903. https://doi.org/10.1038/s41416-019-0717-x, http://www.nature.com/bjc/index.html.

Berod, L., Friedrich, C., Nandan, A., Freitag, J., Hagemann, S., Harmrolfs, K., Sandouk, A., Hesse, C., Castro, C. N., BäHre, H., Tschirner, S. K., Gorinski, N., Gohmert, M., Mayer, C. T., Huehn, J., Ponimaskin, E., Abraham, W. R., MüLler, R., Lochner, M., & Sparwasser, T. (2014). De novo fatty acid synthesis controls the fate between regulatory T and T helper 17 cells. *Nature Medicine, 20*(11), 1327–1333. https://doi.org/10.1038/nm.3704, http://www.nature.com/nm/index.html.

Bharadwaj, U., Kasembeli, M. M., Robinson, P., & Tweardy, D. J. (2020). Targeting janus kinases and signal transducer and activator of transcription 3 to treat inflammation, fibrosis, and cancer: Rationale, progress, and caution. *Pharmacological Reviews, 72*(2), 486–526. https://doi.org/10.1124/pr.119.018440, http://pharmrev.aspetjournals.org/content/pharmrev/72/2/486.full.pdf.

Binnewies, M., Roberts, E. W., Kersten, K., Chan, V., Fearon, D. F., Merad, M., Coussens, L. M., Gabrilovich, D. I., Ostrand-Rosenberg, S., Hedrick, C. C., Vonderheide, R. H., Pittet, M. J., Jain, R. K., Zou, W., Howcroft, T. K., Woodhouse, E. C., Weinberg, R. A., & Krummel, M. F. (2018). Understanding the tumor immune microenvironment (TIME) for effective therapy. *Nature Medicine, 24*(5), 541–550. https://doi.org/10.1038/s41591-018-0014-x, http://www.nature.com/nm/index.html.

Biswas, S. K., & Mantovani, A. (2010). Macrophage plasticity and interaction with lymphocyte subsets: Cancer as a paradigm. *Nature Immunology, 11*(10), 889–896. https://doi.org/10.1038/ni.1937.

Brand, A., Singer, K., Koehl, G. E., Kolitzus, M., Schoenhammer, G., Thiel, A., Matos, C., Bruss, C., Klobuch, S., Peter, K., Kastenberger, M., Bogdan, C., Schleicher, U., Mackensen, A., Ullrich, E., Fichtner-Feigl, S., Kesselring, R., Mack, M., Ritter, U., ... Kreutz, M. (2016). LDHA-associated lactic acid production blunts tumor immunosurveillance by T and NK cells. *Cell Metabolism, 24*(5), 657–671. https://doi.org/10.1016/j.cmet.2016.08.011, http://www.cellmetabolism.org/.

Braun, C., & Weichhart, T. (2021). mTOR-dependent immunometabolism as Achilles' heel of anticancer therapy. *European Journal of Immunology, 51*(12), 3161–3175. https://doi.org/10.1002/eji.202149270, http://onlinelibrary.wiley.com/journal/10.1002/(ISSN)1521-4141.

Bénéteau, M., Zunino, B., Jacquin, M. A., Meynet, O., Chiche, J., Pradelli, L. A., Marchetti, S., Cornille, A., Carles, M., & Ricci, J. E. (2012). Combination of glycolysis inhibition with chemotherapy results in an antitumor immune response. *Proceedings of the National Academy of Sciences of the United States of America, 109*(49), 20071–20076. https://doi.org/10.1073/pnas.1206360109France, http://www.pnas.org/content/109/49/20071.full.pdf+html.

Campesato, L. F., Budhu, S., Tchaicha, J., Weng, C. H., Gigoux, M., Cohen, I. J., Redmond, D., Mangarin, L., Pourpe, S., Liu, C., Zappasodi, R., Zamarin, D., Cavanaugh, J., Castro, A. C., Manfredi, M. G., McGovern, K., Merghoub, T., & Wolchok, J. D. (2020). Blockade of the AHR restricts a Treg-macrophage suppressive axis induced by L-Kynurenine. *Nature Communications, 11*(1). https://doi.org/10.1038/s41467-020-17750-z, http://www.nature.com/ncomms/index.html.

Chang, C. H., Qiu, J., O'Sullivan, D., Buck, M. D., Noguchi, T., Curtis, J. D., Chen, Q., Gindin, M., Gubin, M. M., Van Der Windt, G. J. W., Tonc, E., Schreiber, R. D., Pearce, E. J., & Pearce, E. L. (2015). Metabolic competition in the tumor microenvironment is a driver of cancer progression. *Cell, 162*(6), 1229–1241. https://doi.org/10.1016/j.cell.2015.08.016, https://www.sciencedirect.com/journal/cell.

Chen, J., Huang, Z., Chen, Y., Tian, H., Chai, P., Shen, Y., Yao, Y., Xu, S., Ge, S., & Jia, R. (2025). Lactate and lactylation in cancer. *Signal Transduction and Targeted Therapy, 10*(1). https://doi.org/10.1038/s41392-024-02082-x.

Chi, H. (2012). Regulation and function of mTOR signalling in T cell fate decisions. *Nature Reviews. Immunology, 12*(5), 325–338. https://doi.org/10.1038/nri3198.

Colegio, O. R., Chu, N. Q., Szabo, A. L., Chu, T., Rhebergen, A. M., Jairam, V., Cyrus, N., Brokowski, C. E., Eisenbarth, S. C., Phillips, G. M., Cline, G. W., Phillips, A. J., & Medzhitov, R. (2014). Functional polarization of tumour-associated macrophages by tumour-derived lactic acid. *Nature Publishing Group, United States Nature, 513*(7519), 559–563. https://doi.org/10.1038/nature13490, http://www.nature.com/nature/index.html.

Cruz-Bermúdez, A., Laza-Briviesca, R., Casarrubios, M., Sierra-Rodero, B., & Provencio, M. (2021). The role of metabolism in tumor immune evasion: Novel approaches to improve immunotherapy. *Biomedicines, 9*(4), 361. https://doi.org/10.3390/biomedicines9040361.

Cubillos-Ruiz, J. R., Silberman, P. C., Rutkowski, M. R., Chopra, S., Perales-Puchalt, A., Song, M., Zhang, S., Bettigole, S. E., Gupta, D., Holcomb, K., Ellenson, L. H., Caputo, T., Lee, A. H., Conejo-Garcia, J. R., & Glimcher, L. H. (2015). ER stress sensor XBP1 controls anti tumor immunity by disrupting dendritic cell homeostasis. *Cell, 161*(7), 1527–1538. https://doi.org/10.1016/j.cell.2015.05.025, https://www.sciencedirect.com/journal/cell.

Cui, Y., Chen, J., Zhang, Z., Shi, H., Sun, W., & Yi, Q. (2023). The role of AMPK in macrophage metabolism, function and polarisation. *Journal of Translational Medicine, 21*(1). https://doi.org/10.1186/s12967-023-04772-6, https://translational-medicine.biomedcentral.com.

Deng, M., Gui, X., Kim, J., Xie, L., Chen, W., Li, Z., He, L., Chen, Y., Chen, H., Luo, W., Lu, Z., Xie, J., Churchill, H., Xu, Y., Zhou, Z., Wu, G., Yu, C., John, S., Hirayasu, K., ... Zhang, C. C. (2018). LILRB4 signalling in leukaemia cells mediates T cell suppression and tumour infiltration. *Nature, 562*(7728), 605–609. https://doi.org/10.1038/s41586-018-0615-z, http://www.nature.com/nature/index.html.

Di Conza, G., Tsai, C. H., Gallart-Ayala, H., Yu, Y. R., Franco, F., Zaffalon, L., Xie, X., Li, X., Xiao, Z., Raines, L. N., Falquet, M., Jalil, A., Locasale, J. W., Percipalle, P., Masson, D., Huang, S. C. C., Martinon, F., Ivanisevic, J., & Ho, P. C. (2021). Tumor-induced reshuffling of lipid composition on the endoplasmic reticulum membrane sustains macrophage survival and pro-tumorigenic activity. *Nature Immunology, 22*(11), 1403–1415. https://doi.org/10.1038/s41590-021-01047-4, http://www.nature.com/ni.

Dumauthioz, N., Tschumi, B., Wenes, M., Marti, B., Wang, H., Franco, F., Li, W., Lopez-Mejia, I. C., Fajas, L., Ho, P. C., Donda, A., Romero, P., & Zhang, L. (2021). Enforced PGC-1α expression promotes CD8 T cell fitness, memory formation and antitumor immunity. *Cellular and Molecular Immunology, 18*(7), 1761–1771. https://doi.org/10.1038/s41423-020-0365-3, http://www.nature.com/cmi/archive/index.html.

Erez, N., Truitt, M., Olson, P., & Hanahan, D. (2010). Cancer-associated fibroblasts are activated in incipient neoplasia to orchestrate tumor-promoting inflammation in an NF-κB-dependent manner. *Cancer cell, 17*(2), 135–147. https://doi.org/10.1016/j.ccr.2009.12.041, https://www.journals.elsevier.com/cancer-cell.

Fan, Y., Mao, R., & Yang, J. (2013). NF-κB and STAT3 signaling pathways collaboratively link inflammation to cancer. *Protein & Cell, 4*(3), 176–185. https://doi.org/10.1007/s13238-013-2084-3.

Feng, T., Xie, F., Lyu, Y., Yu, P., Chen, B., Yu, J., Zhang, G., To, K. F., Tsang, C. M., & Kang, W. (2025). The arginine metabolism and its deprivation in cancer therapy. *Cancer Letters, 620*. https://doi.org/10.1016/j.canlet.2025.217680, https://www.sciencedirect.com/science/journal/03043835.

Gabrilovich, D. I., & Nagaraj, S. (2009). Myeloid-derived suppressor cells as regulators of the immune system. *Nature Reviews Immunology, 9*(3), 162–174. https://doi.org/10.1038/nri2506.

Geltink, R. I. K., Kyle, R. L., & Pearce, E. L. (2018). Unraveling the complex Interplay between T cell metabolism and function. *Annual Review of Immunology, 36*, 461–488. https://doi.org/10.1146/annurev-immunol-042617-053019, http://www.annualreviews.org/journal/immunol.

Goldmann, O., & Medina, E. (2024). Metabolic pathways fueling the suppressive activity of myeloid-derived suppressor cells. *Frontiers in Immunology, 15*. https://doi.org/10.3389/fimmu.2024.1461455.

Gu, Q., Wang, Y., Yi, P., & Cheng, C. (2025). Theoretical framework and emerging challenges of lipid metabolism in cancer. *Seminars in Cancer Biology, 108*, 48–70. https://doi.org/10.1016/j.semcancer.2024.12.002, https://www.sciencedirect.com/science/journal/1044579X.

Hao, Z. N., Tan, X. P., Zhang, Q., Li, J., Xia, R., & Ma, Z. (2024). Lactate and lactylation: Dual regulators of T-cell-mediated tumor immunity and immunotherapy. *Biomolecules, 14*(12). https://doi.org/10.3390/biom14121646, http://www.mdpi.com/journal/biomolecules.

Herber, D. L., Cao, W., Nefedova, Y., Novitskiy, S. V., Nagaraj, S., Tyurin, V. A., Corzo, A., Cho, H. I., Celis, E., Lennox, B., Knight, S. C., Padhya, T., McCaffrey, T. V., McCaffrey, J. C., Antonia, S., Fishman, M., Ferris, R. L.,

Kagan, V. E., & Gabrilovich, D. I. (2010). Lipid accumulation and dendritic cell dysfunction in cancer. *Nature Medicine, 16*(8), 880–886. https://doi.org/10.1038/nm.2172.

Hsieh, W. C., Budiarto, B. R., Wang, Y. F., Lin, C. Y., Gwo, M. C., So, D. K., Tzeng, Y. S., & Chen, S. Y. (2022). Spatial multi-omics analyses of the tumor immune microenvironment. *Journal of Biomedical Science, 29*(1). https://doi.org/10.1186/s12929-022-00879-y, https://jbiomedsci.biomedcentral.com.

Hu, Q., Zhu, Y., Mei, J., Liu, Y., & Zhou, G. (2025). Extracellular matrix dynamics in tumor immunoregulation: From tumor microenvironment to immunotherapy. *Journal of Hematology & Oncology, 18*(1). https://doi.org/10.1186/s13045-025-01717-y.

Hu, T., Liu, C. H., Lei, M., Zeng, Q., Li, L., Tang, H., & Zhang, N. (2024). Metabolic regulation of the immune system in health and diseases: Mechanisms and interventions. *Signal Transduction and Targeted Therapy, 9*(1). https://doi.org/10.1038/s41392-024-01954-6, https://www.nature.com/sigtrans.

Huang, C., & Mcconathy, J. (2013). Radiolabeled amino acids for oncologic imaging. *Journal of Nuclear Medicine, 54*(7), 1007–1010. https://doi.org/10.2967/jnumed.112.113100, http://jnm.snmjournals.org/content/54/7/1007.full.pdf+html.

Ikeda, H., Kawase, K., Nishi, T., Watanabe, T., Takenaga, K., Inozume, T., Ishino, T., Aki, S., Lin, J., Kawashima, S., Nagasaki, J., Ueda, Y., Suzuki, S., Makinoshima, H., Itami, M., Nakamura, Y., Tatsumi, Y., Suenaga, Y., Morinaga, T., ... Togashi, Y. (2025). Immune evasion through mitochondrial transfer in the tumour microenvironment. *Nature, 638*(8049), 225–236. https://doi.org/10.1038/s41586-024-08439-0, https://www.nature.com/nature/.

Jennings, M. R., Munn, D., & Blazeck, J. (2021). Immunosuppressive metabolites in tumoral immune evasion: Redundancies, clinical efforts, and pathways forward. *Journal for Immunotherapy of Cancer, 9*(10), e003013. https://doi.org/10.1136/jitc-2021-003013.

Jin, H. R., Wang, J., Wang, Z. J., Xi, M. J., Xia, B. H., Deng, K., & Yang, J. L. (2023). Lipid metabolic reprogramming in tumor microenvironment: From mechanisms to therapeutics. *Journal of Hematology and Oncology, 16*(1). https://doi.org/10.1186/s13045-023-01498-2, https://jhoonline.biomedcentral.com.

Jin, J., Byun, J. K., Choi, Y. K., & Park, K. G. (2023). Targeting glutamine metabolism as a therapeutic strategy for cancer. *Experimental and Molecular Medicine, 55*(4), 706–715. https://doi.org/10.1038/s12276-023-00971-9, https://www.nature.com/emm/.

Kalluri, R. (2016). The biology and function of fibroblasts in cancer. *Nature reviews. Cancer, 16*(9), 582–598. https://doi.org/10.1038/nrc.2016.73.

Karamitopoulou, E., Wenning, A. S., Acharjee, A., Aeschbacher, P., Marinoni, I., Zlobec, I., Gloor, B., & Perren, A. (2024). Spatial heterogeneity of immune regulators drives dynamic changes in local immune responses, affecting disease outcomes in pancreatic cancer. *Clinical Cancer Research, 30*(18), 4215–4226. https://doi.org/10.1158/1078-0432.CCR-24-0368, https://aacrjournals.org/clincancerres/article/30/18/4215/747477/Spatial-Heterogeneity-of-Immune-Regulators-Drives.

Kaymak, I., Williams, K. S., Cantor, J. R., & Jones, R. G. (2021). Immunometabolic interplay in the tumor microenvironment. *Cancer cell, 39*(1), 28–37. https://doi.org/10.1016/j.ccell.2020.09.004, https://www.journals.elsevier.com/cancer-cell.

Kelly, B., & O'Neill, L. A. J. (2015). Metabolic reprogramming in macrophages and dendritic cells in innate immunity. *Cell Research, 25*(7), 771–784. https://doi.org/10.1038/cr.2015.68, http://www.nature.com/cr/index.html.

Koppula, P., Zhuang, L., & Gan, B. (2021). Cystine transporter SLC7A11/xCT in cancer: Ferroptosis, nutrient dependency, and cancer therapy. *Protein and Cell, 12*(8), 599–620. https://doi.org/10.1007/s13238-020-00789-5, http://link.springer.com/journal/13238.

Kornberg, M. D. (2020). The immunologic warburg effect: Evidence and therapeutic opportunities in autoimmunity. *Wiley Interdisciplinary Reviews: Systems Biology and Medicine, 12*(5). https://doi.org/10.1002/wsbm.1486, http://onlinelibrary.wiley.com/journal/10.1002/(ISSN)1939-005X.

Kumagai, S., Koyama, S., Itahashi, K., Tanegashima, T., Lin, Yt, Togashi, Y., Kamada, T., Irie, T., Okumura, G., Kono, H., Ito, D., Fujii, R., Watanabe, S., Sai, A., Fukuoka, S., Sugiyama, E., Watanabe, G., Owari, T., Nishinakamura, H., ... Nishikawa, H. (2022). Lactic acid promotes PD-1 expression in regulatory T cells in highly glycolytic tumor microenvironments. *Cancer cell, 40*(2), 201. https://doi.org/10.1016/j.ccell.2022.01.001, https://www.journals.elsevier.com/cancer-cell.

Leone, R. D., Zhao, L., Englert, J. M., Sun, I. M., Oh, M. H., Sun, I. H., Arwood, M. L., Bettencourt, I. A., Patel, C. H., Wen, J., Tam, A., Blosser, R. L., Prchalova, E., Alt, J., Rais, R., Slusher, B. S., & Powell, J. D. (2019). Glutamine blockade induces divergent metabolic programs to overcome tumor immune evasion. *Science, 366*(6468), 1013–1021. https://doi.org/10.1126/science.aav2588, https://science.sciencemag.org/content/366/6468/1013/tab-pdf.

Li, K., Shi, H., Zhang, B., Ou, X., Ma, Q., Chen, Y., Shu, P., Li, D., & Wang, Y. (2021). Myeloid-derived suppressor cells as immunosuppressive regulators and therapeutic targets in cancer. *Signal Transduction and Targeted Therapy, 6*(1). https://doi.org/10.1038/s41392-021-00670-9.

Li, S., Lu, C. W., Diem, E. C., Li, W., Guderian, M., Lindenberg, M., Kruse, F., Buettner, M., Floess, S., Winny, M. R., Geffers, R., Richnow, H. H., Abraham, W. R., Grassl, G. A., & Lochner, M. (2022). Acetyl-CoA-Carboxylase 1-mediated de novo fatty acid synthesis sustains Lgr5+ intestinal stem cell function. *Nature Communications, 13*(1). https://doi.org/10.1038/s41467-022-31725-2, http://www.nature.com/ncomms/index.html.

Linher-Melville, K., Haftchenary, S., Gunning, P., & Singh, G. (2015). Signal transducer and activator of transcription 3 and 5 regulate system Xc- and redox balance in human breast cancer cells. *Molecular and Cellular Biochemistry, 405*(1-2), 205–221. https://doi.org/10.1007/s11010-015-2412-4, http://www.kluweronline.com/issn/0300-8177/.

Liu, S., Zhang, X., Wang, W., Li, X., Sun, X., Zhao, Y., Wang, Q., Li, Y., Hu, F., & Ren, H. (2024). Metabolic reprogramming and therapeutic resistance in primary and metastatic breast cancer. *Molecular cancer, 23*(1). https://doi.org/10.1186/s12943-024-02165-x.

Liu, Z., Zhang, Z., Zhang, Y., Zhou, W., Zhang, X., Peng, C., Ji, T., Zou, X., Zhang, Z., & Ren, Z. (2024). Spatial transcriptomics reveals that metabolic characteristics define the tumor immunosuppression microenvironment via iCAF transformation in oral squamous cell carcinoma. *International Journal of Oral Science, 16*(1), 9. https://doi.org/10.1038/s41368-023-00267-8.

Llibre, A., Kucuk, S., Gope, A., Certo, M., & Mauro, C. (2025). Lactate: A key regulator of the immune response. *Cell Press, United Kingdom Immunity, 58*(3), 535–554. https://doi.org/10.1016/j.immuni.2025.02.008, https://www.sciencedirect.com/science/journal/10747613.

Long, G. V., Dummer, R., Hamid, O., Gajewski, T. F., Caglevic, C., Dalle, S., Arance, A., Carlino, M. S., Grob, J. J., Kim, T. M., Demidov, L., Robert, C., Larkin, J., Anderson, J. R., Maleski, J., Jones, M., Diede, S. J., & Mitchell, T. C. (2019). Epacadostat plus pembrolizumab versus placebo plus pembrolizumab in patients with unresectable or metastatic melanoma (ECHO-301/KEYNOTE-252): A phase 3, randomised, double-blind study. *The Lancet Oncology, 20*(8), 1083–1097. https://doi.org/10.1016/S1470-2045(19)30274-8, http://www.journals.elsevier.com/the-lancet-oncology/.

Ma, S., Ming, Y., Wu, J., & Cui, G. (2024). Cellular metabolism regulates the differentiation and function of T-cell subsets. *Cellular and Molecular Immunology, 21*(5), 419–435. https://doi.org/10.1038/s41423-024-01148-8, https://www.nature.com/cmi/.

Mantovani, A., Sica, A., Sozzani, S., Allavena, P., Vecchi, A., & Locati, M. (2004). The chemokine system in diverse forms of macrophage activation and polarization. *Trends in Immunology, 25*(12), 677–686. https://doi.org/10.1016/j.it.2004.09.015.

Moreews, M., & Karlsson, M. C. I. (2025). Endoplasmic reticulum stress: A key player in immune cell regulation and autoimmune disorders. *Seminars in Immunology, 78*. https://doi.org/10.1016/j.smim.2025.101954, https://www.sciencedirect.com/science/journal/10445323.

Niu, F., Yu, Y., Li, Z., Ren, Y., Li, Z., Ye, Q., Liu, P., Ji, C., Qian, L., & Xiong, Y. (2022). Arginase: An emerging and promising therapeutic target for cancer treatment. *Biomedicine and Pharmacotherapy, 149*. https://doi.org/10.1016/j.biopha.2022.112840, https://www.journals.elsevier.com/biomedicine-and-pharmacotherapy.

O'Connor, R. S., Guo, L., Ghassemi, S., Snyder, N. W., Worth, A. J., Weng, L., Kam, Y., Philipson, B., Trefely, S., Nunez-Cruz, S., Blair, I. A., June, C. H., & Milone, M. C. (2018). The CPT1a inhibitor, etomoxir induces severe oxidative stress at commonly used concentrations. *Scientific Reports, 8*(1). https://doi.org/10.1038/s41598-018-24676-6, www.nature.com/srep/index.html.

O'Neill, L. A. J., & Pearce, E. J. (2016). Immunometabolism governs dendritic cell and macrophage function. *Journal of Experimental Medicine, 213*(1), 15–23. https://doi.org/10.1084/jem.20151570, http://jem.rupress.org/content/213/1/15.full.pdf.

Olafsen, N. E., Das, S., Gorrini, C., & Matthews, J. (2024). Long-term exposure to BAY2416964 reduces proliferation, migration and recapitulates transcriptional changes induced by AHR loss in PyMT-induced mammary tumor cells. *Frontiers in Oncology, 14*. https://doi.org/10.3389/fonc.2024.1466658.

Park, J., Wang, L., & Ho, P. C. (2022). Metabolic guidance and stress in tumors modulate antigen-presenting cells. *Oncogenesis, 11*(1). https://doi.org/10.1038/s41389-022-00438-y, http://www.nature.com/oncsis/index.html.

Pearce, E. L., Walsh, M. C., Cejas, P. J., Harms, G. M., Shen, H., Wang, L. S., Jones, R. G., & Choi, Y. (2009). Enhancing CD8 T-cell memory by modulating fatty acid metabolism. *Nature, 460*(7251), 103–107. https://doi.org/10.1038/nature08097.

Phan, A. T., & Goldrath, A. W. (2015). Hypoxia-inducible factors regulate T cell metabolism and function. *Molecular Immunology, 68*(2), 527–535. https://doi.org/10.1016/j.molimm.2015.08.004, www.elsevier.com/locate/molimm.

Poznanski, S. M., Singh, K., Ritchie, T. M., Aguiar, J. A., Fan, I. Y., Portillo, A. L., Rojas, E. A., Vahedi, F., El-Sayes, A., Xing, S., Butcher, M., Lu, Y., Doxey, A. C., Schertzer, J. D., Hirte, H. W., & Ashkar, A. A. (2021). Metabolic flexibility determines human NK cell functional fate in the tumor microenvironment. *Cell Metabolism, 33*(6), 1205. https://doi.org/10.1016/j.cmet.2021.03.023, http://www.cellmetabolism.org/.

Rao, D., Verburg, F., Renner, K., Peeper, D. S., Lacroix, R., & Blank, C. U. (2021). Metabolic profiles of regulatory T cells in the tumour microenvironment. *Cancer Immunology, Immunotherapy, 70*(9), 2417–2427. https://doi.org/10.1007/s00262-021-02881-z, link.springer.de/link/service/journals/00262/index.htm.

Saigí, M., Mesía-Carbonell, O., Barbie, D. A., & Guillamat-Prats, R. (2023). Unraveling the intricacies of CD73/adenosine signaling: The pulmonary immune and stromal microenvironment in lung cancer. *Cancers, 15*(23). https://doi.org/10.3390/cancers15235706, http://www.mdpi.com/journal/cancers/.

Saravia, J., & Chi, H. (2025). Immunometabolism of regulatory T cells in cancer. *Oncogene, 44*(25), 2011–2024. https://doi.org/10.1038/s41388-025-03458-1, https://www.nature.com/onc/.

Scharping, N. E., Menk, A. V., Whetstone, R. D., Zeng, X., & Delgoffe, G. M. (2017). Efficacy of PD-1 blockade is potentiated by metformin-induced reduction of tumor hypoxia. *Cancer Immunology Research, 5*(1), 9–16. https://doi.org/10.1158/2326-6066.CIR-16-0103, http://cancerimmunolres.aacrjournals.org/content/5/1/9.full-text.pdf.

Seo, Y., Craig, M. C., Murphy, S. T., Feng, J., Chen, X., & Yuneva, M. (2022). [18 F]-(2S,4R)4-fluoroglutamine PET imaging of glutamine metabolism in murine models of hepatocellular carcinoma (HCC). *Molecular Imaging, 2022*. https://doi.org/10.1155/2022/5185951.

Sharma, D., Singh, M., & Rani, R. (2022). Role of LDH in tumor glycolysis: Regulation of LDHA by small molecules for cancer therapeutics. *Seminars in Cancer Biology, 87*, 184–195. https://doi.org/10.1016/j.semcancer.2022.11.007, http://www.elsevier.com/inca/publications/store/6/2/2/9/4/3/index.htt.

Shi, R., Tang, Y. Q., & Miao, H. (2020). Metabolism in tumor microenvironment: Implications for cancer immunotherapy. *MedComm, 1*(1), 47–68. https://doi.org/10.1002/mco2.6, onlinelibrary.wiley.com/journal/26882663.

Shyer, J. A., Flavell, R. A., & Bailis, W. (2020). Metabolic signaling in T cells. *Cell Research, 30*(8), 649–659. https://doi.org/10.1038/s41422-020-0379-5, http://www.nature.com/cr/index.html.

Steggerda, S. M., Bennett, M. K., Chen, J., Emberley, E., Huang, T., Janes, J. R., Li, W., MacKinnon, A. L., Makkouk, A., Marguier, G., Murray, P. J., Neou, S., Pan, A., Parlati, F., Rodriguez, M. L. M., Van de Velde, L. A., Wang, T., Works, M., Zhang, J., ... Gross, M. I. (2017). Inhibition of arginase by CB-1158 blocks myeloid cell-mediated immune suppression in the tumor microenvironment. *Journal for Immunotherapy of Cancer, 5*(1). https://doi.org/10.1186/s40425-017-0308-4, http://www.immunotherapyofcancer.org/.

Taheri, F., Ochoa, J. B., Faghiri, Z., Culotta, K., Park, H. J., Lan, M. S., Zea, A. H., & Ochoa, A. C. (2001). L-Arginine regulates the expression of the T-cell receptor ζ chain (CD3ζ) in Jurkat cells. *Clinical Cancer Research, 7*(11).

Tang, Y., Chen, Z., Zuo, Q., & Kang, Y. (2024). Regulation of CD8+ T cells by lipid metabolism in cancer progression. *Cellular and Molecular Immunology, 21*(11), 1215–1230. https://doi.org/10.1038/s41423-024-01224-z, https://www.nature.com/cmi/.

Taniguchi, K., & Karin, M. (2018). NF-B, inflammation, immunity and cancer: Coming of age. *Nature Reviews. Immunology, 18*(5), 309–324. https://doi.org/10.1038/nri.2017.142, http://www.nature.com/nri/index.html.

Traba, J., Sack, M. N., Waldmann, T. A., & Anton, O. M. (2021). Immunometabolism at the nexus of cancer therapeutic efficacy and resistance. *Frontiers in Immunology, 12*. https://doi.org/10.3389/fimmu.2021.657293, https://www.frontiersin.org/journals/immunology#.

Tufail, M., Jiang, C.-H., & Li, N. (2024). Altered metabolism in cancer: Insights into energy pathways and therapeutic targets. *Molecular Cancer, 23*(1). https://doi.org/10.1186/s12943-024-02119-3.

Veglia, F., Tyurin, V. A., Mohammadyani, D., Blasi, M., Duperret, E. K., Donthireddy, L., Hashimoto, A., Kapralov, A., Amoscato, A., Angelini, R., Patel, S., Alicea-Torres, K., Weiner, D., Murphy, M. E., Klein-Seetharaman, J., Celis, E., Kagan, V. E., & Gabrilovich, D. I. (2017). Lipid bodies containing oxidatively truncated lipids block antigen cross-presentation by dendritic cells in cancer. *Nature Communications, 8*(1). https://doi.org/10.1038/s41467-017-02186-9, http://www.nature.com/ncomms/index.html.

Vezina, A., Manglani, M., Morris, D. A., Foster, B., McCord, M., Song, H., Zhang, M., Davis, D., Zhang, W., Bills, J., Nagashima, K., Shankarappa, P., Kindrick, J., Walbridge, S., Peer, C. J., Figg, W. D., Gilbert, M. R., McGavern, D. B., Muldoon, L. L., & Jackson, S. (2021). Adenosine A2A receptor activation enhances blood-tumor barrier permeability in a rodent glioma model. *Molecular Cancer Research, 19*(12), 2081–2095. https://doi.org/10.1158/1541-7786.MCR-19-0995, https://mcr.aacrjournals.org/content/19/12/2081.

de Visser, K. E., & Joyce, J. A. (2023). The evolving tumor microenvironment: From cancer initiation to metastatic outgrowth. *Cancer Cell, 41*(3), 374–403. https://doi.org/10.1016/j.ccell.2023.02.016, https://www.journals.elsevier.com/cancer-cell.

Wang, G., Zhang, Z., Zhong, K., Wang, Z., Yang, N., Tang, X., Li, H., Lu, Q., Wu, Z., Yuan, B., Zheng, M., Cheng, P., Tong, A., & Zhou, L. (2023). CXCL11-armed oncolytic adenoviruses enhance CAR-T cell therapeutic efficacy and reprogram tumor microenvironment in glioblastoma. *Molecular Therapy, 31*(1), 134–153. https://doi.org/10.1016/j.ymthe.2022.08.021, https://www.journals.elsevier.com/molecular-therapy.

Wang, R., Dillon, C. P., Shi, L. Z., Milasta, S., Carter, R., Finkelstein, D., McCormick, L. L., Fitzgerald, P., Chi, H., Munger, J., & Green, D. R. (2011). The Transcription Factor Myc controls metabolic reprogramming upon T lymphocyte activation. *Immunity, 35*(6), 871–882. https://doi.org/10.1016/j.immuni.2011.09.021.

Wang, S., Wang, J., Chen, Z., Luo, J., Guo, W., Sun, L., & Lin, L. (2024). Targeting M2-like tumor-associated macrophages is a potential therapeutic approach to overcome antitumor drug resistance. *Npj Precision Oncology, 8*(1). https://doi.org/10.1038/s41698-024-00522-z.

Wang, Y., Huang, T., Gu, J., & Lu, L. (2023). Targeting the metabolism of tumor-infiltrating regulatory T cells. *Trends in Immunology, 44*(8), 598–612. https://doi.org/10.1016/j.it.2023.06.001, www.elsevier.com/locate/it.

Watson, M. J., & Delgoffe, G. M. (2022). Fighting in a wasteland: Deleterious metabolites and antitumor immunity. *Journal of Clinical Investigation, 132*(2). https://doi.org/10.1172/JCI148549, https://www.jci.org/articles/view/148549/pdf.

Wen, X., Hu, A. K., Presnell, S. R., Ford, E. S., Koelle, D. M., & Kwok, W. W. (2025). Longitudinal single cell profiling of epitope specific memory CD4+ T cell responses to recombinant zoster vaccine. *Nature Communications, 16*(1). https://doi.org/10.1038/s41467-025-57562-7, https://www.nature.com/ncomms/.

Wu, C., Spector, S. A., Theodoropoulos, G., Nguyen, D. J. M., Kim, E. Y., Garcia, A., Savaraj, N., Lim, D. C., Paul, A., Feun, L. G., Bickerdike, M., & Wangpaichitr, M. (2023). Dual inhibition of IDO1/TDO2 enhances anti-tumor immunity in platinum-resistant non-small cell lung cancer. *Cancer & Metabolism, 11*(1). https://doi.org/10.1186/s40170-023-00307-1.

Xia, C., Yin, S., To, K. K. W., & Fu, L. (2023). CD39/CD73/A2AR pathway and cancer immunotherapy. *Molecular Cancer, 22*(1). https://doi.org/10.1186/s12943-023-01733-x, https://molecular-cancer.biomedcentral.com.

Xu, S., Chaudhary, O., Rodríguez-Morales, P., Sun, X., Chen, D., Zappasodi, R., Xu, Z., Pinto, A. F. M., Williams, A., Schulze, I., Farsakoglu, Y., Varanasi, S. K., Low, J. S., Tang, W., Wang, H., McDonald, B., Tripple, V., Downes, M., Evans, R. M., ... Kaech, S. M. (2021). Uptake of oxidized lipids by the scavenger receptor CD36 promotes lipid peroxidation and dysfunction in CD8+ T cells in tumors. *Immunity, 54*(7), 1561. https://doi.org/10.1016/j.immuni.2021.05.003, www.immunity.com.

Yan, Y., Huang, L., Liu, Y., Yi, M., Chu, Q., Jiao, D., & Wu, K. (2022). Metabolic profiles of regulatory T cells and their adaptations to the tumor microenvironment: Implications for antitumor immunity. *Journal of Hematology & Oncology, 15*(1). https://doi.org/10.1186/s13045-022-01322-3.

Yi, M., Li, T., Niu, M., Mei, Q., Zhao, B., Chu, Q., Dai, Z., & Wu, K. (2023). Exploiting innate immunity for cancer immunotherapy. *Molecular Cancer, 22*(1). https://doi.org/10.1186/s12943-023-01885-w.

Zeng, H., & Chi, H. (2017). mTOR signaling in the differentiation and function of regulatory and effector T cells. *Current Opinion in Immunology, 46*, 103–111. https://doi.org/10.1016/j.coi.2017.04.005, http://www.journals.elsevier.com/current-opinion-in-immunology/.

Zhu, L., Zhu, X., & Wu, Y. (2022). Effects of glucose metabolism, lipid metabolism, and glutamine metabolism on tumor microenvironment and clinical implications. *Biomolecules, 12*(4), 580. https://doi.org/10.3390/biom12040580.

CHAPTER

8

Personalized medicine utilizing biomarkers

Jingsong Shen[1] *and Zheng Xie*[2]

[1]Department of Cardiology, The Affiliated Hospital of Southwest Medical University, Luzhou, Sichuan, P.R. China [2]Orthopaedics of Zigong Fourth People's Hospital, Zigong, Sichuan, P.R. China

8.1 Introduction

The evolution of cancer therapy is changing from empirical methods to precision approaches aided by molecular profiling using biomarkers that consider tumor genomics, immune signatures, and the inflammatory state of the tumor. Historically, inflammation was seen as an innocent bystander to cancer formation, but accumulating evidence both clinically and experimentally points toward inflammation being actively involved in oncogenic transformation or cancer formation. Inflammatory signals contribute to genome instability, epigenetic reprogramming, angiogenesis, and immune escape—hallmarks of tumorigenesis and progression. The combination of inflammation and precision oncology heralds a change in perspective: inflammation may no longer be simply a bystander process that exists alongside cancer development and might itself be part of the effect of therapy on the tumor microenvironment (TME). Mirroring the clinical success of KEYNOTE and CheckMate, where pretreatment with IL-6, C-reactive protein (CRP), and the neutrophil-to-lymphocyte ratio now guide immunotherapy decisions, chronic inflammation simultaneously sculpts the TME at the molecular level: TNF-α released by tumor-associated macrophage ligation of TNFR1/2 ignites a feedforward NF-κB/MAPK axis that amplifies oncogene transcription and disables apoptotic checkpoints, thereby translating cytokine cues into measurable therapeutic responses (Huseni et al., 2023; Wang, Zhang, et al., 2024). Mechanically, TNF-α–induced NF-κB–RELA complexes recruit the epigenetic coactivator BRD4 to maintain prosurvival genes.

The expression of ephrin B1 and its transmembrane receptor EphB1 in hepatocellular carcinoma, and similarly, IL-6-mediated activation of the JAK–STAT3 axis, drives transcriptional programs that promote cell proliferation (Cyclin D1), angiogenesis Vascular Endothelial

Inflammation in Tumorigenesis and Cancer Treatment
DOI: https://doi.org/10.1016/B978-0-443-36649-9.00012-8

Growth Factor (VEGF), and immune tolerance via the induction of PD-L1 (Huseni et al., 2023). In colorectal cancer (CRC), persistent IL-6/STAT3 signaling provides ferroptosis resistance by inducing GPX4 (Wang, Zhang, et al., 2024). Cytine-driven transcriptional programs do not merely change gene lists—they rewire metabolism: NF-κB–responsive elements increase the expression of glycolytic enzyme-encoding genes while repressing mitochondrial bioxidative genes, thereby locking cells into a Warburg phenotype that satisfies anabolic demand (Huang, Cao, et al., 2025). In pancreatic ductal adenocarcinoma (PDAC) and gastric cancer, this logic becomes constitutive: mutant KRAS signals constitutively activate NF-κB, which in turn sustains autonomous IL-1β expression; the resulting KRAS–NF-κB–IL-1β circuit continuously reinforces stemness signatures (NANOG, OCT4, and SOX2) and concurrently upregulates antioxidant and efflux pathways, conferring cross-resistance to chemotherapy, targeted agents, and even immune attack (Mantsounga et al., 2022). Metabolic inflammatory mediators such as COX-2-produced PGE2 work downstream of G Protein–Coupled Receptor (GPCR) signals through the EP2/EP4 axes to block the maturation of Dendritic Cells (DCs) and impair antitumor immunity (Kulesza et al., 2023). As demonstrated recently in Nature Immunology, blocking COX-2 synergizes with the blockade of PD-1 (Hu et al., 2022).

Although mechanistically well understood, inflammatory cancers display wide clinical variance in outcomes: different cytokine pathways with opposite fates may drive tumorigenesis, which is dependent on the tumor genetic subtype and microenvironmental variations. In CRC, IL-6 hyperactivation indicates poorer outcomes; however, only certain subsets respond favorably to anti-IL-6R therapies (Johnson et al., 2018). Like IL-6 and IL-6R, TNF-α and IL-1β are important contributors to sorafenib resistance in HCC; however, differentially mediated downstream signaling drives HCC tumorigenesis (Cappuyns et al., 2025). The TP53/CTNNB1 mutational status and the COX-2/PGE2–KRAS axis are associated with only some immune exclusion PDACs, although this needs further validation (Di et al., 2024). These observations reflect a dependent relationship between inflammation-driven oncogenesis and context; accurately guiding targeted therapy requires defining personalized, molecular, and inflammatory biomarker-driven therapeutic signatures. Translating these signatures into actionable therapies through biomarker-defined circuit therapeutics provides a future way forward in the field of oncology. This coalescence of ideas can be laid out on a spectrum ranging from proinflammatory signaling and overinflammation related to the progressive severity of disease to therapeutic genotyping, targeted therapy, and patient-specific intervention. Biomarkers for quantifying inflammatory signal activity, transcriptional/metabolic signatures, and circulating inflammatory mediators provide guidance to clinicians. Novel technologies, such as single-cell multiomics, may help to obtain a more exact picture of such markers or their sources in patients.

Spatial transcriptomics and liquid biopsy analyzes enable real-time tracking of the dynamic shifts that characterize inflammation. For example, spatial multiomics in PDAC has revealed that IL-1β- and COX-2-rich fibroblast niches promote immune evasion and predict immunotherapy resistance, which makes such biomarkers perfect for integration with adaptive treatment algorithms (Cappuyns et al., 2025; Di et al., 2024). Thus inflammation itself is both a way of diagnosis and a target of therapy—constituting a dynamic information layer such that precision oncology evolves from a nonpersonalized, fixed-category path of treatment to a self-learned, patient-specific path (Fig. 8.1).

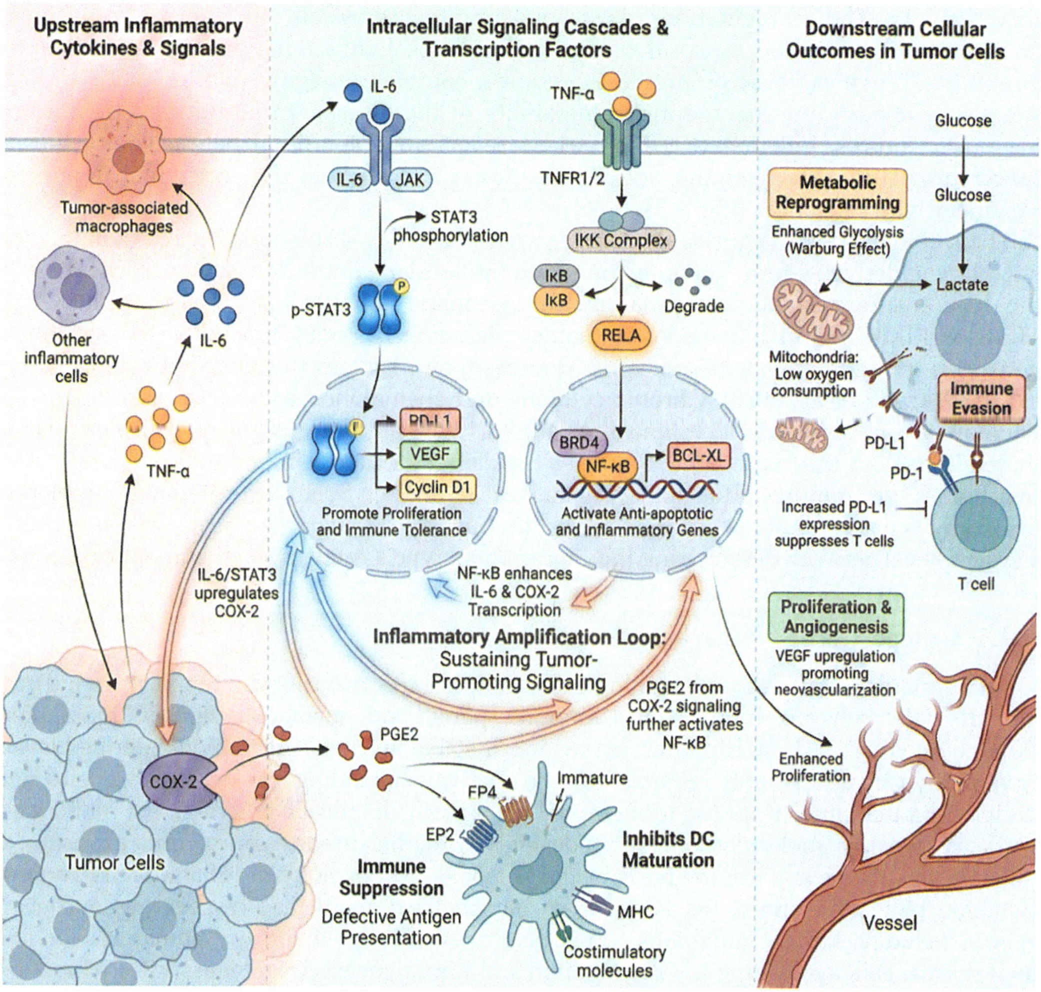

FIGURE 8.1 Inflammation-orchestrated tumorigenic network. Three major inflammatory signaling pathways drive tumor initiation, metabolic reprogramming, and immune evasion.

8.2 The biomarker landscape in inflammatory cancers

The landscape of biomarkers in inflammatory cancers shows a common principle: inflammation is not a mere side effect of cancer; it is an intrinsic, dynamic driver of tumor evolution. Across all forms of cancer, there are unique sets of chronic inflammatory signatures that encode both the order (the relative timing) and activity levels of oncogenic events, immune activation, and metabolic reprogramming. This is achieved via cytokine/T-Cell Receptor (TCR) signaling through transcriptional mechanisms. Tumor cells continuously modulate the cell cycle through oncogenic transcriptional loops, which are associated with proliferative signaling, and rewire metabolism to meet tumor energy requirements. The upregulation of stromal–immune crosstalk that evades antitumor immunity or breaks the mucosal barrier triggers local inflammation and remote autoimmunity. Together, these biomarkers present a complete imaging picture of the disease status and identify the therapeutic vulnerability of the disease. In addition to these static diagnostic indices, inflammatory biomarkers reveal spatiotemporal heterogeneity during cancer progression, recognizing both intratumoral and stromal dynamics that determine treatment responsiveness (Fig. 8.2).

These biomarker categories—genomic, transcriptomic, proteomic, metabolomic, and microbiome-derived—form an interconnected molecular continuum where each layer in this loop creates a situation of inflammation. Genomic mutations, such as those in KRAS, TP53, or PIK3CA, can initiate inflammatory signaling cascades that alter transcriptional networks; transcriptomic and proteomic changes then maintain this aberrant state (Cheung et al., 2014; Xin et al., 2020). Chronic cytokine and chemokine production persists as well, while metabolic shifts produce lipid mediators as well as redox imbalances, which sustain these effects, and the microbiome regulates the degree of cancer inflammation via microbial metabolites or immune education (Zelante et al., 2020). Such layer-by-layer biomarker taxonomy is made up of not separate molecules but rather integrated pathways representing a system-level network determining the cancer phenotype as well as the therapeutic response.

8.2.1 Categories of biomarkers

Inflammatory cancers form a biologically complex spectrum whose biomarkers indicate the crosstalk between tumor cells, immune parts, and metabolic signals. Biomarkers throughout genomic, transcriptomic, proteomic, metabolomic, and microbiome-derived layers have shifted clinicians' and researchers' ways of understanding tumor heterogeneity and deciphering the tumor response to therapy. Unlike static diagnostic criteria, these biomarkers work as dynamic molecular data that develop with the disease course and exposure to different treatments and are the basis of the personalized oncology of inflammatory cancers. Genomic biomarkers form the bedrock of personalized medicine—discovering oncogenic events, including somatic mutations and structural variations—that cause human cells to lose their normal balance, leading to inflammation and tumorigenesis (Ngo et al., 2011). Therefore, canonical oncogenes, such as KRAS, TP53, and PIK3CA, which can perform both proliferative and inflammatory functions, actually underlie tumorigenesis (Mueller et al., 2018). In PDAC, mutant KRAS(G12D) mutations switch on NF-κB and IL-1β autocrine signaling loops, which affect the pancreatic cancer microenvironment (McIntyre et al., 2024). Creating a self-sustained inflammatory niche promotes tumor stemness and makes tumors resistant to therapy (Mahat et al., 2025). Similarly, TP53 loss also increases the levels of proinflammatory cytokines through the NF-κB–IL-6 signaling pathway, which leads to the formation of an autoregulatory system that promotes immune escape (Phelan & Oellerich, 2022). In addition, mutations in a specific gene and single-nucleotide polymorphism mutations in cytokine genes (e.g., IL6–174 G/C, TNF–308 A/G) have been found to be associated with increased susceptibility to psoriasis (Zhao, Wang, et al., 2024).

The assumption that glutamine metabolism can mediate hepatocellular and colorectal carcinogenesis is well substantiated, particularly when it coexists with other risk factors, such as chronic hepatitis or colitis (Lou et al., 2024). Microbial Species Interaction

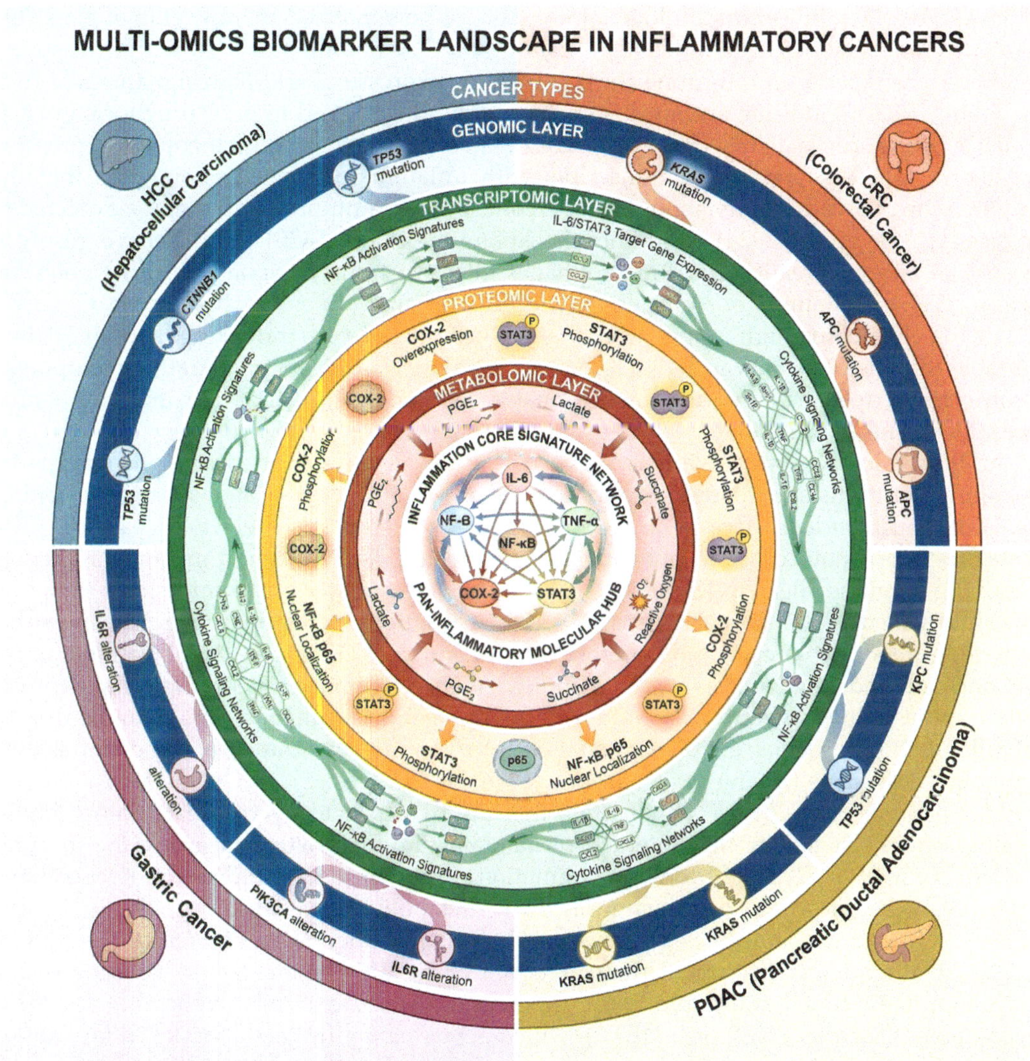

FIGURE 8.2 Multiomics landscape of inflammation-associated biomarkers across cancer types. A systems-level overview illustrating inflammation-related biomarkers in hepatocellular carcinoma (HCC), colorectal cancer (CRC), pancreatic ductal adenocarcinoma (PDAC), and gastric cancer. The concentric rings represent the genomic (outer), transcriptomic, proteomic, and metabolomic layers, converging toward a central inflammation core signature network. The integration of multiomics data highlights how inflammatory signaling pathways such as the IL-6/STAT3, NF-κB, and COX-2/PGE2 pathways collectively shape cancer heterogeneity and the therapeutic response.

Descriptors (MSIDs) are a clinical reflection of mismatch repair deficiencies; Microsatellite Instability (MSI)-high colorectal/gastric cancers present with pronounced accumulation of MSI mutants and increased inherent hypermutability, as well as increased immune cell infiltration and increased sensitivity to immune checkpoint-blocking drugs, which makes them serve as genomic–immunologic biomarkers of personalized therapy (Lin et al., 2020). Transcriptomic biomarkers indicate the status of the inflammatory TME by measuring cytokine, chemokine, and immune checkpoint gene expression, and high signatures of IL-6, IL-8, and CXCL12 indicate an immunosuppressive milieu linked to poor prognosis in HCC and gastric cancer patients (Sui et al., 2022). In contrast, the simultaneous coexpression of PD-L1, CTLA-4, and LAG3 transcripts with inflammatory markers suggests that the suppression of T-cell activity should be overcome before immunotherapy can be expected to succeed (Choi et al., 2024). Immune checkpoint blockade (ICB) studies have resolved colorectal and pancreatic tumor macrophages into two transcriptionally distinct poles: an IL-1β^+/TNF-α^+ inflammatory cluster that forecasts refractoriness to ICB and a CXCL9$^+$/CXCL10$^+$ chemokine-high population that orchestrates T-cell trafficking and predicts a durable response (Zhao, Wang, et al., 2024). This binary classification validates macrophage-centric transcriptomic signatures as actionable biomarkers for adaptive immunotherapy (Boutilier & Elsawa, 2021).

At the omic level, transcript abundance is translated into functional phenotypes by mapping posttranslational modifications (You et al., 2023). CRP and serum amyloid A remain robust, independent sentinels of systemic inflammation; elevated baseline CRP portends inferior outcomes in nonsmall cell lung cancer (NSCLC) and melanoma patients receiving immune therapy (Preianò et al., 2018). Deep-tissue proteomics now identifies phosphorylated STAT3 and acetylated NF-κB p65 as chronic inflammatory gatekeepers that license aggressive colorectal and hepatocellular phenotypes (You et al., 2023). Tandem mass-tag and data-independent Sequential Window Acquisition of All Theoretical Fragment-Ion Spectra Mass Spectrometry (SWATH-MS) multiplexing simultaneously quantify dozens of inflammatory proteins, enabling crystal-clear proteomic cartography of tumor-infiltrating immune ecosystems (Zhang et al., 2024).

Metabonomic biomarkers demonstrate that the two trajectories of inflammatory reprogramming and metabolic flux interact to maintain tumor growth and evade the immune system (Feng et al., 2024). Chronic inflammation results in the accumulation of lactate and AA metabolites, leading to a change in TME metabolism (Vasudevan et al., 2021). The IL-6–STAT3 pathway amplifies glycolysis and lactate production and increases the amount of AA in the microenvironment (Kumar et al., 2025). This creates acidic conditions that impair immune function, inhibiting the function of cytotoxic T cells (Nencini et al., 2025). Eicosanoids (such as PGE2 or 5-HETE), which act as paracrine mediators of inflammation and angiogenesis, are downstream products of the metabolism of AA (Schmelter et al., 2023). Elevated levels of PGE2 driven by COX-2 overexpression can cause DC paralysis and promote Treg expansion, resulting in poor antitumor immunity (Li et al., 2025). Such lipidomic signatures can be quantified on LC–MS platforms, which have become more commonly incorporated into clinical biomarker panels (Monahan et al., 2022). The discovery of such metabolomic fingerprints will enable the design of antiinflammatory metabolic interventions such as COX-2/ALOX inhibitors for certain biomarker-defined subgroups of cancer patients (Preianò et al., 2018).

Ultimately, gut microbiota-derived biomarkers associated with inflammation constitute a new dimension of personalized care. The gut microbiota modifies systemic and localized immune tone via microbial metabolites, including Short-Chain Fatty Acids (SCFAs), bile acid derivatives, and tryptophan catabolites (Arifuzzaman et al., 2024; Su et al., 2022).

An increased abundance of *F. nucleatum* and its metabolite, formylated peptides, was correlated with an increased IL-8–driven neutrophil response in CRC patients (Cong et al., 2024; Liang et al., 2022). Conversely, beneficial microbial metabolites such as butyrate and indole-3-propionic acid dampen NF-κB signaling and potentiate the immunotherapy response. Integrative microbiome–metabolome analyzes now allow clinicians to track these microbial inflammatory biomarkers noninvasively via stool and plasma sampling, marking a major leap in noninvasive inflammatory precision diagnostics.

8.2.2 Case studies in inflammatory cancers

In tumorigenesis, chronic immune activation is inseparable from oncogenesis; each malignancy harbors distinct inflammatory circuits that can simultaneously serve as diagnostic, prognostic, and therapeutic biomarkers. In CRC, the IL-6–STAT3 axis, which governs both tumor initiation and the therapeutic response, is the most intensively studied pathway. Persistent activation of IL-6 signaling—triggered by tumor-associated macrophages and fibroblasts—confers a survival advantage to human cancer cells by activating the STAT3 pathway, which drives the transcription of proliferation (cyclin D1), survival (BCL-XL), and angiogenesis (VEGF) genes. Recently, in two Nature Cancer papers, Patel et al. reported that IL-6–STAT3–GPX4 signaling results in ferroptosis resistance in CRCs, linking inflammation with metabolic adaptation and drug tolerance (Zhang et al., 2022).

Plasma IL-6 and phosphorylated-STAT3 levels in T cells correlate with resistance to immune checkpoint inhibitors (ICIs); paradoxically, patients with high IL-6 expression respond better to anti-IL-6R plus anti-PD-1 therapy than to standard treatment (Nakano et al., 2022). Single-cell transcriptomic analysis revealed a population of $CXCL12^{+}$ stromal cells that chronically activate STAT3 and inhibit $CD8^{+}$T-cell infiltration (Xie, Chen, et al., 2025). Thus this study provides one perspective on how inflamed biomarkers can discriminate among immunotherapy response outcomes within the same microenvironment.

The merging of inflammation with metabolic dysregulation indicates that the induced metabolic signature functions as an accurate precision marker. Chronic hepatitis-associated cytokine exposure, primarily TNF-α and IL-6, causes hepatic JAK-STAT3 and NF-κB signaling to be activated and perturbs hepatic metabolism toward increased aerobic glycolysis and lipogenesis (Xie, Chen, et al., 2025). Relevant metabolomic analyzes identified succinate, lactate, and arachidonic acid derivatives as surrogate markers of cytokine-induced metabolic inflammation (Guo et al., 2024). Mechanistically, IL-6–STAT3 signaling upregulates HK2 and LDHA, promoting lactate accumulation, which acidifies the TME and stabilizes PD-L1 to enable immune evasion (Wang, Zhang, et al., 2024). Concurrently, TNF-α–NF-κB activation induces COX-2 and ALOX5, increasing prostaglandin and leukotriene production. The combination of markers has helped in the development of clinical models that help stratify patients such that profiles of serum PGE2, IL-6, and acyl carnitine predict sorafenib and lenvatinib resistance (Du et al., 2022; Pandey et al., 2024). These metabolites can be used to predict the effective treatment of a highly inflammatory-metabolic patient signature with a combination of JAK inhibitors and Fatty Acid Oxidation (FAO) blockers, resulting in metabolic-immune cotargeting, confirming the utility of metabolite-based, inflammation-driven biomarkers for translation into the clinic.

PDAC is the ultimate disease characterized by interplay between inflammation and the stroma, where a composite of stromal-inflammatory crosstalk markers defines the tumor architecture as well as its response to therapy (Pandey et al., 2024). The abundance of desmoplastic stroma containing cancer-associated fibroblasts (CAFs), along with the infiltration of inflammatory myeloid cells, is a constant release site for IL-1β, CXCL12, and TGF-β, which reciprocally activate NF-κB in both tumor cells and the tumor stroma (Fang et al., 2023). Spatial multiomics analysis of the SPARC platform revealed distinct inflammatory-fibroblast microenvironments in which coenrichment of IL-1β$^+$COX-2$^+$ fibroblasts was associated with immune exclusion and ICI resistance (Qu et al., 2021). Mechanistically, these inflammatory CAFs secrete CXCL12 to form chemokine gradients to capture cytotoxic T cells at the stromal interface and recruit M2 macrophages to establish an "immunological barrier" (Zhang et al., 2023). Typically, targeting this axis with CXCR4 antagonists or IL-1R blockade sensitizes tumors to immunotherapy, presenting clinical biomarkers for breaking up the stromal-inflammatory loop. Furthermore, circulating exosomal markers, such as CXCL12 and soluble IL-1R, are candidates for a minimally invasive biomarker of the inflammatory subtype of PDAC and treatment response (Klaver et al., 2024).

Gastric and lung cancers have long harbored chronic infections that drive chronic tumor-associated inflammation, which generates microbial immune markers in the form of molecular signatures for precision management. *Helicobacter pylori* drives gastric inflammation via NF-kB and IL-8 signaling, leading to COX-2-mediated, chronic epithelial cell renewal and DNA damage (Klaver et al., 2024; Sun et al., 2022). *H. pylori*-positive gastric tumors show increased expression of IL-8, CCL20, and PGE2, making up a biomarker signature that is indicative of intestinal-type histology and resistance to anti-VEGF therapy (Wilson & DuBois, 2022). Furthermore, bacterial virulence factors (including CagA and VacA) not only upregulate the expression of proinflammatory cytokines (IL-1β and TNF-α) but also remodel the tumor immune microenvironment, which links pathogen genotypes with inflammatory signatures and clinical phenotypes (Karbalaei et al., 2022).

Chronic viral inflammation is generally caused by oncogenic viruses such as HPV and EBV, which activate the STAT3–IRF1 axis and lead to the overexpression of PD-L1. In this manner, these viruses act in a similar way to cause disease as the other studies mentioned previously (Liu, Sadaoka, et al., 2020). A 2021 study showed that, compared with NSCLC, HPV+ NSCLC has a more pronounced IL-17–CXCL10–STAT3 inflammatory signature characterized by its responsiveness to PD-1 inhibitors (Eberhardt et al., 2021). These findings further reveal that infection-induced inflammation could be a positive predictive biomarker of immunotherapy response. This infection-derived biomarker panel can also capture the biological consequences of chronic inflammation and be translated into valuable tools for personalized immuno-oncology.

Studies have reported that cancer has inflammation from its conception—and not as an epiphenomenon following the activation of cancer stem cells—that this tumor-associated inflammation is driven by programs that leave molecular hallmarks across all cancers (Kennel et al., 2023; Sohrab et al., 2023). Inflammation manifests itself through patterns of cytokines, metabolic alterations, stromal–immune talk, or alterations in the behavior of microbes; therefore inflammatory biomarkers provide a global view of disease status and therapeutic potential. The incorporation of molecular/cellular inflammatory signatures into clinical settings allows for biomarker-driven segregation that could enable translational moves toward personalized, adaptive medicines whose inflation with learning evolves on the basis of an individual patient's inflammatory landscape.

8.2.3 Emerging technologies for biomarker detection and validation

The rapid progression of the latest high-resolution molecular technology has brought about changes in the detection and interpretation of inflammatory biomarkers while helping doctors better confirm and utilize them in clinical scenarios. Currently, advanced precision oncology is so developed that it requires more types of biodata, such as genomic, transcriptomic, proteomic, and metabolomic data, as well as information on the spatial relationships of tissues, and creates a system to interpret them together. In the last 3 years, tumor biomarker discovery derived through the integration of multiomic approaches, liquid biopsy improvements, AI-driven analyzes, and nanotech-based biosensor technologies has dramatically translated from bench to bedside as a method for detecting, sequencing, analyzing, and tracking tumor-related biomarkers longitudinally, thereby reshaping biomarker-driven precision medicine through noninvasive means and increasing both detection and spatiotemporal sensitivity.

Multiomic integration platforms are at the heart of biomarker research today. These platforms allow scientists to observe a very large part of cancer tumor generation driven by inflammation at various levels in an organism. Multiomics platforms such as genomics, transcriptomics, proteomics, and metabolomics can also provide different views of these molecular circuits that connect inflammation to tumor biology. As an example, an integrated proteogenomic study revealed that the IL-6–JAK–STAT3 metabolic axis in CRC drives coordinated transcriptional activation of inflammatory cytokines, proteomic upregulation of glycolytic enzymes, and lipidomic remodeling of the tumor stroma (Jeong et al., 2025).

A survey of the evolution of oncogenic and immune biomarkers across patient populations revealed that KRAS-mutant pancreatic cancers possess an NF-κB-driven cytokine module that predicts lackluster responses to immunotherapy (Luo, 2021). Broad surveys such as these indicate that inflammatory biomarkers do not exist as stand-alone pieces of molecular evidence but rather exist as parts of a highly layered and integrated system of signaling interactions, thus requiring their simultaneous collection across multiple omic dimensions. Among all these techniques, single-cell multiomics completely transforms our understanding of the inflammatory TME by simultaneously measuring the gene expression level, protein abundance, and state of chromatin accessibility in individual cells (Gao et al., 2022). Single-cell RNA sequencing, in combination with both mass cytometry (CyTOF) and CITE-seq proteomics, revealed that the transcriptional landscape of Tumor-Associated Macrophages (TAMs) is highly heterogeneous, resulting in their functional diversity (Seliger & Massa, 2025).

A seminal cell study revealed that a set of IL-1B+ COX2+ fibroblasts in PDAC creates an immune-exclusion microenvironment by modulating CXCL12 gradients; alongside this finding, parallel single-cell proteomics indicated that an IL-6/STAT3+ macrophage cluster is associated with adaptive resistance to PD-1 blockade (Martínez Fajardo et al., 2024; Yang et al., 2023). In parallel, single-cell ATAC-seq and phosphoproteomic integration highlight the need to incorporate epigenetic priming via NF-κB-dependent enhancers into the modeling of inflammatory transcriptional memory over time in HCC, whereas single-cell multiomics provides the critical level of resolution needed to deconvolve the complex circuitry behind such proinflammatory cells as part of the dissection of inflammation into its cellular and signaling molecular subsets (Hansen & Hodges, 2022). Furthermore, these multiomics studies enable refined, biomarker-based approaches to identify precise targets for therapeutic repositioning.

Spatial transcriptomics incorporates a spatial context into the molecular profile, revealing how different types of inflammatory and immune cells exist in the TME. Advances such as Visium Spatial Gene Expression or MERFISH have recently led to the development of methods capable of producing a transcriptome-wide map of the cytokine gradient, immune infiltrates, and stromal–immune interfaces (Cable et al., 2022). The 1β spatial expression gradient reflects the strong spatial correlation between proinflammatory macrophages (proImm) and exhausted T cells (Wang et al., 2022). This gradient is suggestive of immunotherapy resistance. In lung adenocarcinoma, StTx profiling revealed COX-2-rich niches located around the vasculature and exerting control over angiogenesis via PGF2α/PGES/PGE2 signaling, thus identifying new microanatomical biomarkers correlated with failure to respond to antiangiogenic therapy (Mondal et al., 2024). Thus the spatially resolved view of inflamed tissue leads to more precise typing of "hot," "cold," or "excluded" immune phenotypes, optimizing patient stratification as well as combination therapy design.

Additionally, liquid biopsy has been recognized as a noninvasive means of longitudinally monitoring inflammatory biomarkers in the past few years. Blood or biofluids contain circulating tumor DNA (ctDNA), exosomes, and cytokines that are significant predictors of cancer-associated inflammation (Abbate et al., 2023). Furthermore, exosomal IL-6, miR-21, and PGE2 were shown to indicate resistance to immune checkpoint therapy in HCC and NSCLC patients. Recently, digital droplet PCR, as well as ultradeep sequencing techniques, have been used to detect inflammatory pathway mutations (such as JAK1 and STAT3 mutations) in cttDNA below the sub0.1% allele frequency level, whereas multiplex cytokine assays have been able to simultaneously quantify more than 80 soluble inflammatory factors (Yu et al., 2024). By measuring the above circulatory biomarkers, early diagnosis, prognosis evaluation, and real-time therapeutic effect evaluation can be achieved in the clinic. These inflammatory factors may be used to measure changes in the inflammatory burden and immune status of patients.

AI and deep learning currently offer computing power to unravel the intricacies of inflammatory biomarker networks. Advanced AI frameworks, for example, Graph Neural Networks (GNNs) and transformer-based systems, can merge multicomponent data sources and provide predictions on the basis of novel inflammation-related biomarkers masked within these populations (Sun et al., 2024). One notable report described a study published in Nature Biotechnology, where an Long Short-Term Memory–Convolutional Neural Network (LSTM–CNN)–based combined deep learning network was proposed (Ma et al., 2022). A learning framework integrating histopathological images with transcriptomic inflammation signatures across 14 cancer types was developed, and more than 90% accuracy was obtained in predicting the response to ICIs (Kuenzi et al., 2020). AI clustering analysis of single-cell transcriptome data has revealed unrecognized inflammatory subpopulations in PDAC and gastric cancer, leading to the identification of new biomarker panels (Mercanti et al., 2023). Machine learning models can be used to improve biomarker validation, cross-cohort reproducibility tests, predictive scores, and automatic patient stratification for adaptive clinical trial design.

Complementing the strides made by computers, nanotechnology-based biosensors allow for real-time detection and ultrasensitive quantification of biomarkers of inflammation present in biofluids by detecting cytokines, including IL-6, TNF-α, and CRP, at femtomolar concentrations (Palazuelos et al., 2024). Owing to this, monitoring these markers at the point of care, a service that is normally only available at special laboratory facilities, is now possible. Research has revealed that graphene-based electrochemical biosensors can detect inflammatory cytokines and exosomal miRNAs simultaneously in less than 10 min for the detection of inflammatory cytokines and exosomal miRNAs, suggesting promising clinical applications for monitoring the inflammatory response follow-up of CRC/pancreatic cancer patients treated with immunotherapy (Boroujerdi & Paul, 2022). By applying nanodevices to wearable devices, continuous real-time inflammation monitoring is feasible, achieving a significant step toward personalized and adaptive health care.

8.3 Linking biomarkers to personalized therapeutic strategies

8.3.1 Stratified treatment models

The inclusion of inflammation biomarkers in the therapy selection process has led to the conversion of cancer therapeutics from intuitive strategies to precise and targeted interventions. Inflammation-driven tumors exhibit an extremely complex pattern of immune infiltration, metabolic status, and stromal structure, all of which can now be measured quantitatively via multiplex omic biomarker panels. As such, stratification treatment modalities have emerged. Biomarker-defined subgroups receive targeted therapies that are tuned to fit their unique inflammation dependence profile. In the past 3 years, the integration of multiple types of genomic-, immunologic-, and metabolic-based biomarkers—ranging from PD-L1 expression and Tumor Mutational Burden (TMB) to cytokine-driven immune subtypes—has led clinicians to predict the response to immunotherapy and rational combinations with antiinflammatory agents for blocking immune checkpoint targets to overcome resistance (Rizvi et al., 2018).

Biomarker-guided immunotherapy is the most evolved model of personalized medicine, with immune and inflammatory responses specifically guiding which treatment a patient should receive. PD-L1 remains the canonical biomarker for predicting responsiveness to PD-1/PD-L1 inhibitors, yet its predictive power is context-dependent and modulated by the inflammatory milieu (Yi et al., 2022). Recent studies have shown that PD-L1 positivity is correlated with therapeutic benefit only when accompanied by a proinflammatory cytokine signature, particularly elevated IFN-γ, IL-6, and CXCL9/10 (Lim et al., 2024; Pan et al., 2023). In NSCLC, a high TMB (≥10 mut/Mb) combined with a strong IL-6–STAT3-driven transcriptional program identifies a hyperinflammatory but immunosuppressive subtype that paradoxically responds better to combination therapy than to checkpoint blockade alone (Levy et al., 2023). Similarly, CRCs characterized by MSI-high and IL-1β-enriched profiles exhibit improved sensitivity to PD-1 inhibitors due to an increased neoantigen load and local immune activation, whereas microsatellite-stable CRCs with high IL-8 and TGF-β signatures remain refractory (Lin et al., 2023).

In addition to PD-L1 and TMB, multidimensional inflammatory signatures are emerging as next-generation biomarkers for therapy stratification: a 2024-cell analysis of >1000 solid tumors integrated single-cell transcriptomics and proteomics to delineate three recurrent cytokine-driven immune subtypes—(1) IL-6/STAT3-high tumors enriched for myeloid-derived suppressor cells and T-cell exhaustion programs, (2) TNF-α/NF-κB-active tumors marked by stromal inflammation and angiogenic remodeling, and (3) IFN-γ-dominant tumors harboring robust cytotoxic lymphocyte infiltration—each offering distinct therapeutic vulnerabilities (Shi, Wang, et al., 2024).

Currently, antiinflammatory cotherapies are being increasingly included in immunotherapy treatments as efforts to modulate hostile inflammatory microenvironments that suppress effective immune surveillance intensify. Chronic inflammation can establish immunosuppressive feedback loops via cytokine production, prostaglandin synthesis, and immune checkpoint upregulation, all of which offer potential for pharmacological targeting. COX-2 inhibitors could provide such a possibility. They have recently gained popularity because of their prominent antiinflammatory efficacy, making them an ideal tool for reversing prostaglandin-induced immune paralysis, demonstrating the potential of coadministering them with PD-1 blockade to turn "cold" tumors such as those in PDAC and NSCLC into "cold" immunogenic tumors amenable to T-cell infiltration and antigen presentation (Liu, Yang, et al., 2025). COX-2 inhibition blocks the pathway from PGE2→EP4→β-catenin to inhibit dendritic cell activation and promote Tregs (Liu, Yang, et al., 2025).

IL-6 blockade has been shown to be a promising coadjuvant for immunotherapy, especially for inflammatory types of cancers such as HCC and CRC, where serum IL-6 levels are correlated with checkpoint inhibitor resistance and systemic inflammatory toxicity. Tocilizumab (an anti-IL-6R antibody) or sarilumab combined with PD-1 inhibitors has resulted in significantly improved antitumor immunity (Xie, Yuan, et al., 2025). It has been utilized to treat immune-related adverse effects. IL-6 inhibition interferes with the STAT3–PD-L1–MDSC axis, restores the cytotoxic activity of CD8+ T cells, and reestablishes an inflammatory milieu. Targeted combined therapy with NF-κB or CXCL8/IL-8 signaling and immunotherapy has been explored in early-stage clinical trials, showing that neutralization of IL-8 enhances T-cell recruitment and overcomes stromal resistance to immunotherapy in treatment-refractory gastric cancer or lung cancer (Fabian et al., 2020).

Biomarker-guided immunotherapy coupled with antiinflammatory cotargeting has led to a shift from conventional oncology to precision oncology. In lieu of an effort to increase only immune activation, it is now about precisely modulating inflammation to maximize therapeutic efficacy while minimizing side effects. Multiomics biomarkers track cytokine levels, immune infiltration, and exosomal inflammatory signature changes in real time, allowing adaptive therapies. Patients with persistent increases in circulating IL-6, CRP, or PGE2 levels within the first two cycles of ICB treatment should be potential candidates for the addition of IL-6R or COX-2 inhibitors, as shown in ongoing adaptive clinical trials (Boumelha et al., 2024).

8.3.2 Adaptive clinical trial designs

The tumor-centric clinical research paradigm has been transformed under the impetus of these innovative adaptive trial designs that break from the established, inflexible framework toward flexibility and biomarker-informed strategies. In particular, basket and umbrella trials combine inflammatory biomarker signatures in the context of a large collection of patient data to divide individuals and monitor response across numerous therapies. The accelerated rate of biomarker discoveries, computational analyzes, and real-time monitoring techniques experienced over the last 3 years has enabled the application of adaptive trials from hypotheses and explorations into meaningful, functional instruments for precision clinical immunotherapy and the treatment of inflammation-driven cancers (CRC, Principal Component (PC), and HCC) in the clinic (Bagchi et al., 2024; Jia et al., 2018).

Basket trials are horizontally structured adaptive designs enrolling patients from many different cancer types with shared molecular or inflammation-related biomarkers instead of those with shared tissue origins; this design works well for testing agents targeting inflammation signaling pathways, which can span more than just one type of tissue. For example, the IMPRINT-1 basket trial evaluated a combination IL-6 blockador. This is the result of combining tocilizumab and PD-1 inhibition in a group of patients with increased levels of systemic IL-6 or CRP in 7 different solid tumors, irrespective of cancer type. In early cycles of treatment, if the circulating IL-6 level is reduced consistently, then progression-free survival is much prolonged (Bamane et al., 2021). The INFLAME-BASKET study targeted solid tumors that were overactivated due to hyperactivation of the NF-kB-TNF-α axis (Bakshi et al., 2022). A combination of IKKβ inhibitors and ICB revealed that biomarker-defined inflammation signatures, rather than tumor histology, determine the efficacy of combination therapy. These pantumor, inflammation-based basket designs stratify trials on the basis of molecular phenotype rather than organ system, which is beneficial in accelerating the repurposing of drugs to inflammatory subtypes across multiple malignancies.

In contrast, umbrella trials apply a vertically integrated model within a single tumor type, stratifying patients according to their unique inflammatory biomarker profiles and assigning them to different therapeutic arms. A notable example is the PRECISION-CRC umbrella trial, which classified CRC patients into three inflammation-defined cohorts: (1) IL-6/STAT3-dominant, (2) COX-2/PGE2-high, and (3) IL-1β/TNF-α coactivated. Each subgroup received tailored therapy combinations—IL-6R blockade plus PD-1 inhibition, COX-2 inhibitors with antiangiogenic therapy, and TNF-α inhibitors combined with chemotherapy (Duan et al., 2024). Interim analyzes demonstrated not only increased response rates but also a significant reduction in immune-related adverse events, validating the feasibility of biomarker-guided adaptive therapy allocation. Similarly, the HCC-ADAPT platform trial utilized circulating exosomal PGE2 and serum CRP as real-time biomarkers to dynamically modulate dosing schedules of COX-2 and JAK inhibitors, marking one of the first prospective applications of inflammatory biomarker feedback in trial design (Xiong et al., 2023).

In adaptive trials, the most essential part is real-time biomarker adaptation, which involves tracking molecular and immune signatures over time to dictate real-time changes in treatment. Liquid biopsy techniques such as ctDNA and exosomal cytokines, coupled with the use of AI for predicting changes, help predict changes in a patient's ever-changing inflammation situation to modify the corresponding treatment in an adaptive manner (Al Bakir et al., 2023). The ADAPT-IMMUNE-2025 trial, published in Nature Biotechnology in 2025, employs machine learning models of repeated measurements of IL-6, TNF-α, and PD-L1 levels from the peripheral blood and adjustable combinations of checkpoint inhibitors, JAK blockers, or COX-2 antagonists on the basis of these (Palazuelos et al., 2024). This enables an optimized loop system where biomarker fluctuation is a promptable action to apply predetermined intervention alterations, which leads to a repeating cycle of reduced overtreatment, lower immune toxicity, and long-term efficacy by having a degree of coherence between the therapy burden and the magnitude of the inflammatory response in real time.

From both regulatory and operational points of view, the ability to adopt an adaptive trial design allows the formation of a data-driven and learning healthcare system, such as those already adopted by platforms such as the FDA's CID Program and the EMA's Adaptive Pathways Initiative (Sharpee et al., 2016; Sheban et al., 2025). In addition, decentralized data infrastructure has the ability to incorporate multiomic, radiomic, and immunologic biomarkers from electronic health records (EHRs) in adaptive trial design algorithms. Through the combination of a flexible regulation platform, computational analytics pipeline, and translational biomarker science, an optimal standardization framework for the adaptive trial process of evolving treatments in line with tumor biology is undergoing changes (Román-Villarán et al., 2022).

8.3.3 Precision drug development

Precision oncology has advanced to a stage in which drugs can be developed on the basis of inflammatory biomarker feedback loops, altering the manner in which targets are discovered, validated, and optimized. Inflammation-induced carcinogenesis occurs because cytokines, chemokines, prostaglandins, and immune-modulating molecules inside the TME trigger inflammation-mediated carcinogenesis. In addition, this inflammation not only promotes tumor growth but also induces cell migration and infiltration from blood vessels. Moreover, they direct drug response and resistance mechanisms. Utilization of real-time biomarker analytics allows integration with preclinical models and early-phase trials for the creation of precise drugs that can modulate inflammation levels within the tumor, acting on the evolving state of the tumor's microenvironment on a real-time molecular signal–therapeutic intervention loop, thus forming a positive feedback cycle (Xu et al., 2025). This idea, developed over the last 3 years, has now been developed as a translational framework connecting the TME with inflammation control, multiomic biomarker discovery, and adaptive pharmacological optimization.

At the core of the proposed approach is the targeting of inflammatory factors in the TME, which are believed to drive immune suppression and give rise to resistance to therapy. Key cytokines such as IL-6, IL-1B, and TNF-α and lipid mediators such as PGE2 and leukotrienes orchestrate the recruitment and polarization of MDSCs, Tregs, and TAMs (Yang & Lin, 2017). This is done to form a state where the immune system is not triggered. The combination of dual targeting of inflammatory mediators (COX-2/PGE2 and TNF-α), which was achieved with celecoxib and infliximab, improved the efficacy of checkpoint inhibitors, as reported by Nature Medicine (Yang & Lin, 2017). Furthermore, targeting inflammatory mediators (COX-2/PGE2 and TNF-α) through both inhibitors substantially inhibited the fibroinflammatory microenvironment and promoted fibroinflammatory microenvironment remodeling in patients with PDAC by increasing CD8+ T-cell infiltration and reducing collagen deposition, indicating that targeting inflammatory mediators can also initiate immune restoration, which places inflammation at the core of precise drug design (Zhao, Cheng, et al., 2024).

Another expanding area is the interaction between metabolism and the TME, where crosstalk between inflammation and metabolism impacts tumor maintenance. Approaches targeting inflammation-induced metabolic mediators have been efficacious, as STAT3 inhibitors can ablate STAT3–mediated signaling to disrupt IL-6-induced glycolysis and lactate-driven immune suppression in CRC (Kanarek et al., 2010). Moreover, the inhibition of ALOX5, which blocks the synthesis of leukotrienes, reduces M2 macrophage polarization and angiogenesis (MacE et al., 2018).

In HCC, small-molecule EP4 antagonists are under clinical investigation to block the effect of PGE2-mediated immune exclusion in microsatellite-stable CRC and gastric cancer (Durham et al., 2022; Kang et al., 2024). All of these therapeutic strategies require real-time biomarker surveillance (plasma IL-6, exosomal PGE2, and tumor-infiltrating immune signatures) to inform dosing decisions and optimally time combined therapies for maximum therapeutic efficacy while minimizing the risk of unwanted side effects, such as autoimmunity, and can be validated with cohorts from current PRODIGY trials and additional phase III trials. Current work on a continuous inflammasome-state feedback loop is already advancing as part of the INFLA-PRECISION program, which longitudinally monitors cytokines and metabolites to finely tune the interleukin-6-janus kinase 1, IL-6 antibody, and ICI combinations as determined by IL-6 levels at baseline or during treatment (Liu et al., 2024). A similar level of disruption is likely to be seen with drug design on the basis of a biomarker feedback loop scalable for continuously providing molecular profiles to drive adaptive drugs, thus updating drug information on the basis of real-time data from each patient. This concept is the basis of control theory to develop "intelligent therapeutics" in which therapeutically active molecules monitor and sense biology and then adjust their pharmacodynamic output. Nature Biotechnology reported that such an approach has led to new iterations of these kinds of adaptive dosing systems using IL-6 as input (Igawa et al., 2010).

The use of TNF-α and CRP to modify cytokine-targeting biologic dosing schedules in real time would maximize efficacy and safety in pilot oncology clinical trials. Likewise, biosensor-coupled nanocarriers that are equipped with pH- and cytokine-sensitive release mechanisms can detect inflammation (such as high IL-8 or ROS) in the TME and respond by releasing local antiinflammatory or immunomodulatory cargo (Delhase et al., 1999). They are so-called "smart drug systems" and embody the concept of a closed-loop pharmacotherapy system where biomarker variations work as feedback signals that continually improve therapeutic delivery. Biomarker feedback loops have been used since the beginning of drug discovery and are used in silico/AI-supported pharmacogenomic models to simulate how a certain compound influences inflammatory signaling. Models trained with a combination of both clinical and omic data can be used to determine the best molecules that can block a network with inflammatory signals, making them ineffective at minimizing the risk of immune toxicity (Rupp et al., 2017). A study in 2025 has illustrated the application of this approach. By using a reinforcement learning algorithm to continuously evaluate the impacts of candidate drugs on biomarker trajectories such as IL-1β reduction, NF-κB deactivation, and metabolic normalization, it is possible to perform computer-based "prevalidation" of the effects before resorting to tests on animals or humans (Cao et al., 2025). Combining predictive informatics with adaptive biology decreases the translational cycle from biomarker discovery to use in the clinic and lays the groundwork for the near real-time, biomarker-driven evolution of drug development (Fig. 8.3).

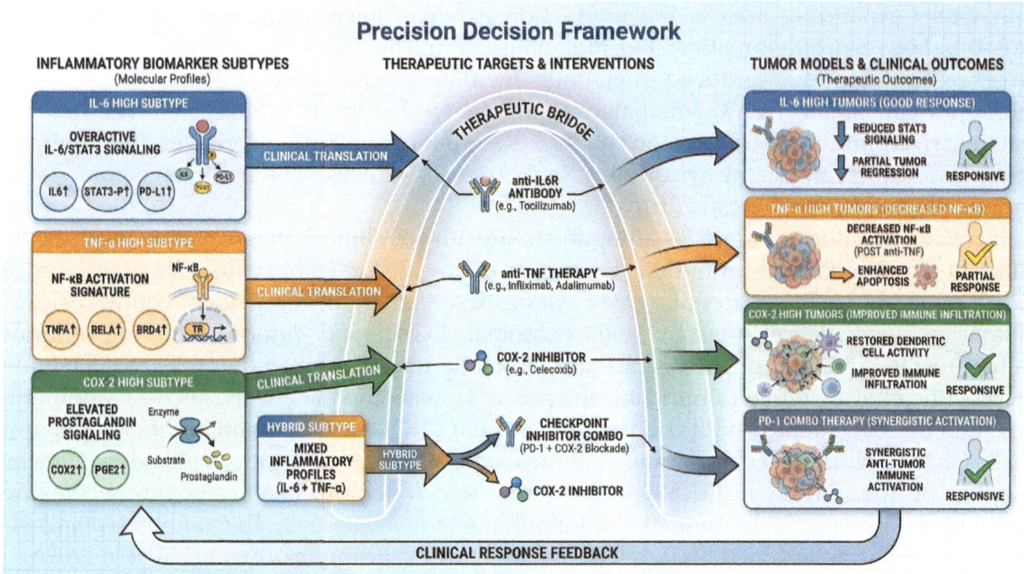

FIGURE 8.3 Translational bridge linking inflammatory biomarkers to precision therapeutic strategies. Schematic representation of biomarker-guided precision oncology. Distinct inflammatory subtypes—IL-6–high, TNF-α–high, and COX-2–high—are mapped to their corresponding targeted interventions (anti-IL6R, anti-TNF, and COX-2 inhibitors) and therapeutic combinations (PD-1 plus COX-2 blockade). The diagram illustrates a closed "diagnosis–subtyping–therapy–response" loop, highlighting how inflammatory signaling profiles inform individualized treatment decisions and clinical outcomes.

8.3.4 Patient monitoring and feedback loops

The crux of personalized medicine is to integrate biomarker dynamics into real-time decision-making processes in clinical settings, transforming cancer from a static, protocol-driven field to an adaptive, feedback-based system. Under the pressure of therapy, the biological behavior of the tumor, as well as the inflammatory environment, changes very quickly, so conventional endpoint-based evaluations (such as imaging) are no longer able to evaluate patients' response to drugs in a timely manner during trials. Pathology often cannot fully represent the molecular or immune patterns that lead to a patient's response or nonresponse to treatment. Patients could greatly benefit from continuously monitoring biomarker trajectories in their circulation or the TME and using these data to modulate treatment on an ongoing basis (Ishizuka et al., 2019). As a result, a constantly adaptable clinical dose will be able to maintain a balance between efficacy and immune toxicity that is far closer to ideal. Over the last 3 years, it has become possible for these concepts to be realized through the integration of real-time multiomic biomarker monitoring, liquid biopsy analysis, AI, and CL-CFS, which can be used to recalibrate therapy in near-real time (Hu et al., 2019; Jia et al., 2022).

The key to evolution is the idea that inflammatory biomarker dynamics represent the biological "pulse" of the tumor-immune ecosystem. Within days after the initiation of therapy, cytokines such as IL-6, TNF-α, and IFN-γ, and lipid mediators such as PGE2, exhibit oscillations that may provide short-term biomarkers for predicting the therapeutic response or developing resistance (Trehan et al., 2025). Nature Medicine has shown that rapid normalization of plasma I is associated with an increased therapeutic response in immuno-oncology therapy (Niu et al., 2022).

Whether the increase in CRP levels within 2 weeks after the start of checkpoint inhibitor therapy correlates with the durability of the response in NSCLC patients, whereas a long-term increase in IL-6 indicates macrophage-mediated immunotherapy resistance. Likewise, in HCC, oscillations in exosomal IL-1β, miR-21, and circulating CD163+ macrophage-derived vesicles correlate with radiological progression several weeks prior (Liu, Yu, et al., 2025). In this respect, the finding is in line with the growing consensus that the actual prognostic value of biomarkers does not rely on static values alone but on biomarker kinetics; thus biomarkers can provide information that is not accessible through static measurements, an insight that will enable future therapeutic decision-making.

To turn this paradigm into a reality, today's medical oncology has already integrated AI-driven biomarker feedback loops into clinical decision-support systems, in which ongoing longitudinal data collection of patient molecular information has become an input stream for AI evaluation. Bayesian modeling and reinforcement learning are used to update the prediction model on the basis of incoming data, for example, cytokines, ctDNA, or metabolite ratios; accordingly, therapeutic inputs such as drug dose, combination, or schedule may also be tuned (Helmink et al., 2020). The INFLA-TRACK program, which was developed by Nature Biotechnology in 2024, uses deep learning methods to read the details of changes in cytokines and ctDNAs to monitor the tumor evolution of patients receiving anti-IL-6/PD-1 combination therapy (Quail et al., 2022). "Adaptive dosing recommendations" for emerging inflammatory toxicity or immune escape may be offered on the basis of changes in these biomarkers. The same model was applied across cancers, where stromal inflammation-driven immune exclusion often depends on a stromal inflammation-regulated model in which the CXCL12-dependent feedback cycle is monitored (Peng et al., 2015).

IL-1β and TGF-β in plasma and the timing of CXCR4 antagonist administration can modify the effects of CXCR4 antagonists on immune penetration. Such a system can predict the therapeutic outcome on the basis of virtual copies that mimic patients' molecular trajectories, making real-world adjustments in patients by modifying the management strategy of existing TAC serum levels and pretreatments of known pathophysiologies, thus avoiding clinical relapse or disease exacerbation (Papalexi & Satija, 2018). By virtue of technological advances, the dynamism of biomarkers can be monitored continuously in a minimally invasive way with the aid of biosensors being either implanted or worn. Nanoplasmonic- or graphene-based microfluidic sensors can now sense cytokines (IL-6, TNF-α, and IFN-γ) at femtomolar levels, whether measured from sweat, saliva, or interstitial fluids, as such information may then be transmitted to cloud-based AI systems to undergo real-time analysis (Liu, Yang, et al., 2020).

A wearable inflammation biosensor patch described in a paper in Nature Nanotechnology can monitor multiple cytokines and exosomal microRNAs at the same time to predict the occurrence of immune hyperactivation and cytokine storms in cancer patients treated with immunotherapy (Wang et al., 2011). When fed into hospital monitoring networks, the data stream from such devices can immediately trigger clinicians to adjust the schedules of corticosteroid prophylaxis, checkpoint inhibitors, or antiinflammatory cotherapy, in hours instead of weeks—an unprecedented improvement in therapeutic agility. It also enables the integration of these data flows into existing EHRs and cloud-based decision support systems so that real-time population-level learning can occur—where biomarker response pattern data across many patients can continuously improve predictive model performance as part of an ongoing cycle of improving clinical intelligence (Wang et al., 2011).

Clinically, this is a biomarker-driven feedback circuit that loops over sensing, prediction, and adaptation. Inflammation-related biomarkers that are terminal diagnostic measures at one point have become dynamic control parameters of a living therapeutic algorithm. For example, multiple trials in CRC (PRECISION-IMMU 2025) and gastric cancer patients will use circulating plasma IL-6/CRP and plasma exosomal PD-L1 for the purpose of turning on or off the therapeutic response by autoswitching systems of anti-IL-6R antibodies, JAK inhibitors, or immune checkpoint therapies on the basis of the real-time threshold of immune activity (Weng et al., 2025). Additionally, real-time toxicities can be detected through machine learning-based real-time predictions, thereby making immune toxicity adjustment feasible when they do not cause any apparent clinical symptoms. Eventually, the integration of biomarker feedback loops in patient monitoring brings a precision oncology full circle and turns it into a fully realized system-level framework wherein each patient's treatment will be an evolving self-learning process from the beginning to the end. This closed loop converts changes in biomarkers into actionable information that synchronizes treatment with the molecular state of the disease at all times. Liquid biopsy platforms are already underway to accommodate biomarker inputs (Yuan et al., 2025). Combining biosensor technology with AI analytics allows cancer therapy to follow an adaptive physiological process that can be constantly adjusted according to the rhythm and timing of inflammation and immune equilibrium; therefore future oncologists could also be clinicians and system engineers to orchestrate therapy based on a cyberbioecological ecosystem where real-time biomarker feedback plays a key role in advancing the intelligence of precision medicine (Yuan et al., 2025).

8.4 Translational challenges and future perspectives: toward systems-level precision oncology

While biomarker-guided precision medicine has grown quickly, translating it from the laboratory to practice poses difficult biological, technical, regulatory, and ethical issues. Inflammatory cancers especially represent a hard problem for translational research; rather than evolving linearly in time, tumors are marked by mutations driven by fluctuating cytokine networks, metabolic reprogramming, and immune modulation, making true system-level precision oncology an area that will benefit greatly from further work to implement molecular, cellular, and digital forms of intelligence in building adaptive multidimensional frameworks continuously feeding back into themselves as a living ecosystem.

Genetic heterogeneity remains the largest barrier to universal biomarker applications. Even if all patients have the same biomarker at the cellular level, intratumoural heterogeneity causes divergent responses to immunotherapy on the basis of clonal differences, such as the inflammatory and genetic subclones present in one patient (Wang, Zhao, et al., 2024).

Gene expression profiling from different single-cell locations revealed that inflammatory pathways such as IL-6-STAT3 or NF-κB activation generate and maintain heterogeneity (Chen et al., 2024).

In addition to interpatient heterogeneity, germline variations, microbiota, and environmental exposures further add variability. The results from a previous study revealed that patients with CRC, hepatocellular cancer, and the same KRAS or TP53 mutation presented distinct cytokine maps and different immunotherapy responses when their microbiota metabolites were altered (Bagchi et al., 2024). Thus it is essential for us to consider the spatial features, metabolic features, and immunological features of biomarkers instead of judging the status with only a single number.

Technical reproducibility and standardization pose considerable difficulties when advancing from the translational study of biomarkers to their use in the clinic. The multifaceted nature of the omics present in the discovery process—such as genomics, proteomics, metabolomics, and spatial transcriptomics—determines various levels of variance. Sample preparation techniques, data standardization methods, and computational procedures all generate somewhat different outputs. Recently, established consortia such as HTAN (Human Tumor Atlas Network) or Immune-Mediated Inflammation (IMI) OncoBioMap have advocated for standardized reference protocols for single-cell or spatial multiomics to ensure consistency between multiple platforms (Shi, Han, et al., 2024). However, even in such groups, robust analytical validation remains scarce, especially in regard to proteomic and metabolomic biomarkers, owing to the wide variation of these measurements over time and their low baselines, making them much harder to measure reproducibly. In the future, regulatory approval may require the use of both validated assays and harmonization across all analytical workflows at different testing sites for any biomarker-aided clinical decision-making to be reproducible in various settings across different healthcare systems globally.

In addition to technological barriers, ethical and data governance problems become more important with the increase in data intensity and algorithmic mediation for biomarker-driven precision medicine. Multiomics biomarker data are composed of genomic, immunologic, and behavioral information to form a molecular "molecular fingerprint" for people, leading to significant concerns about privacy, consent, and algorithmic bias. AI is leveraged to make a precise prediction of the clinical prognosis. Inflammatory trajectories or therapeutic responses to precision medicine require strict data security measures to prevent possible misuse. Furthermore, the lack of equitable access to technology renders data from low- and middle-income countries insufficient, resulting in a lack of data in certain biomarker databases, which may introduce bias into clinical algorithms. In response to this issue, the OECD Global Biomarker Governance Framework and the EU AI Act on Health Data have started defining ethically sound principles of application of algorithmic biomarkers, emphasizing the importance of transparency, interpretability, and obtaining informed consent (Hopf et al., 2024). Nevertheless, as far as system-level oncology is concerned, balancing the interests of patients' privacy with the need for innovations would always be an endless pursuit.

As biomarker science becomes increasingly sophisticated, the regulatory validation pathway is evolving in parallel. Unlike traditional, static, single-endpoint therapeutics—which rely on fixed, solitary diagnostic indices—multiomics inflammatory biomarkers are dynamic and context dependent, leveraging biological heterogeneity (Huang, Wu, et al., 2025).

Adaptive biomarker data can inform critical clinical decisions for patients. Regulators have recently converged on a tiered framework that demands that biological plausibility, analytical performance, and clinical utility be fully validated before integration (Pelka et al., 2021). Adaptive regulatory models such as the "living biomarker dossier" update biomarker data in real time, mirroring the iterative nature of precision oncology. This coevolution of regulatory science and biomarker discovery is shifting the paradigm from one-time, static validation to continuous certification.

Economic sustainability is the major obstacle for developing biomarker-driven therapy from research settings into routine clinical practice. Multiomics approaches, spatial sequencing, and real-time biomarker monitoring require substantial resources, and their applicability is often limited by cost, so cost–benefit analysis tends to favor therapies with the best therapeutic efficiency that can avoid the ineffectiveness of biomarker-stratified therapies as well as reduce adverse events (Gomerdinger et al., 2025). The Lancet Oncology published an article on a new economic model for triple-negative breast cancer in which it was shown that allocating targeted immune therapies for patients with inflammatory signatures may reduce overall treatment cost by up to 27% while increasing median survival by 18% (Fan et al., 2024). These data demonstrate the long-term financial benefits of utilizing precision biomarker-driven therapeutics, although their adoption still depends upon developing cost-effective miniaturized assays and open-source bioinformatics and incorporating digital decentralized platforms that provide real-time analytics in resource-constrained settings.

Looking forward, in the coming decade, studies can integrate biology, computation, and systems engineering toward digital twin-based precision oncology, with the development of patient-specific, continuous updates of digital twin models that emulate individuals and take into account disease trajectories along with the probability of therapeutic success via information on genomics, transcriptomics, proteomics, metabolomics, and various clinical biomarkers. Shifting from reactivity to proactiveness in the clinician's arsenal for preventing inflammation-driven oncogenesis opens up the real opportunity to target those elusive tipping points of irreversible immune exhaustion or premetastatic progression that would be very difficult to target once these stages have progressed far enough.

The field has moved away from static biomarkers toward dynamic biomarker ecosystems that constantly update themselves and become more cognizant of their context as they make real-time adjustments to our biology. In this way, biomarkers are no longer seen as fixed indicators but instead form part of evolving adaptive networks in which biomarkers continually engage with therapy, environmental factors, and host factors. This allows for the creation of closed-loop, continuously learning personalized medicine systems where biomarker data can be automatically piped into AI-driven decision engines that are capable of refining treatment regimens. This will lead to a future world where medicine becomes self-correcting, driven by data, and biosynchronized so that treatment can seamlessly match tumor biology (Fig. 8.4).

Progress toward a more systems-level approach in precision oncology is needed, rather than advanced technology, to guide it through its journey and change its mental perspective on viewing biomarkers as one-time live detection signals for patient-specific disease instead of being a set of unchanging indicators of an inert substance. Additionally, biological heterogeneity, ethical grounds, regulatory understanding, and the economic burden of such innovative medicine should be considered. Integration of the biological heterogeneity,

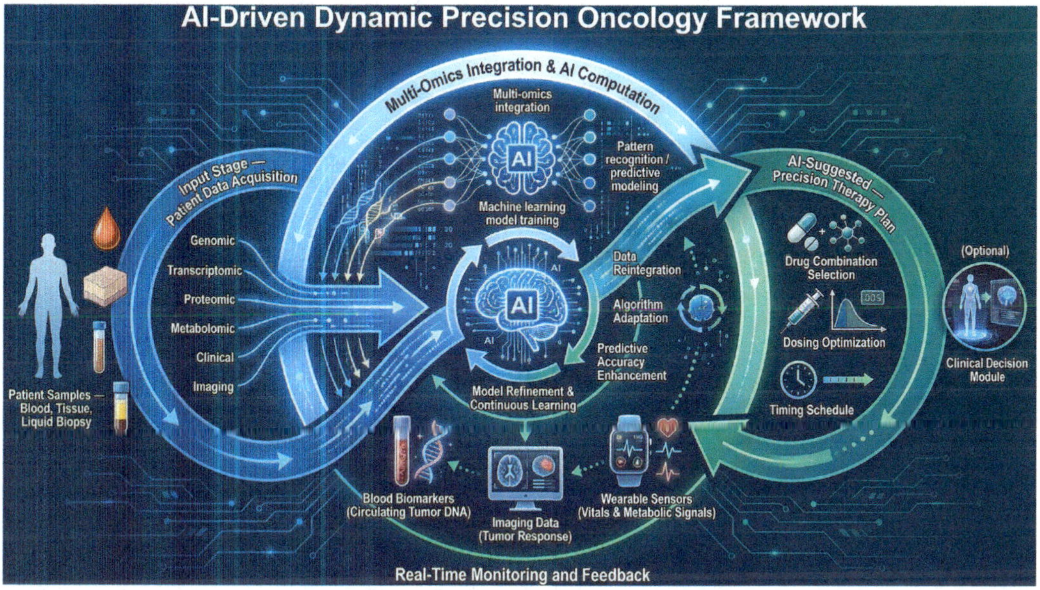

FIGURE 8.4 AI-driven dynamic precision oncology framework. A conceptual model illustrating an AI-guided, closed-loop system for personalized cancer therapy. Patient-derived samples (blood, tissue, and liquid biopsy) undergo multiomics profiling and computational integration through machine learning to generate individualized treatment strategies, including optimized drug combinations, dosing, and timing. Real-time clinical monitoring continuously feeds data back into the AI model, enabling adaptive learning and digital twin–based precision oncology.

ethical responsibility, regulatory understanding, and economic burden of such a personalized treatment would enable the desired real-time learning and result in biomarker-guided precision medicine, where chronic and acute inflammation could serve as important indicators and targets that reveal a person's health or illness status.

8.5 Conclusion

Biomarkers serve as critical junctions between understanding inflammation biology and personalized oncology. They can translate molecular complexity into intelligible and specific targeted treatment methods. As our understanding of cancer evolves, real-time monitoring is important for appropriate therapeutic intervention according to disease progression. This is expected to become one aspect of the coming translational oncology toward a more efficacious biomarker-integrated omics multimodality integrated system powered by machine learning and technology, becoming a system of self-optimization. In this promising era of biomarker-guided precision oncology, tumors will no longer be seen as a single massive disease but as diseases with distinct subtypes that warrant a different therapeutic approach; personalized treatments will then adapt to individual disease conditions accordingly. The contents of inflammatory pathway biomarkers used in precision therapeutics are summarized in Table 8.1.

TABLE 8.1 Inflammatory pathway biomarkers in precision therapeutics.

Material examples	Primary mechanisms	Molecular pathways targeted	Therapeutic outcomes	Advantages/ Innovations	Challenges and limitations	References
IL-6 inhibitors	Neutralize IL-6 signaling to reduce proinflammatory cytokine cascade	IL-6/JAK/ STAT3 axis	Reduces tumor-promoting inflammation and improves immunotherapy response	Target-specific cytokine blockade with clinical applicability	Potential systemic immunosuppression; patient-specific cytokine variability	Huseni et al. (2023), Wang et al. (2024), Johnson et al. (2018)
NF-κB pathway inhibitors	Inhibit transcription of proinflammatory and antiapoptotic genes	NF-κB/IKKβ signaling	Sensitize tumor cells to chemotherapy and apoptosis	Reverses inflammation-induced drug resistance	Broad pathway inhibition may affect normal immune function	Kulesza et al. (2023), Cappuyns et al. (2025)
COX-2 inhibitors	Suppress prostaglandin E2 synthesis to modulate tumor microenvironment	COX-2/PGE2 pathway	Inhibit angiogenesis, tumor proliferation, and immune evasion	Safe repurposing of approved NSAIDs for oncology	Limited selectivity; risk of cardiovascular toxicity	Kulesza et al. (2023), Hu et al. (2022), Di et al. (2024)
miRNA-based biomarkers	Posttranscriptional regulation of inflammatory signaling and tumorigenesis	NF-κB/STAT3/TLR signaling	Early detection and predictive biomarker for therapy response	Noninvasive liquid biopsy potential	Low reproducibility across cohorts	Boutilier and Elsawa (2021), Zhang et al. (2022)
Exosomal biomarkers	Circulating exosomes mediate intercellular inflammation signaling	Exosome–cytokine–STAT3 pathway	Enable real-time monitoring of tumor–immune interactions	Dynamic, minimally invasive diagnostic platform	High heterogeneity; technical standardization required	Jeong et al. (2025), Mercanti et al. (2023)
Multiomics integration models	Combine transcriptomics, proteomics, and metabolomics for patient stratification	Cross-pathway network analysis (IL-6, NF-κB, and COX-2)	Personalized therapeutic optimization and prediction	AI-enhanced modeling for precision medicine	Data integration complexity; computational demand	Jeong et al. (2025), Luo (2021), Gao et al. (2022)
Inflammation-targeted nanoparticles	Controlled delivery of antiinflammatory agents to tumor sites	NF-κB/IL-1β/COX-2 cascade	Enhanced local drug efficacy, reduced systemic toxicity	Smart drug delivery with high specificity	Limited clinical translation thus far	Zhao, Cheng, et al. (2024), Durham et al. (2022), Kang et al. (2024)

References

Abbate, J. M., Arfuso, F., Riolo, K., Giudice, E., Brunetti, B., & Lanteri, G. (2023). Upregulation of miR-21 and pro-inflammatory cytokine genes IL-6 and TNF- α in promoting a pro-tumorigenic microenvironment in canine mammary carcinomas. *Research in Veterinary Science, 164*, 105014. https://doi.org/10.1016/j.rvsc.2023.105014.

Al Bakir, M., Huebner, A., Martínez-Ruiz, C., Grigoriadis, K., Watkins, T. B. K., Pich, O., Moore, D. A., Veeriah, S., Ward, S., Laycock, J., Johnson, D., Rowan, A., Razaq, M., Akther, M., Naceur-Lombardelli, C., Prymas, P., Toncheva, A., Hessey, S., Dietzen, M., ... Swanton, C. (2023). The evolution of non-small cell lung cancer metastases in TRACERx. *Nature, 616*(7957), 534–542. https://doi.org/10.1038/s41586-023-05729-x.

Arifuzzaman, M., Collins, N., Guo, C. J., & Artis, D. (2024). Nutritional regulation of microbiota-derived metabolites: Implications for immunity and inflammation. *Immunity, 57*(1), 14–27. https://doi.org/10.1016/j.immuni.2023.12.009, https://www.sciencedirect.com/science/journal/10747613.

Bagchi, S., Yuan, R., Huang, H.-L., Zhang, W., Chiu, D. K.-C., Kim, H., Cha, S. L., Tolentino, L., Lowitz, J., Liu, Y., Moshnikova, A., Andreev, O., Plevritis, S., & Engleman, E. G. (2024). The acid-sensing receptor GPR65 on tumor macrophages drives tumor growth in obesity. *Science Immunology, 9*(100). https://doi.org/10.1126/sciimmunol.adg6453.

Bakshi, H. A., Quinn, G. A., Nasef, M. M., Mishra, V., Aljabali, A. A. A., El-Tanani, M., Serrano-Aroca, A., Da Silva, M. W., McCarron, P. A., & Tambuwala, M. M. (2022). Crocin Inhibits angiogenesis and metastasis in colon cancer via TNF-α/NF-kB/VEGF pathways. *Cells, 11*(9). https://doi.org/10.3390/cells11091502, https://www.mdpi.com/2073-4409/11/9/1425/pdf.

Bamane, S. D., Bhojwani, V., Balkunde, P. L., Bhattacharya, M., Gupta, I., Mohapatra, A. K., Shekhar, A., & Singh, A. (2021). Smartphone-enabled field monitoring tool for rapid hexavalent chromium detection in water. *Analytical and Bioanalytical Chemistry, 413*(13), 3455–3469. https://doi.org/10.1007/s00216-021-03291-x, https://link.springer.com/journal/216/volumes-and-issues.

Boroujerdi, R., & Paul, R. (2022). Graphene-based electrochemical sensors for psychoactive drugs. *Nanomaterials, 12*(13), 2250. https://doi.org/10.3390/nano12132250.

Boumelha, J., de Castro, A., Bah, N., Cha, H., de Carné Trécesson, S., Rana, S., Tomaschko, M., Anastasiou, P., Mugarza, E., Moore, C., Goldstone, R., East, P., Litchfield, K., Lee, S.-H., Molina-Arcas, M., & Downward, J. (2024). CRISPR–Cas9 screening identifies KRAS-Induced COX2 as a driver of immunotherapy resistance in lung cancer. *Cancer Research, 84*(14), 2231–2246. https://doi.org/10.1158/0008-5472.can-23-2627.

Boutilier, A. J., & Elsawa, S. F. (2021). Macrophage polarization states in the tumor microenvironment. *International Journal of Molecular Sciences, 22*(13), 6995. https://doi.org/10.3390/ijms22136995.

Cable, D. M., Murray, E., Shanmugam, V., Zhang, S., Zou, L. S., Diao, M., Chen, H., Macosko, E. Z., Irizarry, R. A., & Chen, F. (2022). Cell type-specific inference of differential expression in spatial transcriptomics. *Nature Methods, 19*(9), 1076–1087. https://doi.org/10.1038/s41592-022-01575-3.

Cao, J., Wang, Y., Lin, Q., Wang, S., Shen, Y., Zhang, L., Li, W., Chen, L., Liu, C., Yao, S., Shuai, L., Chen, X., Li, Z., & Chang, Y. (2025). IL-1β stimulates ADAMTS9 expression and contributes to preterm prelabor rupture of membranes. *Cell Communication and Signaling, 23*(1). https://doi.org/10.1186/s12964-025-02120-3, https://biosignaling.biomedcentral.com/.

Cappuyns, S., Piqué-Gili, M., Esteban-Fabró, R., Philips, G., Balaseviciute, U., Pinyol, R., Gris-Oliver, A., Vandecaveye, V., Abril-Fornaguera, J., Montironi, C., Bassaganyas, L., Peix, J., Zeitlhoefler, M., Mesropian, A., Huguet-Pradell, J., Haber, P. K., Figueiredo, I., Ioannou, G., Gonzalez-Kozlova, E., ... Llovet, J. M. (2025). Single-cell RNA sequencing-derived signatures define response patterns to atezolizumab + bevacizumab in advanced hepatocellular carcinoma. *Journal of Hepatology, 82*(6), 1036–1049. https://doi.org/10.1016/j.jhep.2024.12.016.

Chen, S., Zhang, P., Duan, X., Bao, A., Wang, B., Zhang, Y., Li, H., Zhang, L., & Liu, S. (2024). Lesion localization and pathological diagnosis of ovine pulmonary adenocarcinoma based on MASK R-CNN. *Animals, 14*(17), 2488. https://doi.org/10.3390/ani14172488.

Cheung, K. L., Lee, J. H., Khor, T. O., Wu, T. Y., Li, G. X., Chan, J., Yang, C. S., & Kong, A. N. T. (2014). Nrf2 knockout enhances intestinal tumorigenesis in Apcmin/+ mice due to attenuation of anti-oxidative stress pathway while potentiates inflammation. *Molecular Carcinogenesis, 53*(1), 77–84. https://doi.org/10.1002/mc.21950.

Choi, H., Baek, J. H., Seo, A. N., Park, S. Y., Kim, H. J., Park, J. S., Choi, G. S., Kim, J. G., & Kang, B. W. (2024). Systemic inflammatory response following preoperative chemoradiotherapy can affect oncologic outcomes in MSI-H/dMMR rectal cancer. *Chonnam Medical Journal, 60*(2), 105. https://doi.org/10.4068/cmj.2024.60.2.105.

Cong, J., Liu, P., Han, Z., Ying, W., Li, C., Yang, Y., Wang, S., Yang, J., Cao, F., Shen, J., Zeng, Y., Bai, Y., Zhou, C., Ye, L., Zhou, R., Guo, C., Cang, C., Kasper, D. L., Song, X., ... Zhu, S. (2024). Bile acids modified by the intestinal microbiota promote colorectal cancer growth by suppressing CD8+ T cell effector functions. *Immunity, 57*(4), 876. https://doi.org/10.1016/j.immuni.2024.02.014.

Delhase, M., Hayakawa, M., Chen, Y., & Karin, M. (1999). Positive and negative regulation of IκB kinase activity through IKKβ subunit phosphorylation. *Science (New York, N.Y.), 284*(5412), 309–313. https://doi.org/10.1126/science.284.5412.309.

Di, D., Zhou, H., Cui, Z., Zhang, J., Liu, Q., Yuan, T., Zhou, T., Luo, X., Ling, D., & Wang, Q. (2024). Frailty phenotype as mediator between systemic inflammation and osteoporosis and fracture risks: A prospective study. *Journal of Cachexia, Sarcopenia and Muscle, 15*(3), 897–906. https://doi.org/10.1002/jcsm.13447.

Du, P., Zhang, Q., & Zhang, Y. (2022). The role of IL-6, IL-10, and PGE2 in the treatment of intervertebral disc herniation by dual-channel endoscopic lumbar discectomy. *Cellular and Molecular Biology, 67*(5), 188–195. https://doi.org/10.14715/cmb/2021.67.5.26.

Duan, X. P., Qin, B. D., Jiao, X. D., Liu, K., Wang, Z., & Zang, Y. S. (2024). New clinical trial design in precision medicine: Discovery, development and direction. *Signal Transduction and Targeted Therapy, 9*(1). https://doi.org/10.1038/s41392-024-01760-0, https://www.nature.com/sigtrans.

Durham, P. G., Kim, J., Eltz, K. M., Caskey, C. F., & Dayton, P. A. (2022). Polyvinyl alcohol cryogels for acoustic characterization of phase-change contrast agents. *Ultrasound in Medicine & Biology, 48*(5), 954–960.

Eberhardt, C. S., Kissick, H. T., Patel, M. R., Cardenas, M. A., Prokhnevska, N., Obeng, R. C., Nasti, T. H., Griffith, C. C., Im, S. J., Wang, X., Shin, D. M., Carrington, M., Chen, Z. G., Sidney, J., Sette, A., Saba, N. F., Wieland, A., & Ahmed, R. (2021). Functional HPV-specific PD-1+ stem-like CD8 T cells in head and neck cancer. *Nature, 597*(7875), 279–284. https://doi.org/10.1038/s41586-021-03862-z, http://www.nature.com/nature/index.html.

Fabian, K. P., Padget, M. R., Donahue, R. N., Solocinski, K., Robbins, Y., Allen, C. T., Lee, J. H., Rabizadeh, S., Soon-Shiong, P., Schlom, J., & Hodge, J. W. (2020). PD-L1 targeting high-affinity NK (t-haNK) cells induce direct antitumor effects and target suppressive MDSC populations. *Journal for ImmunoTherapy of Cancer, 8*(1). https://doi.org/10.1136/jitc-2019-000450, http://www.immunotherapyofcancer.org/.

Fan, L., Wang, Z.-H., Ma, L.-X., Wu, S.-Y., Wu, J., Yu, K.-D., Sui, X.-Y., Xu, Y., Liu, X.-Y., Chen, L., Zhang, W.-J., Jin, X., Xiao, Q., Shui, R.-H., Xiao, Y., Wang, H., Yang, Y.-S., Huang, X.-Y., Cao, A.-Y., ... Shao, Z.-M. (2024). Optimising first-line subtyping-based therapy in triple-negative breast cancer (FUTURE-SUPER): A multi-cohort, randomised, phase 2 trial. *The Lancet Oncology, 25*(2), 184–197. https://doi.org/10.1016/s1470-2045(23)00579-x.

Fang, P., Liu, X., Qiu, Y., Wang, Y., Wang, D., Zhao, J., Ding, H., & Bao, N. (2023). Exploring causal correlations between inflammatory cytokines and ankylosing spondylitis: A bidirectional mendelian-randomization study. *Frontiers in Immunology, 14*. https://doi.org/10.3389/fimmu.2023.1285106.

Feng, X., Wu, W., & Liu, F. (2024). AH-6809 mediated regulation of lung adenocarcinoma metastasis through NLRP7 and prognostic analysis of key metastasis-related genes. *Frontiers in Pharmacology, 15*. https://doi.org/10.3389/fphar.2024.1486265.

Gao, J., Liang, Y., & Wang, L. (2022). Shaping polarization of tumor-associated macrophages in cancer immunotherapy. *Frontiers in Immunology, 13*. https://doi.org/10.3389/fimmu.2022.888713.

Gomerdinger, V. F., Nabar, N., & Hammond, P. T. (2025). Advancing engineering design strategies for targeted cancer nanomedicine. *Nature Reviews. Cancer, 25*(9), 657–683. https://doi.org/10.1038/s41568-025-00847-2, https://www.nature.com/cancer/.

Guo, C. L., Wang, C. S., Wang, Z. C., Liu, F. F., Liu, L., Yang, Y., Li, X., Guo, B., Lu, R. Y., Liao, B., Liu, J. X., Wang, H., Song, J., Yao, Y., Zhu, L. P., Yu, D., & Liu, Z. (2024). Granzyme K+CD8+ T cells interact with fibroblasts to promote neutrophilic inflammation in nasal polyps. *Nature Communications, 15*(1). https://doi.org/10.1038/s41467-024-54685-1, https://www.nature.com/ncomms/.

Hansen, T. J., & Hodges, E. (2022). ATAC-STARR-seq reveals transcription factor–bound activators and silencers within chromatin-accessible regions of the human genome. *Genome Research, 32*(8), 1529–1541. https://doi.org/10.1101/gr.276766.122, https://genome.cshlp.org/content/32/8/1529.full.pdf+html.

Helmink, B. A., Reddy, S. M., Gao, J., Zhang, S., Basar, R., Thakur, R., Yizhak, K., Sade-Feldman, M., Blando, J., Han, G., Gopalakrishnan, V., Xi, Y., Zhao, H., Amaria, R. N., Tawbi, H. A., Cogdill, A. P., Liu, W., LeBleu, V. S., Kugeratski, F. G., ... Wargo, J. A. (2020). B cells and tertiary lymphoid structures promote immunotherapy response. *Nature, 577*(7791), 549–555. https://doi.org/10.1038/s41586-019-1922-8, http://www.nature.com/nature/index.html.

Hopf, N. B., Rousselle, C., Poddalgoda, D., Lamkarkach, F., Bessems, J., Schmid, K., Jones, K., Takaki, K., Casteleyn, L., Zare Jeddi, M., Bader, M., Koller, M., Browne, P., FitzGerald, R., Viegas, S., Göen, T., Santonen, T., Väänänen, V., Duca, R.-C., & Pasanen-Kase, R. (2024). A harmonized occupational biomonitoring approach. *Environment International, 191*, 108990. https://doi.org/10.1016/j.envint.2024.108990.

Hu, H., Kang, L., Zhang, J., Wu, Z., Wang, H., Huang, M., Lan, P., Wu, X., Wang, C., Cao, W., Hu, J., Huang, Y., Huang, L., Wang, H., Shi, L., Cai, Y., Shen, C., Ling, J., Xie, X., ... Deng, Y. (2022). Neoadjuvant PD-1 blockade with toripalimab, with or without celecoxib, in mismatch repair-deficient or microsatellite instability-high, locally advanced, colorectal cancer (PICC): A single-centre, parallel-group, non-comparative, randomised, phase 2 trial. *The Lancet Gastroenterology & Hepatology, 7*(1), 38–48. https://doi.org/10.1016/s2468-1253(21)00348-4.

Hu, W., Zi, Z., Jin, Y., Li, G., Shao, K., Cai, Q., Ma, X., & Wei, F. (2019). CRISPR/Cas9-mediated PD-1 disruption enhances human mesothelin-targeted CAR T cell effector functions. *Cancer Immunology, Immunotherapy, 68*(3), 365–377. https://doi.org/10.1007/s00262-018-2281-2, link.springer.de/link/service/journals/00262/index.htm.

Huang, F., Cao, X., Mei, J., Wu, C., Zhu, W., Sun, L., Dai, C., & Wang, M. (2025). Gastric cancer cells shuttle lactate to induce inflammatory CAF-like phenotype and function in bone marrow-derived mesenchymal stem cells. *Molecular Immunology, 183*, 93–103. https://doi.org/10.1016/j.molimm.2025.05.002.

Huang, L., Wu, X., You, J., Jin, Z., He, W., Sun, J., Shen, H., Liu, X., Yue, X., Cai, W., Zhang, S., & Zhang, B. (2025). Artificial intelligence can predict personalized immunotherapy outcomes in cancer. *Cancer Immunology Research, 13*(7), 964–977. https://doi.org/10.1158/2326-6066.CIR-24-1270, https://aacrjournals.org/cancerimmunolres/article/13/7/964/763126/Artificial-Intelligence-Can-Predict-Personalized.

Huseni, M. A., Wang, L., Klementowicz, J. E., Yuen, K., Breart, B., Orr, C., Liu, L.-fen, Li, Y., Gupta, V., Li, C., Rishipathak, D., Peng, J., Şenbabaoğlu, Y., Modrusan, Z., Keerthivasan, S., Madireddi, S., Chen, Y.-J., Fraser, E. J., Leng, N., ... West, N. R. (2023). CD8+ T cell-intrinsic IL-6 signaling promotes resistance to anti-PD-L1 immunotherapy. *Cell Reports Medicine, 4*(1), 100878. https://doi.org/10.1016/j.xcrm.2022.100878.

Igawa, T., Ishii, S., Tachibana, T., Maeda, A., Higuchi, Y., Shimaoka, S., Moriyama, C., Watanabe, T., Takubo, R., Doi, Y., Wakabayashi, T., Hayasaka, A., Kadono, S., Miyazaki, T., Haraya, K., Sekimori, Y., Kojima, T., Nabuchi, Y., Aso, Y., ... Hattori, K. (2010). Antibody recycling by engineered pH-dependent antigen binding improves the duration of antigen neutralization. *Nature Biotechnology, 28*(11), 1203–1207. https://doi.org/10.1038/nbt.1691.

Ishizuka, J. J., Manguso, R. T., Cheruiyot, C. K., Bi, K., Panda, A., Iracheta-Vellve, A., Miller, B. C., Du, P. P., Yates, K. B., Dubrot, J., Buchumenski, I., Comstock, D. E., Brown, F. D., Ayer, A., Kohnle, I. C., Pope, H. W., Zimmer, M. D., Sen, D. R., Lane-Reticker, S. K., ... Haining, W. N. (2019). Loss of ADAR1 in tumours overcomes resistance to immune checkpoint blockade. *Nature, 565*(7737), 43–48. https://doi.org/10.1038/s41586-018-0768-9, http://www.nature.com/nature/index.html.

Jeong, H., Koh, J., Kim, S., Yim, J., Song, S. G., Kim, H., Li, Y., Lee, S. H., Chung, Y. K., Kim, H., Lee, C.-H., Kim, H. Y., Keam, B., Lee, S.-H., Chung, D. H., & Jeon, Y. K. (2025). Cell-intrinsic PD-L1 signaling drives immunosuppression by myeloid-derived suppressor cells through IL-6/Jak/Stat3 in PD-L1-high lung cancer. *Journal for ImmunoTherapy of Cancer, 13*(3), e010612. https://doi.org/10.1136/jitc-2024-010612.

Jia, Chu, Jin, Long, & Zhu (2022). High-throughput single-cell sequencing in cancer research. *Signal Transduction and Targeted Therapy, 7*(1). https://doi.org/10.1038/s41392-022-00990-4.

Jia, W., Xie, G., & Jia, W. (2018). Bile acid–microbiota crosstalk in gastrointestinal inflammation and carcinogenesis. *Nature Reviews Gastroenterology & Hepatology, 15*(2), 111–128. https://doi.org/10.1038/nrgastro.2017.119.

Johnson, D. E., O'Keefe, R. A., & Grandis, J. R. (2018). Targeting the IL-6/JAK/STAT3 signalling axis in cancer. *Nature Reviews Clinical Oncology, 15*(4), 234–248. https://doi.org/10.1038/nrclinonc.2018.8, http://www.nature.com/nrclinonc/archive/index.html.

Kanarek, N., London, N., Schueler-Furman, O., & Ben-Neriah, Y. (2010). Ubiquitination and degradation of the inhibitors of NF-kappaB. *Cold Spring Harbor perspectives in biology, 2*(2), a000166. https://doi.org/10.1101/cshperspect.a000166.

Kang, Y. K., Kim, H. D., Yook, J. H., et al. (2024). Neoadjuvant docetaxel, oxaliplatin, and S-1 plus surgery and adjuvant S-1 for resectable advanced gastric cancer: Updated overall survival outcomes from phase III PRODIGY. *Journal of Clinical Oncology: Official Journal of the American Society of Clinical Oncology, 42*(25), 2961–2965.

Karbalaei, M., Talebi Bezmin Abadi, A., & Keikha, M. (2022). Clinical relevance of the cagA and vacA s1m1 status and antibiotic resistance in Helicobacter pylori: A systematic review and meta-analysis. *BMC Infectious Diseases, 22*(1). https://doi.org/10.1186/s12879-022-07546-5.

Kennel, K. B., Bozlar, M., De Valk, A. F., & Greten, F. R. (2023). Cancer-associated fibroblasts in inflammation and antitumor immunity. *Clinical Cancer Research, 29*(6), 1009–1016. https://doi.org/10.1158/1078-0432.CCR-22-1031, https://watermark.silverchair.com/1009.pdf.

Klaver, D., Gander, H., Frena, B., Amato, M., & Thurnher, M. (2024). Crosstalk between purinergic receptor P2Y11 and chemokine receptor CXCR7 is regulated by CXCR4 in human macrophages. *Cellular and Molecular Life Sciences, 81*(1). https://doi.org/10.1007/s00018-024-05158-7.

Kuenzi, B. M., Park, J., Fong, S. H., Sanchez, K. S., Lee, J., Kreisberg, J. F., Ma, J., & Ideker, T. (2020). Predicting drug response and synergy using a deep learning model of human cancer cells. *Cancer Cell, 38*(5), 672. https://doi.org/10.1016/j.ccell.2020.09.014, https://www.journals.elsevier.com/cancer-cell.

Kulesza, A., Paczek, L., & Burdzinska, A. (2023). The role of COX-2 and PGE2 in the regulation of immunomodulation and other functions of mesenchymal stromal cells. *Biomedicines, 11*(2), 445. https://doi.org/10.3390/biomedicines11020445.

Kumar, R., Panda, S. P., Abomughaid, M. M., Lakhanpal, S., Avinash, D., Kumar Jha, N., & Gupta, R. (2025). Microglial pyroptosis in neurological disorders: Mechanistic crosstalk, metabolic triggers, and therapeutic frontiers. *Metabolic Brain Disease, 40*(7). https://doi.org/10.1007/s11011-025-01685-9.

Levy, B. P., Felip, E., Reck, M., Yang, J. C. H., Cappuzzo, F., Yoneshima, Y., Zhou, C., Rawat, S., Xie, J., Basak, P., Xu, L., & Sands, J. (2023). TROPION-Lung08: Phase III study of datopotamab deruxtecan plus pembrolizumab as first-line therapy for advanced NSCLC. *Future Oncology, 19*(21), 1461–1472. https://doi.org/10.2217/fon-2023-0230, http://www.futuremedicine.com/loi/fon.

Li, T., Li, X., Kang, P., & Zhao, J. (2025). Exploring CX3CR1 as a prognostic biomarker and immunotherapeutic target in sarcoma. *Translational Oncology, 53*, 102283. https://doi.org/10.1016/j.tranon.2025.102283.

Liang, L., Liu, L., Zhou, W., Yang, C., Mai, G., Li, H., & Chen, Y. (2022). Gut microbiota-derived butyrate regulates gut mucus barrier repair by activating the macrophage/WNT/ERK signaling pathway. *Clinical Science, 136*(4), 291–307. https://doi.org/10.1042/cs20210778.

Lim, R. J., Salehi-Rad, R., Tran, L. M., Oh, M. S., Dumitras, C., Crosson, W. P., Li, R., Patel, T. S., Man, S., Yean, C. E., Abascal, J., Huang, Z. L., Ong, S. L., Krysan, K., Dubinett, S. M., & Liu, B. (2024). CXCL9/10-engineered dendritic cells promote T cell activation and enhance immune checkpoint blockade for lung cancer. *Cell Reports Medicine, 5*(4), 101479. https://doi.org/10.1016/j.xcrm.2024.101479.

Lin, A., Zhang, J., & Luo, P. (2020). Crosstalk between the MSI status and tumor microenvironment in colorectal cancer. *Frontiers in Immunology, 11*. https://doi.org/10.3389/fimmu.2020.02039.

Lin, K. X., Istl, A. C., Quan, D., Skaro, A., Tang, E., & Zheng, X. (2023). PD-1 and PD-L1 inhibitors in cold colorectal cancer: Challenges and strategies. *Cancer Immunology, Immunotherapy, 72*(12), 3875–3893. https://doi.org/10.1007/s00262-023-03520-5, https://www.springer.com/journal/262.

Liu, S. J., Yang, R., Zuo, Y., Qiao, C., Jiang, W., Cheng, W., Wei, W., Liu, Z., Geng, Y., & Dong, Y. (2024). The association of circulating systemic inflammation with premature death and the protective role of the Mediterranean diet: A large prospective cohort study of UK biobank. *BMC Public Health, 24*(1). https://doi.org/10.1186/s12889-024-18888-x.

Liu, X., Sadaoka, T., Krogmann, T., & Cohen, J. I. (2020). Epstein–Barr Virus (EBV) tegument protein BGLF2 suppresses type I interferon signaling to promote EBV reactivation. *Journal of Virology, 94*(11) e00258-20.

Liu, Y., Yang, M., Deng, Y., Su, G., Enninful, A., Guo, C. C., Tebaldi, T., Zhang, D., Kim, D., Bai, Z., Norris, E., Pan, A., Li, J., Xiao, Y., Halene, S., & Fan, R. (2020). High-spatial-resolution multi-omics sequencing via deterministic barcoding in tissue. *Cell, 183*(6), 1665. https://doi.org/10.1016/j.cell.2020.10.026, https://www.sciencedirect.com/journal/cell.

Liu, Y., Yu, Y., Hu, C., Jiang, M., Zhao, C., Li, X., Cheng, L., & Zhou, C. (2025). ZEB2 upregulation modulates the polarization of TAMs toward the immunosuppressive state in EGFR-TKI-resistant NSCLC. *Journal of Cancer Metastasis and Treatment, 8*. https://doi.org/10.20517/cdr.2024.206, jcmtjournal.com/.

Liu, Z., Yang, Z., Wu, J., Zhang, W., Sun, Y., Zhang, C., Bai, G., Yang, L., Fan, H., Chen, Y., Zhang, L., Jiang, B., Liu, X., Ma, X., Tang, W., Liu, C., Qu, Y., Yan, L., Zhao, D., ... Zhang, Z. (2025). A single-cell atlas reveals immune heterogeneity in anti-PD-1-treated non-small cell lung cancer. *Cell, 188*(11), 3081. https://doi.org/10.1016/j.cell.2025.03.018.

Lou, E., Xiu, J., Baca, Y., Saeed, A., Prakash, A., Gholami, S., Subramanian, S., Starr, T. K., Fontana, E., Pandey, R., Lenz, H.-J., Shields, A. F., Nabhan, C., Oberley, M., Seeber, A., & El-Deiry, W. (2024). Differential landscape of immune evasion in oncogenic RAS-driven primary and metastatic colorectal cancers. *Molecular Therapy: Oncology, 32*(1), 200786. https://doi.org/10.1016/j.omton.2024.200786.

Luo, J. (2021). KRAS mutation in pancreatic cancer. *Seminars in Oncology, 48*(1), 10–18. https://doi.org/10.1053/j.seminoncol.2021.02.003.

Ma, Y., Guo, Z., Xia, B., Zhang, Y., Liu, X., Yu, Y., Tang, N., Tong, X., Wang, M., Ye, X., Feng, J., Chen, Y., & Wang, J. (2022). Identification of antimicrobial peptides from the human gut microbiome using deep learning. *Nature Biotechnology, 40*(6), 921–931. https://doi.org/10.1038/s41587-022-01226-0.

MacE, T. A., Shakya, R., Pitarresi, J. R., Swanson, B., McQuinn, C. W., Loftus, S., Nordquist, E., Cruz-Monserrate, Z., Yu, L., Young, G., Zhong, X., Zimmers, T. A., Ostrowski, M. C., Ludwig, T., Bloomston, M., Bekaii-Saab, T., & Lesinski, G. B. (2018). IL-6 and PD-L1 antibody blockade combination therapy reduces tumour progression in murine models of pancreatic cancer. *Gut, 67*(2), 320–332. https://doi.org/10.1136/gutjnl-2016-311585, http://gut.bmj.com/content/by/year.

Mahat, D. B., Kumra, H., Castro, S. A., Metcalf, E., Nguyen, K., Morisue, R., Ho, W. W., Chen, I., Sullivan, B., Yim, L. H., Singh, A., Fu, J., Waterton, S. K., Cheng, Y. C., Moiso, E., Chauhan, V. P., Silva, H. M., Spranger, S., Jain, R. K., & Sharp, P. A. (2025). Mutant p53 exploits enhancers to elevate immunosuppressive chemokine expression and impair immune checkpoint inhibitors in pancreatic cancer. *Immunity, 58*(7), 1688. https://doi.org/10.1016/j.immuni.2025.06.005, https://www.sciencedirect.com/science/journal/10747613.

Mantsounga, C. S., Lee, C., Neverson, J., Sharma, S., Healy, A., Berus, J. M., Parry, C., Ceneri, N. M., López-Giráldez, F., Chun, H. J., Lu, Q., Sellke, F., Choudhary, G., & Morrison, A. R. (2022). Macrophage IL-1β promotes arteriogenesis by autocrine STAT3- and NF-κB-mediated transcription of pro-angiogenic VEGF-A. *Cell Reports, 38*(5), 110309. https://doi.org/10.1016/j.celrep.2022.110309.

Martínez Fajardo, C., Morote, L., Moreno-Giménez, E., López-López, S., Rubio-Moraga, Á., Díaz-Guerra, M. J. M., Diretto, G., López Jiménez, A. J., Ahrazem, O., & Gómez-Gómez, L. (2024). Exosome-like nanoparticles from *Arbutus unedo* L. mitigate LPS-induced inflammation via JAK-STAT inactivation. *Food & Function, 15*(22), 11280–11290. https://doi.org/10.1039/d4fo03646h.

McIntyre, C. A., Grimont, A., Park, J., Meng, Y., Sisso, W. J., Seier, K., Jang, G. H., Walch, H., Aveson, V. G., Falvo, D. J., Fall, W. B., Chan, C. W., Wenger, A., Ecker, B. L., Pulvirenti, A., Gelfer, R., Zafra, M. P., Schultz, N., Park, W., ... Chandwani, R. (2024). Distinct clinical outcomes and biological features of specific KRAS mutants in human pancreatic cancer. *Cancer Cell, 42*(9), 1614. https://doi.org/10.1016/j.ccell.2024.08.002, https://www.sciencedirect.com/science/journal/15356108.

Mercanti, L., Sindaco, M., Mazzone, M., Di Marcantonio, M. C., Piscione, M., Muraro, R., & Mincione, G. (2023). PDAC, the influencer cancer: Cross-talk with tumor microenvironment and connected potential therapy strategies. *Cancers, 15*(11), 2923. https://doi.org/10.3390/cancers15112923.

Monahan, R. C., van den Beukel, M. D., Borggreven, N. V., Fronczek, R., Huizinga, T. W. J., Kloppenburg, M., Steup-Beekman, G. M., & Trouw, L. A. (2022). Autoantibodies against specific post-translationally modified proteins are present in patients with lupus and associate with major neuropsychiatric manifestations. *RMD Open, 8*(1), e002079. https://doi.org/10.1136/rmdopen-2021-002079.

Mondal, S., Mor, A., Reddy, I. J., Nandi, S., & Gupta, P. S. P. (2024). Effect of heat exposure on prostaglandin production and expression of COX-2, PGES, PGFS, ITGAV and LGALS15 mRNAs in endometrial epithelial cells of buffalo (*Bubalus bubalis*). *Molecular Biology Reports, 51*(1). https://doi.org/10.1007/s11033-024-09361-4, https://www.springer.com/journal/11033.

Mueller, S., Engleitner, T., Maresch, R., Zukowska, M., Lange, S., Kaltenbacher, T., Konukiewitz, B., Öllinger, R., Zwiebel, M., Strong, A., Yen, H.-Y., Banerjee, R., Louzada, S., Fu, B., Seidler, B., Götzfried, J., Schuck, K., Hassan, Z., Arbeiter, A., ... Rad, R. (2018). Evolutionary routes and KRAS dosage define pancreatic cancer phenotypes. *Nature, 554*(7690), 62–68. https://doi.org/10.1038/nature25459.

Nakano, R., Shiomi, H., Fujiwara, A., Yoshihara, K., Yoshioka, R., Kawata, S., Ota, S., Yuri, Y., Takashima, T., Aizawa, N., Ikeda, N., Nishimura, T., Enomoto, H., & Iijima, H. (2022). Clinical characteristics of ICI-related pancreatitis and cholangitis including radiographic and endoscopic findings. *Healthcare, 10*(5), 763. https://doi.org/10.3390/healthcare10050763.

Nencini, F., Borghi, S., Giurranna, E., Barbaro, I., Taddei, N., Fiorillo, C., & Becatti, M. (2025). Reactive nitrogen species and fibrinogen: Exploring the effects of nitration on blood clots. *Antioxidants, 14*(7), 825. https://doi.org/10.3390/antiox14070825.

Ngo, V. N., Young, R. M., Schmitz, R., Jhavar, S., Xiao, W., Lim, K.-H., Kohlhammer, H., Xu, W., Yang, Y., Zhao, H., Shaffer, A. L., Romesser, P., Wright, G., Powell, J., Rosenwald, A., Muller-Hermelink, H. K., Ott, G., Gascoyne,

R. D., Connors, J. M., ... Staudt, L. M. (2011). Oncogenically active MYD88 mutations in human lymphoma. *Nature, 470*(7332), 115–119. https://doi.org/10.1038/nature09671.

Niu, L., Thiele, M., Geyer, P. E., Rasmussen, D. N., Webel, H. E., Santos, A., Gupta, R., Meier, F., Strauss, M., Kjaergaard, M., Lindvig, K., Jacobsen, S., Rasmussen, S., Hansen, T., Krag, A., & Mann, M. (2022). Noninvasive proteomic biomarkers for alcohol-related liver disease. *Nature Medicine, 28*(6), 1277–1287. https://doi.org/10.1038/s41591-022-01850-y, http://www.nature.com/nm/index.html.

Palazuelos, C. E. M., Medina, E. M. A., Felix, M. M. A., Payan, R. R., Cortes, M. B., Avila, L. L., Salazar, A. H., Llanes, J. M., Sanchez-Schmitz, G., & Quintana, J. G. R. (2024). IL-6, IL-10 and TNF-α gene polymorphisms in preeclampsia: A case-control study in a Mexican population. *Ginekologia Polska, 95*(2), 108–113. https://doi.org/10.5603/gpl.94272, https://journals.viamedica.pl/ginekologia_polska.

Pan, M., Wei, X., Xiang, X., Liu, Y., Zhou, Q., & Yang, W. (2023). Targeting CXCL9/10/11–CXCR3 axis: An important component of tumor-promoting and antitumor immunity. *Clinical and Translational Oncology, 25*(8), 2306–2320. https://doi.org/10.1007/s12094-023-03126-4.

Pandey, V. K., Premkumar, K., Kundu, P., & Shankar, B. S. (2024). PGE2 induced miR365/IL-6/STAT3 signaling mediates dendritic cell dysfunction in cancer. *Life Sciences, 350*, 122751. https://doi.org/10.1016/j.lfs.2024.122751.

Papalexi, E., & Satija, R. (2018). Single-cell RNA sequencing to explore immune cell heterogeneity. *Nature Reviews. Immunology, 18*(1), 35–45. https://doi.org/10.1038/nri.2017.76, http://www.nature.com/nri/index.html.

Pelka, K., Hofree, M., Chen, J. H., Sarkizova, S., Pirl, J. D., Jorgji, V., Bejnood, A., Dionne, D., Ge, W. H., Xu, K. H., Chao, S. X., Zollinger, D. R., Lieb, D. J., Reeves, J. W., Fuhrman, C. A., Hoang, M. L., Delorey, T., Nguyen, L. T., Waldman, J., ... Hacohen, N. (2021). Spatially organized multicellular immune hubs in human colorectal cancer. *Cell, 184*(18), 4734. https://doi.org/10.1016/j.cell.2021.08.003, https://www.sciencedirect.com/journal/cell.

Peng, D., Kryczek, I., Nagarsheth, N., Zhao, L., Wei, S., Wang, W., Sun, Y., Zhao, E., Vatan, L., Szeliga, W., Kotarski, J., Tarkowski, R., Dou, Y., Cho, K., Hensley-Alford, S., Munkarah, A., Liu, R., & Zou, W. (2015). Epigenetic silencing of TH1-type chemokines shapes tumour immunity and immunotherapy. *Nature, 527*(7577), 249–253. https://doi.org/10.1038/nature15520, http://www.nature.com/nature/index.html.

Phelan, J. D., & Oellerich, T. (2022). BCL10 mutants: Architects of oncogenic signaling provide a blueprint for precision medicine. *Cancer Discovery, 12*(8), 1844–1846. https://doi.org/10.1158/2159-8290.CD-22-0614, https://aacrjournals.org/cancerdiscovery/article-pdf/12/8/1844/3183563/1844.pdf.

Preianò, M., Maggisano, G., Murfuni, M. S., Villella, C., Pelaia, C., Montalcini, T., Lombardo, N., Pelaia, G., Savino, R., & Terracciano, R. (2018). An analytical method for assessing optimal storage conditions of gingival crevicular fluid and disclosing a peptide biomarker signature of gingivitis by MALDI-TOF MS. *PROTEOMICS – Clinical Applications, 12*(5). https://doi.org/10.1002/prca.201800005.

Qu, Q. C., Shen, H. H., Wang, C. J., Zhang, X. Y., Wu, J. N., Lu, H. C., Qiu, X. M., Ding, J. Y., Tan, X. F., Liu, L. B., & Li, M. Q. (2021). A positive COX-2/IL-1β loop promotes decidualization by upregulating CD82. *Reproduction (Cambridge, England), 162*(3), 227–236. https://doi.org/10.1530/REP-21-0204, https://rep.bioscientifica.com/view/journals/rep/162/3/REP-21-0204.xml.

Quail, D. F., Amulic, B., Aziz, M., Barnes, B. J., Eruslanov, E., Fridlender, Z. G., Goodridge, H. S., Granot, Z., Hidalgo, A., Huttenlocher, A., Kaplan, M. J., Malanchi, I., Merghoub, T., Meylan, E., Mittal, V., Pittet, M. J., Rubio-Ponce, A., Udalova, I. A., van den Berg, T. K., ... Kubes, P. (2022). Neutrophil phenotypes and functions in cancer: A consensus statement. *Journal of Experimental Medicine, 219*(6). https://doi.org/10.1084/jem.20220011, https://rupress.org/jem/article-pdf/219/6/e20220011/1434099/jem_20220011.pdf.

Rizvi, H., Sanchez-Vega, F., La, K., Chatila, W., Jonsson, P., Halpenny, D., Plodkowski, A., Long, N., Sauter, J. L., Rekhtman, N., Hollmann, T., Schalper, K. A., Gainor, J. F., Shen, R., Ni, A., Arbour, K. C., Merghoub, T., Wolchok, J., Snyder, A., ... Hellmann, M. D. (2018). Molecular determinants of response to anti–programmed cell death (PD)-1 and anti–programmed death-ligand 1 (PD-L1) blockade in patients with non–small-cell lung cancer profiled with targeted next-generation sequencing. *Journal of Clinical Oncology, 36*(7), 633–641. https://doi.org/10.1200/jco.2017.75.3384.

Román-Villarán, E., Ammenwerth, E., Wijayaratne, J., & Parra-Calderón, C. L. (2022). Desiderata for a new generation of EHRs for inclusive healthcare. *Yearbook of Medical Informatics, 31*(1), 88–93. https://doi.org/10.1055/s-0042-1742507, https://www.thieme-connect.com/products/ejournals/journal/10.1055/s-00034612.

Rupp, L. J., Schumann, K., Roybal, K. T., Gate, R. E., Ye, C. J., Lim, W. A., & Marson, A. (2017). CRISPR/Cas9-mediated PD-1 disruption enhances anti-tumor efficacy of human chimeric antigen receptor T cells. *Scientific Reports, 7*(1). https://doi.org/10.1038/s41598-017-00462-8, www.nature.com/srep/index.html.

Schmelter, C., Brueck, A., Perumal, N., Qu, S., Pfeiffer, N., & Grus, F. H. (2023). Lectin-based affinity enrichment and characterization of N-glycoproteins from human tear film by mass spectrometry. *Molecules (Basel, Switzerland), 28*(2), 648. https://doi.org/10.3390/molecules28020648.

Seliger, B., & Massa, C. (2025). CyTOF as a suitable tool for stratification and monitoring of cancer patients. *Journal of Translational Medicine, 23*(1). https://doi.org/10.1186/s12967-025-06764-0.

Sharpee, T. O., Destexhe, A., Kawato, M., Sekulić, V., Skinner, F. K., Wójcik, D. K., Chintaluri, C., Cserpán, D., Somogyvári, Z., Kim, J. K., Kilpatrick, Z. P., Bennett, M. R., Josić, K., Elices, I., Arroyo, D., Levi, R., Rodriguez, F. B., Varona, P., Hwang, E., ... Chhabria, K. (2016). 25th annual computational neuroscience meeting: CNS-2016. *BMC Neuroscience, 17*(S1). https://doi.org/10.1186/s12868-016-0283-6.

Sheban, F., Phan, T. S., Xie, K., Ingelfinger, F., Gur, C., Shapir Itai, Y., Blecher-Gonen, R., Yu, C., Avellino, R., Chalan, P., Freitag, K., Yofe, I., Yutkin, V., Boyeau, P., Ergen, C., Hong, J., Mazuz, K., Liu, Y., Chen, K., ... Amit, I. (2025). ZEB2 is a master switch controlling the tumor-associated macrophage program. *Cancer Cell, 43*(7), 1227. https://doi.org/10.1016/j.ccell.2025.03.021, https://www.sciencedirect.com/science/journal/15356108.

Shi, P., Han, J., Zhang, Y., Li, G., & Zhou, X. (2024). IMI-driver: Integrating multilevel gene networks and multiomics for cancer driver gene identification. *PLoS Computational Biology, 20*(8), e1012389.

Shi, S., Wang, Y., Wu, J., Zha, B., Li, P., Liu, Y., Yang, Y., Kong, J., Gao, S., Cui, H., Huangfu, L., Sun, X., Li, Z., Liang, I., Zheng, Y., & Yang, D. (2024). Predictive value of PD-L1 and TMB for short-term efficacy prognosis in non-small cell lung cancer and construction of prediction models. *Frontiers in Oncology, 14*. https://doi.org/10.3389/fonc.2024.1342262.

Sohrab, Raj, Nagar, et al. (2023). Chronic inflammation's transformation to cancer: A nanotherapeutic paradigm. *Molecules (Basel, Switzerland), 28*(11).

Su, X., Gao, Y., & Yang, R. (2022). Gut microbiota-derived tryptophan metabolites maintain gut and systemic homeostasis. *Cells, 11*(15), 2296. https://doi.org/10.3390/cells11152296.

Sui, Q., Zhang, X., Chen, C., Tang, J., Yu, J., Li, W., Han, K., Jiang, W., Liao, L., Kong, L., Li, Y., Hou, Z., Zhou, C., Zhang, C., Zhang, L., Xiao, B., Mei, W., Xu, Y., Qin, J., ... Ding, P.-R. (2022). Inflammation promotes resistance to immune checkpoint inhibitors in high microsatellite instability colorectal cancer. *Nature Communications, 13*(1). https://doi.org/10.1038/s41467-022-35096-6.

Sun, E., Motolani, A., Campos, L., & Lu, T. (2022). The pivotal role of NF-kB in the pathogenesis and therapeutics of Alzheimer's disease. *International Journal of Molecular Sciences, 23*(16), 8972. https://doi.org/10.3390/ijms23168972.

Sun, J., Hwang, P., Sakkas, E. D., Zhou, Y., Perez, L., Dave, I., Kwon, J. B., McMahon, A. E., Wichman, M., Raval, M., Scopino, K., Krizanc, D., Thayer, K. M., & Weir, M. P. (2024). GNN codon adjacency tunes protein translation. *International Journal of Molecular Sciences, 25*(11), 5914. https://doi.org/10.3390/ijms25115914.

Trehan, R., Huang, P., Zhu, X. B., Wang, X., Soliman, M., Strepay, D., Nur, A., Kedei, N., Arhin, M., Ghabra, S., Rodríguez-Matos, F., Benmebarek, M. R., Ma, C., Korangy, F., & Greten, T. F. (2025). SPP1 + macrophages cause exhaustion of tumor-specific T cells in liver metastases. *Nature Communications, 16*(1). https://doi.org/10.1038/s41467-025-59529-0, https://www.nature.com/ncomms/.

Vasudevan, V., Agnihotri, P., & Biswas, S. (2021). Post translational modification and its pathologic association in rheumatoid arthritis: A brief perspective. *Current Protein & Peptide Science, 22*(7), 548–558. https://doi.org/10.2174/1389203722666210215152433.

Wang, J., Yang, P., Yu, T., Gao, M., Liu, D., Zhang, J., Lu, C., Chen, X., Zhang, X., & Liu, Y. (2022). Lactylation of PKM2 suppresses inflammatory metabolic adaptation in pro-inflammatory macrophages. *International Journal of Biological Sciences, 18*(16), 6210–6225. https://doi.org/10.7150/ijbs.75434.

Wang, L., Zhang, R.-K., Sang, P., Xie, Y.-X., Zhang, Y., Zhou, Z.-H., Wang, K.-K., Zhou, F.-M., Ji, X.-B., Liu, W.-J., Qiu, J.-G., & Jiang, B.-H. (2024). HK2 and LDHA upregulation mediate hexavalent chromium-induced carcinogenesis, cancer development and prognosis through miR-218 inhibition. *Ecotoxicology and Environmental Safety, 279*, 116500. https://doi.org/10.1016/j.ecoenv.2024.116500.

Wang, X., Zhao, J., Marostica, E., Yuan, W., Jin, J., Zhang, J., Li, R., Tang, H., Wang, K., Li, Y., Wang, F., Peng, Y., Zhu, J., Zhang, J., Jackson, C. R., Zhang, J., Dillon, D., Lin, N. U., Sholl, L., ... Yu, K.-H. (2024). A pathology foundation model for cancer diagnosis and prognosis prediction. *Nature, 634*(8035), 970–978. https://doi.org/10.1038/s41586-024-07894-z.

Wang, Y., Zheng, D., Tan, Q., Wang, M. X., & Gu, L. Q. (2011). Nanopore-based detection of circulating microRNAs in lung cancer patients. *Nature Nanotechnology, 6*(10), 668–674. https://doi.org/10.1038/nnano.2011.147, http://www.nature.com/nnano/index.html.

Wang, Z., Zong, H., Liu, W., Lin, W., Sun, A., Ding, Z., Chen, X., Wan, X., Liu, Y., Hu, Z., Zhang, H., Li, H., Liu, Y., Li, D., Zhang, S., & Zha, X. (2024). Augmented ERO1α upon mTORC1 activation induces ferroptosis resistance and tumor progression via upregulation of SLC7A11. *Journal of Experimental & Clinical Cancer Research, 43*(1). https://doi.org/10.1186/s13046-024-03039-2.

Weng, Y., Jia, R., & Ning, P. (2025). Mechanisms of synergistic regulation of the tumor microenvironment by fibroblasts and keratinocytes in esophageal squamous cell carcinoma. *Discover Oncology, 16*(1). https://doi.org/10.1007/s12672-025-03877-2.

Wilson, D. J., & DuBois, R. N. (2022). Role of prostaglandin E2 in the progression of gastrointestinal cancer. *Cancer Prevention Research, 15*(6), 355–363. https://doi.org/10.1158/1940-6207.capr-22-0038.

Xie, M., Yuan, K., Zhang, Y., Zhang, Y., Zhang, R., Gao, J., Wei, W., Jiang, L., Li, T., Ding, Y., Wang, L., Lin, Y., Wong, C. C., & Yu, J. (2025). Tumor-resident probiotic *Clostridium butyricum* improves aPD-1 efficacy in colorectal cancer models by inhibiting IL-6-mediated immunosuppression. *Cancer Cell, 43*(10), 1885. https://doi.org/10.1016/j.ccell.2025.07.012.

Xie, Y., Chen, C., Wu, F., Peng, Y., Su, J., Zhao, Y., Huang, H., Li, Z. A., Pei, Y., Li, W., He, Y., Xue, T., Cao, C., Peng, S., Zhang, X., & Song, W. (2025). Single-cell analysis clarifies pathological heterogeneity in tenosynovial giant cell tumor and identifies biomarkers for predicting disease recurrence. *Advanced Science, 12*(26). https://doi.org/10.1002/advs.202415835, http://onlinelibrary.wiley.com/journal/10.1002/(ISSN)2198-3844.

Xin, P., Xu, X., Deng, C., Liu, S., Wang, Y., Zhou, X., Ma, H., Wei, D., & Sun, S. (2020). The role of JAK/STAT signaling pathway and its inhibitors in diseases. *International Immunopharmacology, 80*, 106210. https://doi.org/10.1016/j.intimp.2020.106210.

Xiong, Z., Chan, S. L., Zhou, J., Vong, J. S. L., Kwong, T. T., Zeng, X., Wu, H., Cao, J., Tu, Y., Feng, Y., Yang, W., Wong, P. P. C., Si-Tou, W. W. Y., Liu, X., Wang, J., Tang, W., Liang, Z., Lu, J., Li, K. M., ... Cheng, A. S. L. (2023). Targeting PPAR-gamma counteracts tumour adaptation to immune-checkpoint blockade in hepatocellular carcinoma. *Gut, 72*(9), 1758–1773. https://doi.org/10.1136/gutjnl-2022-328364, http://gut.bmj.com/content/by/year.

Xu, J., Ding, L., Mei, J., Hu, Y., Kong, X., Dai, S., Bu, T., Xiao, Q., & Ding, K. (2025). Dual roles and therapeutic targeting of tumor-associated macrophages in tumor microenvironments. *Signal Transduction and Targeted Therapy, 10*(1). https://doi.org/10.1038/s41392-025-02325-5.

Yang, L., & Lin, P. C. (2017). Mechanisms that drive inflammatory tumor microenvironment, tumor heterogeneity, and metastatic progression. *Seminars in Cancer Biology, 47*, 185–195. https://doi.org/10.1016/j.semcancer.2017.08.001, http://www.elsevier.com/inca/publications/store/6/2/2/9/4/3/index.htt.

Yang, Y., Li, J., Lei, W., Wang, H., Ni, Y., Liu, Y., Yan, H., Tian, Y., Wang, Z., Yang, Z., Yang, S., Yang, Y., & Wang, Q. (2023). CXCL12-CXCR4/CXCR7 axis in cancer: From mechanisms to clinical applications. *International Journal of Biological Sciences, 19*(11), 3341–3359. https://doi.org/10.7150/ijbs.82317.

Yi, M., Zheng, X., Niu, M., Zhu, S., Ge, H., & Wu, K. (2022). Combination strategies with PD-1/PD-L1 blockade: Current advances and future directions. *Molecular Cancer, 21*(1). https://doi.org/10.1186/s12943-021-01489-2.

You, Y., Tsai, C.-F., Patel, R., Sarkar, S., Clair, G., Zhou, M., Liu, T., Metz, T. O., Das, C., & Nakayasu, E. S. (2023). Analysis of a macrophage carbamylated proteome reveals a function in post-translational modification crosstalk. *Cell Communication and Signaling, 21*(1). https://doi.org/10.1186/s12964-023-01257-3.

Yu, Z., Zhang, Q., Wei, S., Zhang, Y., Zhou, T., Zhang, Q., Shi, R., Zinovkin, D., Pranjol, Z. I., Zhang, J., & Wang, H. (2024). CD146+CAFs promote progression of endometrial cancer by inducing angiogenesis and vasculogenic mimicry via IL-10/JAK1/STAT3 pathway. *Cell Communication and Signaling, 22*(1). https://doi.org/10.1186/s12964-024-01550-9.

Yuan, L., Wang, Q., Sun, F., & Shi, H. (2025). Deep learning and inflammatory markers predict early response to immunotherapy in unresectable NSCLC: A multicenter study. *Biomolecules and Biomedicine, 25*(10), 2252–2268. https://doi.org/10.17305/bb.2025.12324.

Zelante, T., Costantini, C., & Romani, L. (2020). Microbiome-mediated regulation of anti-fungal immunity. *Current Opinion in Microbiology, 58*, 8–14. https://doi.org/10.1016/j.mib.2020.05.002.

Zhang, X., Fu, Z., Wang, H., & Sheng, L. (2024). Metabolic pathways, genomic alterations, and post-translational modifications in pulmonary hypertension and cancer as therapeutic targets and biomarkers. *Frontiers in Pharmacology, 15*. https://doi.org/10.3389/fphar.2024.1490892.

Zhang, Z., Tang, J., Song, J., Xie, M., Liu, Y., Dong, Z., Liu, X., Li, X., Zhang, M., Chen, Y., Shi, H., & Zhong, J. (2022). Elabela alleviates ferroptosis, myocardial remodeling, fibrosis and heart dysfunction in hypertensive mice by modulating the IL-6/STAT3/GPX4 signaling. *Free Radical Biology and Medicine, 181*, 130–142. https://doi.org/10.1016/j.freeradbiomed.2022.01.020.

Zhang, Z., Yu, Y., Zhang, Z., Li, D., Liang, Z., Wang, L., Chen, Y., Liang, Y., & Niu, H. (2023). Cancer-associated fibroblasts-derived CXCL12 enhances immune escape of bladder cancer through inhibiting P62-mediated autophagic degradation of PDL1. *Journal of Experimental & Clinical Cancer Research, 42*(1). https://doi.org/10.1186/s13046-023-02900-0.

Zhao, M., Cheng, X., Shao, P., Dong, Y., Wu, Y., Xiao, L., Cui, Z., Sun, X., Gao, C., Chen, J., Huang, Z., & Zhang, J. (2024). Bacterial protoplast-derived nanovesicles carrying CRISPR-Cas9 tools re-educate tumor-associated macrophages for enhanced cancer immunotherapy. *Nature Communications, 15*(1). https://doi.org/10.1038/s41467-024-44941-9.

Zhao, M., Wang, T., Gleber-Netto, F. O., Chen, Z., McGrail, D. J., Gomez, J. A., Ju, W., Gadhikar, M. A., Ma, W., Shen, L., Wang, Q., Tang, X., Pathak, S., Raso, M. G., Burks, J. K., Lin, S. Y., Wang, J., Multani, A. S., Pickering, C. R., ... Zhou, G. (2024). Mutant p53 gains oncogenic functions through a chromosomal instability-induced cytosolic DNA response. *Nature Communications, 15*(1). https://doi.org/10.1038/s41467-023-44239-2, https://www.nature.com/ncomms/.

SECTION V

Clinical implications and therapeutic strategies

CHAPTER

9

Inflammation and tumor microenvironment

Meng Xia

Department of Cardiology, The Affiliated Hospital of Southwest Medical University, Luzhou, Sichuan, P.R. China

9.1 Introduction

Immunometabolism has experienced significant progress in recent years, notably with regard to its relevance in cancer biology. Specifically, immunometabolism concerns the metabolic phenotypes of immune cells and their modulation to mediate immune responses. The emergence of this field of study has demonstrated how metabolic pathways modulate the functions of immune cells and how these immune cells interact with tumor cells in the tumor microenvironment (TME). Concerning cancer, the metabolic reprogramming of both tumor and immune cells is a focus of study, as it is recognized that metabolic reprogramming may determine the response to treatment, as well as the effectiveness of treatment, including immunotherapy. For example, energy demands of rapidly dividing cancer cells create a nutrient-deficient immune suppressive TME, which may limit the activation and function of immune cells, particularly T cells (Leone & Powell, 2020).

The relationship between cancer cell metabolism and immune cell activity is complicated and multifactorial. Tumor cells often have disrupted metabolic pathways, specifically enhanced glycolysis and glutaminolysis, which promote their growth and change the metabolic status of the TME. This metabolic competition between tumor and immune cells can lead to immune evasion; immune cells can become dysfunctional when deprived of their nutrients and dependent on the accumulation of immunosuppressive metabolites produced by the tumor like lactate, adenosine, and others (Ricci, 2025). The scope of these metabolic interactions needs to be clarified and evaluated to inform the design of novel therapeutic strategies designed to bypass immune suppression and promote antitumor immunity.

Recent discoveries have identified essential metabolic pathways that modulate the immune response to tumors. In particular, the metabolic pathways of glucose and glutamine have been shown to support T cell activation and function. Thus altered metabolism of glucose or glutamine can lead to T cell exhaustion, a state of impaired effector function with

Inflammation in Tumorigenesis and Cancer Treatment
DOI: https://doi.org/10.1016/B978-0-443-36649-9.00001-3

increased expression of inhibitory receptors like PD-1 (Wei, Wang, et al., 2021). Furthermore, metabolic reprogramming of immune cells also provides the ability to differentiate into particular subsets with specific functional roles, meaning the immune response to tumors is more complex than we think. The identification of metabolic pathways and accessibility to modify these pathways highlights an opportunity to reestablish or enhance immune function in patients with cancer.

In addition, the TME is not simply a passive place but a dynamic environment that interacts with infiltrating immune cells to shape their metabolic profiles. For instance, tumor-associated macrophages (TAMs) and myeloid-derived suppressor cells (MDSCs) can drastically modify the metabolic environment and induce immune tolerance on the part of the immune cells and ultimately promote tumor progression (Khameneh et al., 2024). The metabolic interplay between tumor cells and immune cells represents a unique opportunity for detecting potential new therapeutic targetable strategies that may improve the efficacy of current immunotherapies.

The field of immunometabolism is constantly changing, and one area of future research is the implementation of metabolic interventions as adjunct therapies in cancer treatment. The inclusion of metabolic modulators to restore immune cell functionality by modifying metabolic pathways in conjunction with targeting the metabolic weaknesses of cancer cells can allow for innovative therapeutic approaches. The better we understand the metabolic competition and interplay in the TME, the better we can develop cancer immunotherapy based on advances in immunometabolism that can promote tumor targeting antitumor immunity while possibly also reducing the adverse effects associated with conventional therapeutic options (Zhao et al., 2025).

In conclusion, the study of immunometabolism provides an exciting opportunity for improving cancer therapy. By providing insight into the relationship between metabolic reprogramming, immune responses, and tumor progression, investigators can develop new approaches to battle the challenges of TME. Understanding this relationship will be invaluable in developing next-generation immunotherapies that capitalize on and enhance the immune response to effectively treat cancer.

9.2 Main body

9.2.1 Immune metabolism: basic concepts and core pathways

9.2.1.1 Major metabolic characteristics of immune cells

T cell subtype metabolic preferences: Effector T cells (Teff) utilize glycolysis; memory T cells (Tmems) prefer oxidative phosphorylation (OXPHOS). Cells utilize different metabolic adaptations that are important for their function and longevity. Teff utilize glycolysis mainly to support their high energy requirements when they rapidly proliferate and perform their effector function, which includes any aspect of their sudden and acute new immune response. This metabolic process, commonly termed the Warburg effect, enables Teff cells to rapidly generate ATP while simultaneously providing metabolic intermediates that will be processed for the biosynthetic pathways needed for the cell to grow and function

(Butterfield et al., 2020). Tmems, in contrast to Teff cells, use OXPHOS primarily, which helps Tmem maintain energy homeostasis while remaining in a quiescent state for long periods (Wei, Ding, et al., 2021). These two modes of ATP production are cyclical in the T cell subset and thus allow for a more flexible immune system that can respond and replicate when encountering pathogens again and provide rest time when subjected to inactivity. The balance of the different energy production pathways is important not only to type of T cell differentiation, but also determines the T cell functional potential. Metabolic pathways represent a fundamental set of processes that can shape how adaptive immunity looks.

Macrophage polarization and metabolic reprogramming: Increased glycolysis in M1 macrophages, OXPHOS in M2 macrophages. Macrophages are extremely versatile immune cells, capable of polarizing into either of two functional states, M1 and M2, and each macrophage state corresponds to a different metabolic profile. M1 macrophages are associated with proinflammatory responses and exhibit increased glycolysis to help support the rapid activation of macrophages and production of inflammatory cytokines (Tabas & Bornfeldt, 2020). This metabolic reprogramming is necessary to fight pathogens and protect of a host. M2 macrophages, responsible for tissue repair, or that exhibit antiinflammatory responses, rely upon OXPHOS and fatty acid oxidation for their energy production (Su et al., 2024). While the metabolic similarities between M1 and M2 macrophages complements their role in response function, they also highlight that metabolism is part of the pathway to reprogram macrophage polarization and modulate the immune responses to complex diseases, such as cancer or chronic inflammation. Fig. 9.1 provides a schematic

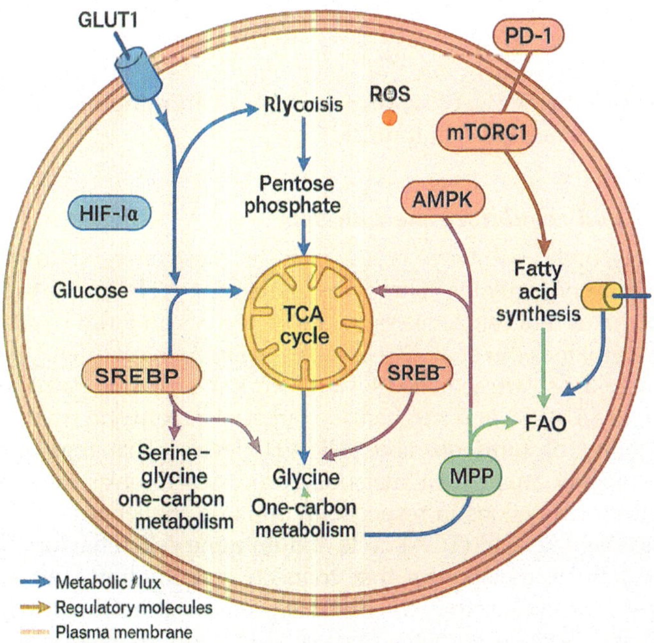

FIGURE 9.1 Immunometabolic pathway overview schematic. This figure provides a schematic illustration of the immune metabolic pathways.

TABLE 9.1 Summary of immunometabolic phenotypes of key immune cell subsets.

Immune cell type	Dominant metabolic pathway	Functional phenotype	Key regulatory molecules
$CD8^+$ effector T cells	Aerobic glycolysis	Cytotoxic effector function	mTORC1, HIF-1α
$CD4^+$ memory T cells	Oxidative phosphorylation and fatty acid oxidation	Long-term memory	AMPK, PGC-1α
M1-like macrophages	Aerobic glycolysis	Proinflammatory phenotype	NF-κB, IRF5
M2-like macrophages	Fatty acid oxidation and oxidative phosphorylation	Antiinflammatory phenotype	PPARγ, STAT6

illustration of the immune metabolic pathways. Table 9.1 provides a summary of the immunometabolic phenotypes related to the major immune cell subsets. The role of dendritic cell (DC) metabolic adaptation in antigen presentation function.

DCs are important linkers of the innate and adaptive immunity, and the metabolic landscape of DCs determines their ability to present antigens and stimulate T cells upon activation. Activated DCs reprogram their metabolism and increase OXPHOS and glycolysis as transitional states prior to full maturation and function (Kazmi et al., 2022). This metabolic shift supports the production of proinflammatory cytokines and improves their ability to present antigens. Finally, the metabolic mode taken by DCs can also affect the DC-stimulated T cell response. Increased glycolytic activity in DCs supports a downstream Th17 response to inflammation, while relying on OXPHOS favored regulatory T cell (Treg) differentiation (Spangenberg et al., 2024). Clarifying the metabolic needs of DCs will be critical to designing new methods to improve vaccine responses, new immunotherapeutic approaches, and other strategies to enhance local immunity.

9.2.1.2 Key metabolic pathways and regulatory mechanisms

The immunoregulatory role of glycolytic pathways is not only the most energy-releasing pathway but also an important immunoregulator. Glycolysis generates ATP in activated immune cells and produces intermediates that can act as signaling molecules and also regulate the expression of key inflammatory cytokines (Su et al., 2024). Furthermore, glycolytic enzymes such as hexokinase and phosphofructokinase are activated by a network of signaling pathways such as AMP-activated protein kinase (AMPK) and mechanistic target of rapamycin (mTOR), which will respond to the availability of nutrients and cell ATP levels. This regulatory landscape allows immune cells to quickly adapt their metabolic processes to environmental signals and greatly amplify their effector functions in response to immune challenges.

The relationship between the tricarboxylic acid (TCA) cycle and immune cell behavior: The TCA cycle is a key component of cellular metabolism that connects carbohydrate, fat, and protein metabolism. In immune cells, TCA cycle activity is critical to producing metabolites that will be used to generate energy and for biosynthetic purposes (Butterfield et al., 2020). Additionally, not only do T cells and macrophages rely on the activity of the TCA cycle, but continued TCA cycle activity also indirectly serves to support the generation of acetyl-CoA. In T cells, once TCA cycle activity produces citrate, citrate can be converted to acetyl-CoA, a substrate for both fatty acid synthesis and histone acetylation, thus making significant contributions to T cell function and differentiation. The role of the TCA cycle in regulating immune cell behavior is illustrative of the important functions of metabolic processes on immune function and their ability to create homeostatic or defensive immune responses. The two sides of fatty acid metabolism in immune cells represent two sides of the same coin in immune function: energy source (catabolic) versus second messenger (anabolic). In macrophages, fatty acid oxidation (a catabolic role of fatty acid metabolism) serves to drive M2 polarization and antiinflammatory profiles, whereas mediating excess amounts of fatty acids as an energy source leads to increased proinflammatory M1 polarization (Su et al., 2024). Key transcription factors (e.g., PPARs, SREBP) regulate the use of fatty acid metabolism depending upon different stimuli in the cellular environment and availability of nutrients. Furthermore, understanding how metabolic pathways regulate fatty acid metabolism in immune cells is vital to developing therapeutic strategies that can impact immune responses relevant to human disease (including cancer and autoimmune disorders).

9.2.1.3 Crosstalk between metabolic sensors and signaling pathways

9.2.1.3.1 The role of the mechanistic target of rapamycin pathway in immune metabolism

The mTOR is an important regulator of cellular metabolism and immune cell function. mTOR integrates signals regarding nutrients, growth factors, and cellular energy levels to regulate metabolic pathways (e.g., glycolysis, TCA cycle, fatty acid metabolism), ultimately impacting cellular function (Butterfield et al., 2020). In T cells, mTOR activity drives glycolytic catabolism and enhances the T cell effector functions that protect against infection, while mTOR inhibition allows reprogramming to a metabolism that favors memory formation. mTOR activity is intricately regulated by a variety of upstream signal transduction pathways (e.g., PI3K/Akt, AMPK) that respond to nutrient availability and cellular stress. This complexity further emphasizes the significance of mTOR to support immune responses and provides compelling rationale for utilizing it as a potential therapeutic target in cancer and autoimmune disease.

9.2.1.3.2 AMPK-activated protein kinase regulation of energy balance in immune cells

AMPK functions as a key energy sensor in cells that regulates metabolic pathways in response to a changing cellular energy state. AMPK activation in immune cells stimulates catabolic processes (that generate ATP) and inhibits anabolic processes (that consume ATP) (Butterfield et al., 2020). This important regulatory function is critical for immune cell function under metabolic stress, as can occur during immunity, infection, or inflammation. The relationship between AMPK and mTOR pathways illustrates the complexity of immune metabolism; AMPK can also exert inhibitory effects on the mTOR pathway under low energy conditions, promoting metabolic flexibility and maintaining immune homeostasis.

Hypoxia-inducible factor-1α (HIF-1α) and metabolic modulation in hypoxia: HIF-1α is a transcription factor that modulates cellular responses to low oxygen levels. In immune cells, HIF-1α activation leads to metabolic reprogramming that supports glycolysis and facilitates proinflammatory responses (Butterfield et al., 2020). Overall, metabolic adaptation of immune cell function in hypoxic environments surrounding tumors or inflamed tissues is important. HIF-1α interacts with many metabolic pathways, including the TCA cycle and fatty acid metabolism, to coordinate immune responses and maintain balance within cellular energy levels. Evaluating the role of HIF-1α in immune metabolism reveals important information on ways to manipulate immune responses in cancer and chronic inflammatory disease to develop potential or novel therapies.

9.2.2 Metabolic reprogramming in the tumor microenvironment

9.2.2.1 Metabolic characteristics of tumor cells

The Warburg effect, or the preference by cancer cells for aerobic glycolysis in lieu of OXPHOS, is a defined trait of tumor metabolism, even in the presence of sufficient oxygen. Tumor cells preferentially operate from aerobic glycolysis, which supports several processes, including ATP generation, enabling proliferative survival in the TME (Tan et al., 2023). There is a byproduct of aerobic glycolysis, and that is lactic acid, which establishes an acidic microenvironment initially, but lactic acid also acts as an immunosuppressive agent that inhibits cytotoxic T lymphocytes, as well as natural killer cells from functioning (Guo et al., 2024). Furthermore, the Warburg effect fuels tumor growth via angiogenesis and provides adequate niches for tumor growth to be sustained. The ability of tumor cells to adapt metabolically is usually synonymous with changes in gene expression and signaling pathways, which can confer resistant and survival advantages for the tumor (Zeng et al., 2025). Thus targeting by way of the Warburg effect may present an alternative therapy approach when addressing the distribution of these unique metabolic advantages for maximizing the effects of immunity.

Tumor cells possess competitive strategies for nutrient acquisition that are vital for their growth and survival in a nutrient-poor TME. They often take over the nutrient-handling pathways of neighboring stroma cells and immune cells through a process called "nutritional competition" (Li et al., 2025). For example, tumor cells can upregulate glucose transporters and downstream enzymes in glycolysis to out-compete immune cells for glucose, which is critical for the activation and function of immune cells (Zhou et al., 2023). In addition, tumor cells can alter the metabolism of amino acids and lipids and continue to deprive immune cells of the substrates required for immune functions (Li et al., 2024). Nutritional competition not only supports tumor growth but is an aspect of immune evasion, in which the absence of nutrients can drive severe dysfunction and exhaustion in T cells (Guo et al., 2024). Therefore understanding how nutritional competition occurs in the TME is an important consideration for developing approaches that can restore immune function and improve outcomes in the face of tumor nutrition.

As a major metabolic byproduct of the Warburg effect, lactate is an important factor in forming an immunosuppressive TME. Lactate can also inhibit T cell activation and proliferation, promote Treg differentiation, and enhance the suppressive functions of MDSCs (Barba et al., 2024). Increasing lactate concentrations induced an acidic environment, which can hinder the cytotoxic capacity of Teff and natural killer cells and help drive immune escape (Liang et al., 2025). Lactate can directly influence levels of immune checkpoint molecules such as PD-L1 (Guo et al., 2024). These findings suggest that targeting lactate metabolism and its influence on immune cells may provide a promising strategy to increase the effectiveness of immunotherapies and resistance in cancer treatment.

9.2.2.2 *The tumor microenvironment and immune cell metabolism*

Hypoxia alters immune cell metabolism and is a major feature of the TME. Immune cells, including T cell and macrophages that develop under hypoxic conditions, will experience metabolic reprogramming that impacts survival and functionality (Tan et al., 2023). For example, the pathway of OXPHOS will be inhibited in hypoxic conditions, limiting the energy production pathway to glycolysis, which, although less efficient overall, allows T cells to produce ATP in a rapid manner (Guo et al., 2024). Therefore the metabolic changes that occur in cells exposed to hypoxic conditions will impact T cell effector function, such as cytokine production and cytotoxicity, which will lead to tumor promotion. Notably, hypoxia causes increased expression of immune checkpoints that inhibit immune responses and promote tumor immune escape (Liang et al., 2025). The influence of hypoxia on immune cell metabolism is finely tuned and provides a strong rationale for exploring strategies to promote antitumor immunity and potentially improve the efficacy of immunotherapies. Within the TME, nutrient deprivation (i.e., hypoglycemia, hypolipidemia) and prolonged nutrient deprivation frequently develop as rapidly proliferative tumor cells increase their external metabolic demand (Li et al., 2025). It is well known that immune cells require sufficient nutrients, including glucose, amino acids, and lipids, for activation and function. In the absence of nutrient availability, waste recovery using endogenous nutrients that contribute to metabolism causes T cell dysfunction, decreased cytokine production, and progressively increased expression of IL-6, PD-1, and CTLA-4 (Barba et al., 2024). T cell dysfunction is associated with diminished ability to control tumor growth and ultimately poor patient responses to the treatment/maintenance care of immunotherapy. Restoring nutrients from the microenvironment to utilize in bioenergetic metabolism or providing alternative nutrients to increase metabolic fitness of T cells may also be important for reinvigorating antitumor immune responses to nutrient-depleted TME.

The acidic TME produced by tumor metabolism, largely due to the accumulation of lactic acid, alters the function and activation of immune cells. Evolving acidic microenvironments limit T cell, macrophage, and DC activation and proliferation, thus limiting the overall ability of those cells to initiate antitumor responses (Barba et al., 2024). Low pH can also affect surface receptor and cytokine expression by immune cells, further limiting function. For example, T cells proliferated in an acidic environment can show elevated expression of inhibitory receptors, which inhibit the cytotoxicity of the T cells (Liang et al., 2025). As such, targeting the acidic TME to restore immune cell function represents a viable therapeutic strategy to maximize immunotherapy efficacy and improve patient outcomes.

9.2.2.3 *The role and importance of metabolic checkpoints*

The PD-1/PD-L1 pathway is an important checkpoint in immune regulation as well as metabolic reprogramming in tumor and immune cells. PD-1 engagement on T cells leads to a metabolic reprogramming that facilitates glycolytic processes and inhibits OXPHOS, which together diminish T cell activation and function (Liang et al., 2025). This metabolic reprogramming is associated with increased lactate production and acidifying the TME that now established a positive feedback loop that inhibits antitumor immunity. The relationship between PD-1 signaling and metabolic pathways is vital to understanding how combination therapies will work to target immune checkpoints and metabolic liabilities for therapeutic treatment.

CTLA-4 is an important immune checkpoint associated with T cell metabolism and activity. Similar to PD-1, binding of CTLA-4 may inhibit T cell activity and promote a suppressive immunosuppressive environment (Zeng et al., 2025). By influencing the metabolic signals, CTLA-4 can influence the ratio of regulatory and Teff, and therefore impact the antitumor immune activity. These findings suggest that CTLA-4 in combination with metabolic inhibitors may improve T cell optimizations and eventually an intended end therapeutic state of T cell adoptive transfer in cancer immunotherapy (Ding et al., 2025). Recently, metabolic checkpoints have been identified that regulate immune activity in the TME. Fig. 9.2 depicts the collective metabolic processes involving tumor cells, immune cells, and extracellular matrix. These metabolic checkpoints consist of different metabolic enzymes and pathways that characterize TME and dictate the immune landscape and function of immunotherapy (Barba et al., 2024). For example, inhibition of metabolic enzymes involved in either glycolysis or lipid metabolism has shown improvement in

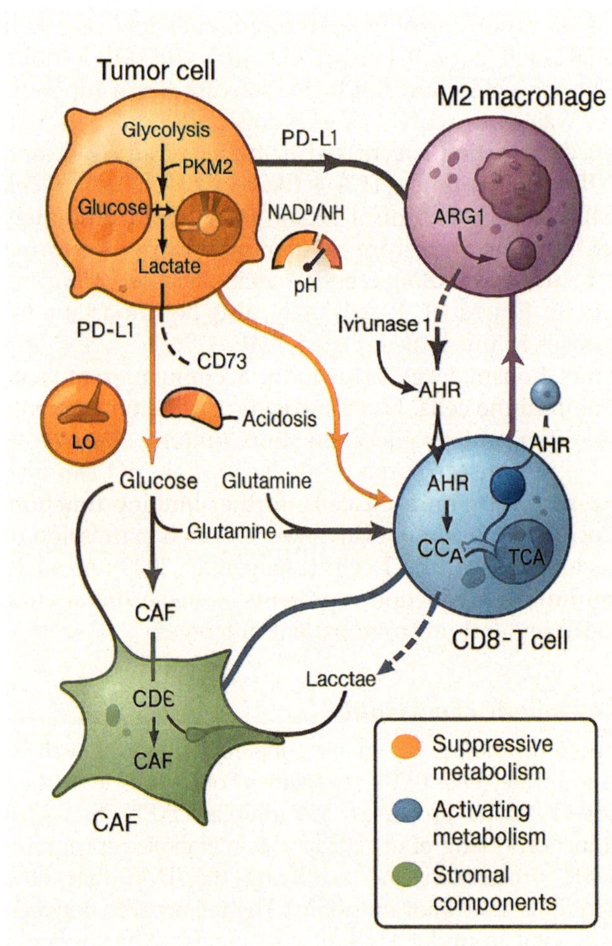

FIGURE 9.2 Comprehensive tumor–immune–stroma metabolic interaction network. The figure depicts the collective metabolic processes involving tumor cells, immune cells, and extracellular matrix. These metabolic checkpoints consist of different metabolic enzymes and pathways that characterize TME and dictate the immune landscape and function of immunotherapy.

reversing immune suppression and restoring T cell function. Continued identification and validation of novel metabolic checkpoints positively enhance our understanding of tumor immunology and led to previously unidentifiable therapeutic assets for the treatment of cancer.

9.2.3 Immune metabolic abnormalities and tumor immune evasion

9.2.3.1 Metabolic basis of T cell exhaustion

Mitochondrial dysfunction has been identified as a major driver of T cell exhaustion in a TME. Energy production and competent immune responses, particularly in CD8+ cytotoxic T lymphocytes, rely on mitochondrial OXPHOS. Following persistently elevated tumor antigens, such as in cancer, T cells undergo metabolic reprogramming, which is evidenced by a shift from OXPHOS to glycolysis. T cells also experience general mitochondrial impairment as demonstrated by decreased mitochondrial function, increased production of reactive oxygen species (ROS), and reduced ATP production. The shift from OXPHOS causes T cell effector functions, including cytokine production and cytotoxicity, to decline as observed in exhausted T cells. Studies have shown that mitochondrial dysfunction leads to both decreased ATP production and reduced mitochondrial membrane potential, which further propagates T cell dysfunction. For example, mitochondrial complex I inhibition has been shown to propagate T cell exhaustion. The increasing accumulation of damaged or dysfunctional mitochondria in exhausted T cells precedes the manifestation of their own feed-forward loop, as increased levels of ROS and deteriorating metabolism, along with continued increased tumor antigens, create a proinflammatory environment that can drive tumor progression (Huldani et al., 2024; Wang, Chen, et al., 2025).

In the TME, metabolic stress can lead to critical epigenetic changes in T cells and perpetual exhaustion. The altered metabolism of T cells, including aberrant metabolic pathways like kynurenine, generates more kynurenine, which contributes to the T cell's epigenetics. Kynurenine epigenetic changes include alterations of patterns of histone acetylation and patterns of methylation that affect specific gene expression patterns essential to T cell differentiation and T cell activation. To illustrate, metabolic stress could lead to increased levels of histone deacetylases that will repress certain genes necessary for T cell effector functions. Additionally, certain epigenetic regulators that interact with metabolic stress, such as c-Myc and transcription factors, can negatively influence T cell exhaustion. This relationship between metabolism and epigenetics illustrates the multilayered complexity of T-cell exhaustion and how therapeutic interventions aimed at changing the epigenetic changes made by T cells would improve T-cell responses in cancer (Liu, Li, et al., 2025; Tomar et al., 2025).

The concept of Tmems is critical for persistent immunity, but metabolic dysfunction in the surrounding TME can interfere with their differentiation. Tmems require a different metabolic signature consisting of potent oxidative metabolism and fatty acid oxidation for differentiation and abilities to function. A high lactate and other metabolic byproducts found in tumors, however, inhibit Teff from becoming Tmems, as lactate has been shown to stunt mitochondrial function and promote glycolytic burnout—both of which deter memory cell differentiation. Also, T cells must compete with tumors for substrates such as glucose and amino acids, which also impedes Tmems from developing. The ability to develop

Tmems after exhaustion stems from the role of the TME, on T cell metabolism, and any approach that modifies the metabolic state of the tumor, including reducing lactate and utilizing more substrates, has the potential to resume Tmem formation and efficacy in immunotherapy (Lawton et al., 2024; Tao et al., 2023).

9.2.3.2 Metabolic reprogramming of myeloid cells

TAMs have metabolic profiles that affect their function in the TME. M2 macrophages depend on OXPHOS and fatty acids to meet their energy needs, and they are often associated with tumor progression. Whereas M1 macrophages represent the proinflammatory and antitumor function of macrophages. The shift from utilizing glucose for energy to fatty acid oxidation allows M2 macrophages to sustain tumor growth and angiogenesis and suppress antitumor immunity. A recent review of the TAMs shows that in many different cancers, the macrophages had an increased ability to utilize fatty acids, which in turn altered their glucose metabolism to promote immune suppression. For example, TAMs can utilize fatty acids derived from the TME to fuel their metabolism, which, in turn, leads to the production of more immunosuppressive cytokines such as IL-10 and TGF-β. TAMs' propensity to undergo metabolic reprogramming promotes their survival and proliferation as macrophages while allowing them to continue in the pathway that leads to the generation of a protumor microenvironment that promotes immune evasion (Jiang et al., 2024; Tomar et al., 2025).

MDSCs are also an important factor in the TME. MDSCs possess powerful immunosuppressive abilities. Due to the tissue microenvironment and various tumor-associated stimuli, MDSCs undergo significant metabolic reprogramming that contributes to their ability to suppress T cell responses. MDSCs appear to have increased glycolysis rates and altered amino acid metabolites (especially the catabolism of arginine and tryptophan). The increased arginase activity leads to low arginine concentrations, which is important for T cell activation and proliferation. MDSCs also possess metabolic plasticity that enables them to adapt to fluctuating tumor-associated nutrient conditions, which further enhances their suppressive capabilities. Targeting the metabolic pathways that contribute to MDSC immunosuppression (inhibition of arginase and specific regulation of glycolysis) is a novel strategy to enhance antitumor immunity and/or increase the effectiveness of immunotherapies (Flory et al., 2024; Iu et al., 2024).

Tumor-associated neutrophils (TANs) are being studied for their simultaneous roles in tumor progression and immune suppression. TANs can undergo metabolic adaptations as a part of their function in the TME. For example, TANs typically have increased rates of glycolysis that convert glucose into pyruvate, which provides energy for TAN migration to the tumor sites and proliferation. Another metabolic adaptation of TANs is their ability to make ROS and secrete proinflammatory cytokines, which establish or maintain a tumor-supporting inflammation. With respect to T cell responses, TANs can promote T cell immune responses in some tumor contexts as well, so TANs are not always protumor agents. The metabolic state of TANs will dictate the balance between these opposing functions, and the metabolic state of TANs can depend on factors such as hypoxia and nutrient availability. It is important to determine the metabolic adaptations of TANs specifically in the TME and the effect of those adaptations on tumor immunity to formulate strategies to harness the function of TANs to promote antitumor immunity (Flory et al., 2024; Lawton et al., 2024).

9.2.3.3 Metabolism-mediated immune suppression networks

The IDO (indoleamine 2,3-dioxygenase) pathway is an important immune modulation mechanism related to tumor immune evasion by altering tryptophan metabolism to form kynurenine. Fig. 9.3 shows a schematic to demonstrate the metabolic checkpoint and inhibitory network. IDO is frequently expressed in high amounts in TMEs to generate an increased level of kynurenine. Kynurenine is an immunosuppressive metabolite that drives the differentiation of Tregs and inhibits the proliferation and function of Teff. In doing this, this metabolic pathway essentially induces T cell exhaustion, that is thereby enhancing tumor growth. Additionally, kynurenine enhances the function of Tregs and myeloid cells by activating the aryl hydrocarbon receptor. The IDO/kynurenine metabolic pathway has potential to reverse immune suppression in tumors and has possible synergism with immunotherapies (Flory et al., 2024; Wang, Zhuang, et al., 2025).

Another crucial metabolic pathway that is important for immune regulation in the TME is arginine metabolism. Arginase, produced primarily by myeloid cells such as TAMs and MDSCs, converts arginine to ornithine, decreasing arginine's availability for T cell activation. The importance of arginine metabolism in immune regulation is twofold: both the depletion of arginine diminishes T cell function and increases additional

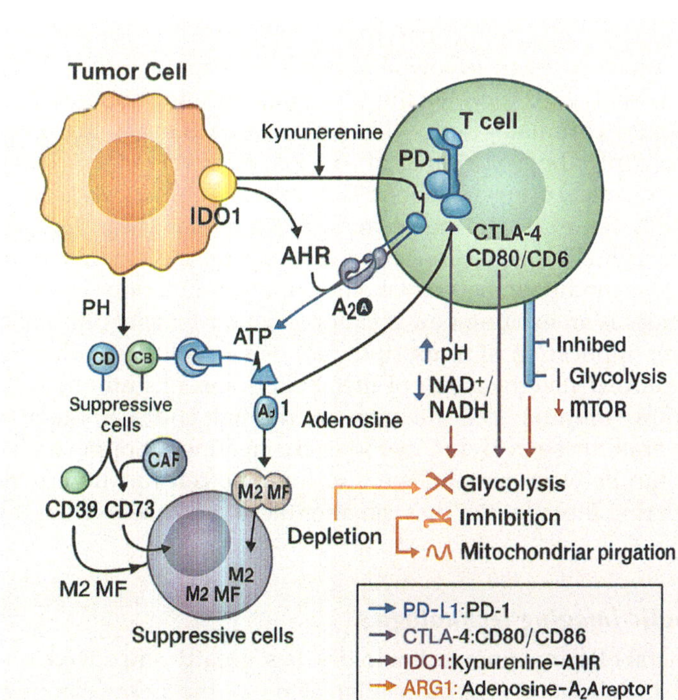

FIGURE 9.3 **Metabolic checkpoints and suppressive network schematic.** This figure shows a schematic to demonstrate the metabolic checkpoint and inhibitory network.

immunosuppressive cell populations. Additionally, depletion of arginine can also lead to accumulation of polyamines, which exacerbate the suppression of T cell activity. Approaches to block arginase functionality or to supplement levels of arginine in the TME could improve T cell activation and strengthen the body's antitumor immunity (Flory et al., 2024; Lawton et al., 2024).

The adenosine signaling pathway is also an important pathway mediating immune suppression in the TME. The presence of adenosine in the TME established by ecto-nucleotidases CD39 and CD73 acts to establish immune suppressive context through inhibiting T cell activation and allowing for Treg type differentiation. Adenosine receptors, A2A and A2B, are expressed on immune cells, and the downstream signaling associated with activating those receptors inhibits proinflammatory signaling events. Strategies that target the adenosine pathway by inhibiting adenosine production or adenosine receptor blockade have been a very promising avenue for enhancing antitumor immunity and increasing the success of immunotherapy (Flory et al., 2024; Lawton et al., 2024).

9.2.4 Immunometabolism research experimental methods and technological advances

9.2.4.1 *Applications of metabolomics in immunometabolism research*

Metabolomics has rapidly grown into an important approach within immunometabolism, allowing us to study the metabolic changes in immune cells during activation and their effector functions. The greatest strength of metabolomics is the use of mass spectrometry (MS) due to its high sensitivity and specificity, which permits the assessment of a number of metabolites, including those that can be present in low abundance. Metabolomics can also utilize the MS phase with additional ionization methods to measure metabolites and separation techniques, such as liquid chromatography (LC–MS) and gas chromatography (GC–MS), to provide full metabolic profiling of biological samples (Carbone et al., 2021). Mike Tull's recent developments on measuring metabolic flux expand our knowledge of metabolic pathways in immune cells. For example, the Seahorse Extracellular Flux Analyzer provides valuable readouts from cellular respiration and real-time measurements from glycolysis to show how immune cells modulate their metabolism upon stimulation (Huldani et al., 2024). Single-cell metabolomics is an exciting new area for examining metabolites and metabolic changes with the further application of transcriptomics. Single-cell metabolomics approaches may reveal the intracellular heterogeneity of metabolic states of immune cells that are integral to understanding immune cell function in normal and pathological conditions (Maas et al., 2022). Overall, these evolving methods are creating an opportunity to study and assess the relationship between metabolism and immune cell function, with important implications for discovering therapeutics that can alter these processes within the field of immunometabolism.

9.2.4.2 *Development of metabolic imaging technologies*

In recent years, growth in metabolic imaging technologies has greatly improved our capacity to visualize and study metabolic processes in vivo. One of the more common imaging modalities for studying in vivo metabolism (particularly related to cancer) is positron emission tomography–computed tomography (PET–CT). PET–CT allows for noninvasive assessment of metabolic activity through tracking the uptake of radiolabeled glucose analogs, such as 18F-FDG, which is taken up by metabolically active cells- tumor and immune cells (Chen, Han, et al., 2023). PET imaging has therefore emerged as a highly relevant and powerful tool to assess both tumor metabolism and effects of immunotherapy through metabolic pathways in the TME. In addition to PET imaging, the development of metabolic fluorescent probes has enabled new real-time imaging approaches to evaluate specific metabolic processes. Metabolic fluorescent probes can be developed to target specific metabolic pathways, which provides insight into the dynamic changes taking place in cells throughout immune responses (Brydges et al., 2022). Superresolution microscopy technologies also have great promise in research on metabolism by enabling researchers to visualize metabolic processes at the nanoscale level. This technology enables researchers to visualize structures and characterize the cellular interactions and metabolic fluxes that were undetectable previously and develop a greater level of understanding of the spatial organization of metabolism in tissues (Povo-Retana et al., 2023). Together, these advances in metabolic imaging technologies will continue to revolutionize our ability to study immunometabolism and provide new ideas for innovative therapies.

9.2.4.3 *Gene editing and metabolism research*

The emergence of gene editing technologies—most notably CRISPR–Cas9—has fundamentally changed how we study immunometabolism by allowing us to more precisely alter metabolic genes and pathways. CRISPR technology allows researchers to directly question the functional roles of specific metabolic genes in immune cell activation→differentiation to determine how downstream metabolic reprogramming has an impact on immune responses (Mikaeloff et al., 2025). As an example, researchers can generate conditional gene knockout models, which can be used to study the effects of deleting metabolic genes in specific immune cell populations (Zhang et al., 2024). These studies allow us to better understand how metabolic genes support their contributions to immune function and disease progression. Additionally, metabolic enzyme reporter gene systems help researchers study real-time metabolic activity in live cells, leading to a better understanding of how metabolic enzymes control immune cell fate and function, especially in the context of cancer immunotherapy (Verheijen et al., 2024). Overall, the convergence of gene editing and metabolic studies is opening up new therapies to target metabolic pathways to activate immune responses against tumors. As we continue to unravel the metabolic and immunological library of knowledge→our new tools and tools will support the new directions of studying and manipulating immune cells' metabolism to provide better therapeutic outcomes for cancer and other maladies.

9.2.5 Targeting immunometabolism in cancer therapy

9.2.5.1 *Development of metabolic intervention drugs*

The idea of metabolic intervention drugs has gained traction in cancer therapy by focusing on targeting key metabolic pathways that are regulated abnormally in tumors. Glycolysis inhibitors are promising because many tumors rely on aerobic glycolysis, otherwise known as the Warburg effect. Studies provide evidence that glycolysis inhibitors such as 2-deoxy-D-glucose (2-DG) can curb the glycolytic pathway, reduce tumor cell proliferation, and increase apoptosis. For example, studies indicate that lactate production was decreased following the 2-DG treatment, which reversed the immunosuppressive impact of the TME and enhanced the efficacy of immune checkpoint inhibitors (ICIs) (Sasaki et al., 2021). Additionally, glutaminase inhibitors may have fulfillment based on early clinical trials; for example, CB-839 could attenuate glutamine metabolism a metabolic dependency that is critical to tumor growth and survival, and not only target the metabolic vulnerabilities of cancer cells, but possibly, progressive reprogram the immune landscape to encourage a more favorable immune landscape to enable T cell infiltration and activities (Chen, Tan, et al., 2023). IDO inhibitors were examined to enhance antitumor immunity by targeting immunosuppressive effects of the tryptophan metabolic pathway. Although there is inspiration from preclinical studies using IDO inhibitors, the clinical data are less promising; thus there requires emphasis on approaches integrating existing drugs and treatment combinations (Guo et al., 2021). Overall, there are a few more metabolic intervention drugs being developed that are anticipated to take advantage of tumor-specific metabolic dependencies to improve cancer therapy efficacy.

9.2.5.2 *Combination therapy with immune checkpoint inhibitors and metabolic modulation*

The use of ICIs and metabolic modulation approaches is a favorable strategy to increase antitumor responses. Recently is has been demonstrated that there is a synergistic effect of PD-1 blockade with metabolic modulation aimed at targeting tumor metabolism. For example, PD-1 blockade can enhance T cell responses in the context of metabolic reprogramming using glycolytic inhibitors. In animal models, increasing glycolysis using 2-DG and PD-1 inhibitors enhanced T cell activation and inhibited tumor growth compared to either alone (Sasaki et al., 2021). Also, glutaminase inhibitors in conjunction with ICIs restored T cell function and improved treatment in multiple cancer models (Chen, Tan, et al., 2023). Overall, metabolic reprogramming involving alterations in not only glycolysis (through modulation of fatty-acid oxidation and OXPHOS) enhances the efficacy of ICIs via enhancing the immune microenvironment. Therefore combining drug effects with metabolic modulators to overcome metabolic barriers imposed by helping T cell effector cells persist and function posttherapy probably improves the overall clinical outcome. Combinational treatment highlights the need to integration of metabolism and immune response, which needs to be more than ancillary, not just in the context of the TME. The summarization of the research concerning the combination of metabolic intervention approaches with immune checkpoint blockade therapies is found in Table 9.2.

9.2.5.3 *Metabolic engineering in cell therapy*

Metabolic engineering is quickly emerging as an important mechanism to improve efficacy of cell therapies, such as chimeric antigen receptor (CAR) T cell therapies. The metabolic requirements of CAR T cells are significantly affected by the TME, which can impose a metabolic stress that negatively influences T cell function and persistence. While there are a number of advances that have been made in metabolic engineering to facilitate

TABLE 9.2 Summary of metabolic intervention strategies combined with immune checkpoint blockade.

Pharmacologic agent	Checkpoint inhibitor combination	Mechanistic rationale	Clinical development status
2-Deoxy-D-glucose	Anti-PD-1 mAb	Competitive inhibition of hexokinase reduces lactate accumulation in TME, restoring $CD8^+$ T-cell function	Preclinical (murine)
Telaglenastat (CB-839)	Anti-PD-1 mAb	GLS1 inhibition deprives tumor cells of glutamine, enhances TIL proliferation, and cytotoxicity	Phase Ib
Epacadostat (INCB024360)	Anti-PD-1/Anti-CTLA-4 mAb	Blocks Trp→Kyn catabolism, lowering Kyn-mediated Treg expansion and reversing local immunosuppression	Phase II/III
AZD4635	Anti-PD-L1 mAb	A2A receptor antagonism prevents adenosine-driven T-cell anergy and enhances effector cytokine release	Phase Ib
CB-1158 (INCB001158)	Anti-PD-1 mAb	Arginase inhibition increases L-arginine availability, promoting T-cell receptor ζ-chain expression	Phase I

TME, Tumor microenvironment.

better metabolic regulation of CAR T cells, it has been shown that genetic modifications that preferentially favor OXPHOS vs glycolytic metabolism have been able to enhance both the survival and function of CAR T cells in solid tumors (Wang, Liao, et al., 2025). The use of metabolic modifiers of ACT, such as IL-15, for example, has also been shown to improve the memory phenotype of CAR T cells, enhance their persistence, and induce an antitumor effect (Xia et al., 2024). Similar metabolic checkpoints, such as mTOR inhibition, have been classified under the approaches designed to enhance metabolic fitness and revitalize exhausted T cells (Ramapriyan et al., 2024). These strategies are generating novel ways to maximize the effectiveness of CAR T cells while reducing the damaging effects of the immunosuppressive TME. As such, there is a growing interest among researchers to discover and integrate metabolic engineering strategies into CAR T cell manufacturing and clinical developments as a way to evolve more effective and durable cancer therapies.

9.2.6 Clinical translation challenges in immunometabolism research

9.2.6.1 Adverse effects of metabolic interventions

The safety of systemic metabolic modifications is a key consideration in immunometabolism advances and translating to the clinic. Metabolic interventions may lead to improvement of immune responses against cancer; however, deleterious effects warrant consideration. Systemic metabolic modifications can lead to unwanted effects and dysregulation of glucose homeostasis and/or lipid metabolism that may worsen existing disorders or lead to novel metabolic disorders (Su et al., 2024). Further, metabolic pathways are intricately linked; therefore interfering with one pathway may affect another and cause additional metabolic effects. For example, modifying the glycolytic pathways to enhance T cell functionality may influence lactate production, leading to increased lactate, which may contribute to an immunoinhibitory TME (Spangenberg et al., 2024). Thus tissue-specific delivery is of utmost importance to limit adverse effects of systemic metabolic intervention. Targeted metabolic therapy could manipulate the metabolic dynamics of immune cells in the TME without systemic exposure, optimizing the chance for therapeutic efficacy while minimizing the opportunity for unwanted or potentially harmful effects (Wei, Ding, et al., 2021). Considering dose escalation and potential therapeutic windows are also important factors in ensuring metabolic modifications provide therapeutic benefits without reaching a threshold that is toxic or may impair immune functionality (Liu, Wu, et al., 2025).

9.2.6.2 *Development of personalized treatment strategies*

Personalized therapeutic strategies based upon metabolic profiling are a notable advancement in immunometabolism research. Metabolic characteristics may serve as potential biomarkers, allowing for the specific therapeutic strategies we use with them to inform patient stratification strategies relative to patients' metabolic profiles (Kazmi et al., 2022). For instance, patients with certain metabolic signatures might respond differently to the daily immunotherapies, which should be those precision medicine approaches, similarly considering patients' metabolic states in addition to their genetic and phenotypic states (Su et al., 2024). Metabolic profiles can vary widely in TMEs, and should similarly think of representing their metabolic profiles as patients receiving therapeutic interventions, which also vary relative to one another. The metabolic heterogeneity that is associated with tumors underscores that metabolic reprogramming will be different when viewed as individuals apart from clinical molecular consequences potentially taking place even within the tumor of one patient (Spangenberg et al., 2024). Incorporating metabolic profiling would better facilitate clinical patient stratification of patients undergoing immunotherapies which would translate to increased efficacy and decreased side effects; however, there are obstacles, such as establishing increasingly better standards of metabolic assay performance and interpreting some metabolic data in clinical patient populations, threatening these future directions of research aimed at improving these methods and demonstrating its clinical utility will remain (Su et al., 2024).

9.2.6.3 *Overcoming drug resistance mechanisms*

Overcoming drug resistance within cancer treatment represents a significant challenge in immunometabolism. Tumor cells, in response to therapeutic pressures, have the ability to reprogram their metabolic pathways, which can result in resistance to treatment (Su et al., 2024). For example, an increase in OXPHOS would be an adaptation at the tumor level, or simply using different nutrients than the commonly used glucose, leading to enhanced tumor cell survival despite the presence of the chemotherapeutic agent (Su et al., 2024). Therefore combination therapy targeted at both metabolic pathways and immune responses is being considered to preempt the development of resistant phenotypes (Su et al., 2024). In addition, dynamic monitoring technologies in the field of metabolic imaging or real-time monitoring of metabolism changes are being developed to provide insight into tumor responsiveness to therapy and changes in therapy regimens if necessary (Su et al., 2024). All of these avenues provide the potential for improved response to immunotherapies and improved development of resistance mechanisms. Ultimately, the transition of any of these approaches to clinical use will need to be validated by developing clinical trials focused on safety, efficacy, and validating outcomes on heterogeneous populations of patients with cancer (Su et al., 2024).

9.2.7 Future research directions and perspectives

9.2.7.1 Research on emerging metabolic pathways

Recent reports have established that ketone body metabolism plays a role in tumor immunity, particularly in cancer therapies. Ketone bodies (i.e., acetoacetate, beta-hydroxybutyrate, and acetone) are acquired from the breakdown of fatty acids, and act as alternative energy substrates for immune cells- particularly CD8+ T effector cells. Numerous reports have demonstrated that at least ketone bodies like β-hydroxybutyrate can positively affect the metabolic considerations leading to improving the metabolic fitness of Teff and subsequent improvements in usage of proliferation and cytotoxicity against tumor cells (Luda et al., 2023). Furthermore, ongoing deliveries of dietary-based initiatives such as the ketogenic diet are described to be able to sensitize tumors to existing therapies such as chemotherapy by transforming the TME in the form of perturbations in the metabolic state of the tumor, with subsequent improvements in immune efficacy (Yang et al., 2022). This suggests that there may be longer term opportunities moving cancer immunotherapy forward based on the dependency of tumors on ketone bodies as a mechanism of metabolism, and potentially improving patient outcomes. One-carbon metabolites also remain an important regulator of immune responses, especially in the context of cancer. One-carbon metabolism relates primarily to nucleotide and amino acid synthesis and energy allocation for proliferating immune cells. Recent work indicates that observing modulation of one-carbon metabolism may play a role in maintaining differentiation and function of a number of immune cell types (i.e., T cells and macrophages) (Xiao et al., 2023). Furthermore, dietary interventions related to one-carbon metabolism (i.e., folate, methionine) may reprogram the immune landscape within a tumor, as well as consider the impact interrelatedly on newly defined immune interventions resonating from dietary influences (Lyon et al., 2020). Future reports should evaluate the role of one-carbon metabolism in regulating immune function and cancer, and assess future opportunities to integrate altered delivery of one-carbon metabolism targeted approaches to create long-term approaches to intervention in immuno-metabolic therapy.

The relationship between the microbiome (and its metabolism) and immune responses may also represent a new area of research opportunity for cancer treatment. We know the gut microbiome can affect systemic metabolism and immune modulation (Luda et al., 2023), and their potential roles in tumor propagation and cancer treatment response. Recent studies have established that some bacteria-specific metabolites can accelerate or dampen immune responses, which affect immunotherapy efficacy (Zhu et al., 2024). By delineating how microbiota affect metabolic pathways, we may also be able to determine therapeutic pathways that use microbes to beneficially temper or improve antitumor immunity. Future studies should focus on characterizing microbial influences on metabolic reprogramming in tumors and their potential as a pharmacological target for treatment.

9.2.7.2 *Technological innovations and multiomics integration*

Spatial metabolomics is a novel strategy that enables the visualization of metabolites in tissues to describe the metabolic heterogeneity present in tumors. This technology integrates advanced imaging strategies and MS to visualize and quantify metabolites in their native state (Min et al., 2024). Investigating the spatial distribution of metabolic activity in a tumor's microenvironment can increase our understanding of tumor biology and tumor responses to therapy. Future studies will identify best practices for integrating spatial metabolomics with other omics technologies, such as genomics and transcriptomics, to further characterize tumor metabolism and its impact on therapy. With increasing details of tumor metabolic activity and its impact on therapy, new biomarkers and treatment targets may be found, thus improving patient outcomes. The incorporation of artificial intelligence (AI) is changing the analysis of metabolic activity. AI algorithms can analyze many human samples derived from multiomics studies in minutes and highlight patterns that could predict responses to treatment (Zhou et al., 2025). Researchers have developed machine learning models designed to predict responses to immunotherapy treatments derived from metabolic profiles, improving stratification of patients and subsequent personalized therapy (Zhao et al., 2024). Future research can include investigations into the integration of a "one framework AI" structured to collate the diverse strands of multiomics data to generate new ways of discovering potentially new therapeutic strategies, as well as developing a more precise approach to therapy for patients. Likewise, the use of AI to extract information from spatial metabolomics data may also deepen our knowledge of tumors and the metabolism associated with the immune system.

Integrating multiomics is critical to understanding the complicated relationship between metabolic pathways and immune responses in cancer. New computational tools now allow researchers to integrate multiomics data from genomics, transcriptomics, proteomics, and metabolomics, giving researchers a complete view of tumor biology (Zhou et al., 2025). However, developing standardized protocols for data collection, data analysis, and modeling still poses challenges. Future research endeavors should be aimed at building integrated frameworks that allow multiomics data to be harmonized, thus allowing prediction of treatment response and clinician outcomes related to disease progression to be more accurate and meaningful. The emphasis on multiomics necessitates that research institutions will need to work collaboratively to develop usable databases and standardized methodologies to better enable multiomics research and clinical applications.

9.2.7.3 *Breakthrough directions for clinical translation*

The identification and exploration of new metabolic modulators is a valuable way to enhance cancer therapies. Recent evidence shows that metabolic pathways can be targeted to potentially sensitize tumors to existing therapies (at or near a therapeutic dose), including chemotherapy and immunotherapy (Luda et al., 2023). For example, compounds that stimulate the production of ketone bodies or modulate one-carbon metabolism could induce more powerful immune responses and lower tumor growth. The literature supports new research that identifies these and other metabolic modulators, and tests their effects in preclinical and clinical studies, as a means of generating new therapeutic approaches to treat cancer. Importantly, the timing and duration of the associate metabolic intervention could be incredibly impactful for the use of these in cancer treatment. Some literature suggests that a more potent therapeutic effect can be achieved by time-adjusting dietary or lifestyle intervention schedules to coincide with treatment schedules (Li et al., 2023). In the same context, some studies have suggested that time-restricted feeding may improve metabolic health and treatment responses in cancer population. Future studies that identify not just the research questions associated with timing and duration of metabolic treatment, but that recognize individual patient factors such as circadian rhythm or metabolic profiles, may be beneficial to maximize the effects of metabolic treatments and preservation of health.

The advancement of metabolism-based predictive models to predict immunotherapy response is a nascent area of research that could yield improved patient outcomes. If metabolic profiles were correlated with clinical and genomic data, researchers could create predictive models that would result in accurate prediction of patient response and identify those that would benefit from specific immunotherapies (Liu et al., 2024). Future research should aim to validate predictive models in multiple patient populations and examine impact on clinical decision-making. Predictive models based on these methods may lend itself to personalized treatment approaches, allowing patients to seek therapies that each individual is metabolically and immunologically expected to respond to.

9.3 Conclusion

The study of immunometabolism has become an exciting new frontier in determining how tumors evade the immune system and how those insights are reformulating the field of cancer therapy. There is a rapidly accumulating body of evidence that provides a primary approach to systematically study the metabolic features of immune cells and the dynamic changes occurring within the TME. Researchers are just starting to identify multiple potential therapeutic targets for cancer therapy based on immunometabolic outcomes that may be exploited to the benefit of promoting an effective antitumor immune response. The study of immunometabolism raises important questions about the interplay and relative contributions of metabolism and immune function, as well as its implications for the development of new cancer therapies that may change the clinical course of the disease.

However, the application of immunometabolic approaches for therapy in the clinic is challenged by unique complexities of both the TME and cancer heterogeneity. As we consider different avenues for pursuing research agendas in the field of immunometabolism, it is apparent that competing perspectives and data will lead to greater diversity in future research; despite these differences, the reality is that one size does not fit all. Further research needs to be concerned with specificity of the metabolic intervention to minimize any unplanned consequences that may arise as a result of broad metabolic interventions targeting specific metabolic pathways.

Furthermore, metabolic regulation may interact with other biological processes, such as epigenetics and the microbiome. Exploring the interactions between these may complete our understanding of the immunometabolic network during the initiation and progression of cancer. Continuing our investigations into these multiple intertwined processes may give us more layers of regulation that can be targeted therapeutically, opening up more avenues for prevention and alleviation of the effects of cancer.

In conclusion, while immunometabolism is a rapidly advancing and emerging discipline, it represents a unique opportunity for the development of cancer immunotherapy. Targeting metabolic pathways for therapeutics will represent a significant paradigm shift in how we may treat cancer. This will entail recognizing the unique metabolic characteristics of tumors and how we, as practitioners, characterize our therapeutic response to them, practically in mind, of course. We have much to learn about the immune response and immune metabolism more generally, and we will have to rely on others who have more experience in this area. We see genuine opportunities here for having a cancer biology learning opportunity become a learning opportunity about cancer in a broader sense, and using insights about immunometabolism to inform where novel treatment opportunities may arise, and an individualized approach for cancer care. Ultimately, we may be able to develop successful cancer therapies through learning from immunometabolism in the context of their being other contextual biological processes involved.

References

Barba, I., Carrillo-Bosch, L., & Seoane, J. (2024). Targeting the Warburg Effect in Cancer: Where Do We Stand? *International Journal of Molecular Sciences, 25*(6). https://doi.org/10.3390/ijms25063142, http://www.mdpi.com/journal/ijms.

Brydges, C. R., Bhattacharyya, S., Dehkordi, S. M., Milaneschi, Y., Penninx, B., Jansen, R., Kristal, B. S., Han, X., Arnold, M., Kastenmüller, G., Bekhbat, M., Mayberg, H. S., Craighead, W. E., Rush, A. J., Fiehn, O., Dunlop, B. W., & Kaddurah-Daouk, R. (2022). Metabolomic and inflammatory signatures of symptom dimensions in major depression. *Brain, Behavior, and Immunity, 102*, 42–52. https://doi.org/10.1016/j.bbi.2022.02.003.

Butterfield, T. R., Landay, A. L., & Anzinger, J. J. (2020). Dysfunctional Immunometabolism in HIV Infection: Contributing Factors and Implications for Age-Related Comorbid Diseases. *Current HIV/AIDS Reports, 17*(2), 125–137. https://doi.org/10.1007/s11904-020-00484-4, http://www.springerlink.com/content/1548-3568/8/1/.

Carbone, F., Bruzzaniti, S., Fusco, C., Colamatteo, A., Micillo, T., De Candia, P., Bonacina, F., Norata, G. D., & Matarese, G. (2021). Metabolomics, lipidomics, and immunometabolism. *Methods in Molecular Biology, 2285*, 319–328. https://doi.org/10.1007/978-1-0716-1311-5_24, http://www.springer.com/series/7651.

Chen, P., Han, Y., Wang, L., Zheng, Y., Zhu, Z., Zhao, Y., Zhang, M., Chen, X., Wang, X., & Sun, C. (2023). Spatially Resolved Metabolomics Combined with the 3D Tumor-Immune Cell Coculture Spheroid Highlights Metabolic Alterations during Antitumor Immune Response. *Analytical Chemistry, 95*(41), 15153–15161. https://doi.org/10.1021/acs.analchem.2c05734.

Chen, Y., Tan, L., Gao, J., Lin, C., Wu, F., Li, Y., & Zhang, J. (2023). Targeting glutaminase 1 (GLS1) by small molecules for anticancer therapeutics. *European Journal of Medicinal Chemistry, 252*, 115306. https://doi.org/10.1016/j.ejmech.2023.115306.

Ding, C. H., Yan, F. Z., Xu, B. N., Qian, H., Hong, X. L., Liu, S. Q., Luo, Y. Y., Wu, S. H., Cai, L. Y., Zhang, X., & Xie, W. F. (2025). PRMT3 drives PD-L1-mediated immune escape through activating PDHK1-regulated glycolysis in hepatocellular carcinoma. *Cell Death and Disease, 16*(1). https://doi.org/10.1038/s41419-025-07482-7, https://www.nature.com/cddis/.

Flory, M., Bravo, P., & Alam, A. (2024). Impact of gut microbiota and its metabolites on immunometabolism in colorectal cancer. *Immunometabolism, 6*(4), e00050. https://doi.org/10.1097/in9.0000000000000050.

Guo, Y., Hu, P., & Shi, J. (2024). Nanomedicine Remodels Tumor Microenvironment for Solid Tumor Immunotherapy. *Journal of the American Chemical Society, 146*(15), 10217–10233. https://doi.org/10.1021/jacs.3c14005.

Guo, Y., Liu, Y., Wu, W., Ling, D., Zhang, Q., Zhao, P., & Hu, X. (2021). Indoleamine 2,3-dioxygenase (Ido) inhibitors and their nanomedicines for cancer immunotherapy. *Biomaterials, 276*, 121018. https://doi.org/10.1016/j.biomaterials.2021.121018.

Huldani, H., Malviya, J., Rodrigues, P., Hjazi, A., Deorari, M. M., Al-Hetty, H. R. A. K., Qasim, Q. A., Alasheqi, M. Q., & Ihsan, A. (2024). Discovering the strength of immunometabolism in cancer therapy: Employing metabolic pathways to enhance immune responses. *Cell Biochemistry and Function, 42*(2). https://doi.org/10.1002/cbf.3934, http://onlinelibrary.wiley.com/journal/10.1002/(ISSN)1099-0844.

Iu, D. S., Maya, J., Vu, L. T., Fogarty, E. A., McNairn, A. J., Ahmed, F., Franconi, C. J., Munn, P. R., Grenier, J. K., Hanson, M. R., & Grimson, A. (2024). Transcriptional reprogramming primes CD8+ T cells toward exhaustion in Myalgic encephalomyelitis/chronic fatigue syndrome. *Proceedings of the National Academy of Sciences, 121*(50). https://doi.org/10.1073/pnas.2415119121.

Jiang, Q., Qiao, B., Zheng, J., Song, W., Zhang, N., Xu, J., Liu, J., Zhong, Y., Zhang, Q., Liu, W., You, L., Wu, N., Liu, Y., Li, P., Ran, H., Wang, Z., & Guo, D. (2024). Potentiating dual-directional immunometabolic regulation with nanomedicine to enhance anti-tumor immunotherapy following incomplete photothermal ablation. *Journal of Nanobiotechnology, 22*(1). https://doi.org/10.1186/s12951-024-02643-w.

Kazmi, S., Khan, M. A., Shamma, T., Altuhami, A., Assiri, A. M., & Broering, D. C. (2022). Therapeutic nexus of T cell immunometabolism in improving transplantation immunotherapy. *International Immunopharmacology, 106*, 108621. https://doi.org/10.1016/j.intimp.2022.108621.

Khameneh, S. C., Razi, S., Lashanizadegan, R., Akbari, S., Sayaf, M., Haghani, K., & Bakhtiyari, S. (2024). MicroRNA-mediated metabolic regulation of immune cells in cancer: an updated review. *Frontiers in Immunology, 15*. https://doi.org/10.3389/fimmu.2024.1424909, https://www.frontiersin.org/journals/immunology#.

Lawton, M. L., Inge, M. M., Blum, B. C., Smith-Mahoney, E. L., Bolzan, D., Lin, W., McConney, C., Porter, J., Moore, J., Youssef, A., Tharani, Y., Varelas, X., Denis, G. V., Wong, W. W., Padhorny, D., Kozakov, D., Siggers, T., Wuchty, S., Snyder-Cappione, J., ... Bhandoola, A. (2024). Multiomic profiling of chronically activated CD4+ T cells identifies drivers of exhaustion and metabolic reprogramming. *PLOS Biology, 22*(12), e3002943. https://doi.org/10.1371/journal.pbio.3002943.

Leone, R. D., & Powell, J. D. (2020). Metabolism of immune cells in cancer. *Nature Reviews Cancer, 20*(9), 516–531. https://doi.org/10.1038/s41568-020-0273-y, http://www.nature.com/cancer/.

Li, J., Xu, P., & Chen, S. (2024). Research progress on mitochondria regulating tumor immunity. *Zhejiang Da Xue Xue Bao Yi Xue Ban, 53*(1), 1–14. https://doi.org/10.3724/zdxbyxb-2023-0484.

Li, S., Han, H., Yang, K., Li, X., Ma, L., Yang, Z., & Zhao, Y.-xun (2025). Emerging role of metabolic reprogramming in the immune microenvironment and immunotherapy of thyroid cancer. *International Immunopharmacology, 144*, 113702. https://doi.org/10.1016/j.intimp.2024.113702.

Li, X., Jiang, O., & Wang, S. (2023). Molecular mechanisms of cellular metabolic homeostasis in stem cells. *International Journal of Oral Science, 15*(1). https://doi.org/10.1038/s41368-023-00262-z, https://www.nature.com/ijos/.

Liang, L., Kuang, X., He, Y., Zhu, L., Lau, P., Li, X., Luo, D., Gong, L., Zhou, W., Zhang, F., Liang, X., Li, Z., Hu, B., Liu, D., Ding, T., Li, H., Zhao, S., Su, J., Hung, M.-C., ... Chen, X. (2025). Alterations in PD-L1 succinylation shape anti-tumor immune responses in melanoma. *Nature Genetics, 57*(3), 680–693. https://doi.org/10.1038/s41588-025-02077-6.

Liu, J., Li, X., Li, Y., Gong, Q., & Luo, K. (2025). Metformin-based nanomedicines for reprogramming tumor immune microenvironment. *Theranostics, 15*(3), 993–1016. https://doi.org/10.7150/thno.104872.

Liu, Y., Wu, Z., Li, Y., Chen, Y., Zhao, X., Wu, M., & Xia, Y. (2025). Metabolic reprogramming and interventions in angiogenesis. *Journal of Advanced Research, 70*, 323–338. https://doi.org/10.1016/j.jare.2024.05.001.

Liu, Y., Zou, X., Tong, H. H. Y., Ji, Y., Tan, L., & Hao, J. (2024). Protocol for using scCURE to construct an immunotherapy outcome prediction model. *STAR Protocols, 5*(4), 103476. https://doi.org/10.1016/j.xpro.2024.103476.

Luda, K. M., Longo, J., Kitchen-Goosen, S. M., Duimstra, L. R., Ma, E. H., Watson, M. J., Oswald, B. M., Fu, Z., Madaj, Z., Kupai, A., Dickson, B. M., DeCamp, L. M., Dahabieh, M. S., Compton, S. E., Teis, R., Kaymak, I., Lau, K. H., Kelly, D. P., Puchalska, P., ... Jones, R. G. (2023). Ketolysis drives CD8+ T cell effector function through effects on histone acetylation. *Immunity, 56*(9), 2021. https://doi.org/10.1016/j.immuni.2023.07.002, www.immunity.com.

Lyon, P., Strippoli, V., Fang, B., & Cimmino, L. (2020). B vitamins and one-carbon metabolism: Implications in human health and disease. *Nutrients, 12*(9), 1–24. https://doi.org/10.3390/nu12092867, https://www.mdpi.com/2072-6643/12/9/2867/pdf.

Maas, P., den Hartog, I., Kindt, A., Boman, S., Hankemeier, T., van Hasselt, C., & Hernandez-Lemus, E. (2022). The Immunometabolic Atlas: A tool for design and interpretation of metabolomics studies in immunology. *PLOS ONE, 17*(5), e0268408. https://doi.org/10.1371/journal.pone.0268408.

Mikaeloff, F., Gelpi, M., Escós, A., Wang, T., Gupta, S., Olofsson, A., Akusjärvi, S. S., Schuster, S., Naval, P., Sood, V., Nikouyan, N., Knudsen, A. D., Vestad, B., Høgh, J., Hov, J. R., Benfield, T., Trøseid, M., Pawar, V., Rucevic, M., ... Neogi, U. (2025). Host Plasma Microenvironment in Immunometabolically Impaired HIV Infection Leads to Dysregulated Monocyte Function and Synaptic Transmission Ex Vivo. *Advanced Science, 12*(16). https://doi.org/10.1002/advs.202416453.

Min, X., Zhao, Y., Yu, M., Zhang, W., Jiang, X., Guo, K., Wang, X., Huang, J., Li, T., Sun, L., & He, J. (2024). Spatially resolved metabolomics: From metabolite mapping to function visualising. *Clinical and Translational Medicine, 14*(11). https://doi.org/10.1002/ctm2.70031.

Povo-Retana, A., Fariñas, M., Landauro-Vera, R., Mojena, M., Alvarez-Lucena, C., Fernández-Moreno, M. A., Castrillo, A., de la Rosa Medina, J. V., Sánchez-García, S., Foguet, C., Mas, F., Marin, S., Cascante, M., & Boscá, L. (2023). Immunometabolic actions of trabectedin and lurbinectedin on human macrophages: relevance for their anti-tumor activity. *Frontiers in Immunology, 14*. https://doi.org/10.3389/fimmu.2023.1211068.

Ramapriyan, R., Vykunta, V. S., Vandecandelaere, G., Richardson, L. G. K., Sun, J., Curry, W. T., & Choi, B. D. (2024). Altered cancer metabolism and implications for next-generation CAR T-cell therapies. *Pharmacology & Therapeutics, 259*, 108667. https://doi.org/10.1016/j.pharmthera.2024.108667.

Ricci, J.-E. (2025). Tumor-induced metabolic immunosuppression: Mechanisms and therapeutic targets. *Cell Reports, 44*(1), 115206. https://doi.org/10.1016/j.celrep.2024.115206.

Sasaki, K., Nishina, S., Yamauchi, A., Fukuda, K., Hara, Y., Yamamura, M., Egashira, K., & Hino, K. (2021). Nanoparticle-Mediated Delivery of 2-Deoxy-D-Glucose Induces Antitumor Immunity and Cytotoxicity in Liver Tumors in Mice. *Cellular and Molecular Gastroenterology and Hepatology, 11*(3), 739–762. https://doi.org/10.1016/j.jcmgh.2020.10.010.

Spangenberg, H., Ramklint, M., Cunningham, J. L., & Ramirez, A. (2024). Correlations between personality traits, personality disorders, and immunometabolic markers. *Scientific Reports, 14*(1). https://doi.org/10.1038/s41598-024-62214-9, https://www.nature.com/srep/.

Su, R., Shao, Y., Huang, M., Liu, D., Yu, H., & Qiu, Y. (2024). Immunometabolism in cancer: basic mechanisms and new targeting strategy. *Cell Death Discovery, 10*(1). https://doi.org/10.1038/s41420-024-02006-2.

Tabas, I., & Bornfeldt, K. E. (2020). Intracellular and Intercellular Aspects of Macrophage Immunometabolism in Atherosclerosis. *Circulation Research, 126*(9), 1209–1227. https://doi.org/10.1161/CIRCRESAHA.119.315939, https://www.ovid.com/product-details.454.html.

Tan, S., Yang, Y., Yang, W., Han, Y., Huang, L., Yang, R., Hu, Z., Tao, Y., Liu, L., Li, Y., Oyang, L., Lin, J., Peng, Q., Jiang, X., Xu, X., Xia, L., Peng, M., Wu, N., Tang, Y., ... Zhou, Y. (2023). Exosomal cargos-mediated metabolic reprogramming in tumor microenvironment. *Journal of Experimental & Clinical Cancer Research, 42*(1). https://doi.org/10.1186/s13046-023-02634-z.

Tao, H., Zhong, X., Zeng, A., & Song, L. (2023). Unveiling the veil of lactate in tumor-associated macrophages: a successful strategy for immunometabolic therapy. *Frontiers in Immunology, 14*. https://doi.org/10.3389/fimmu.2023.1208870.

Tomar, M. S., Mohit, Kumar, A., & Shrivastava, A. (2025). Circadian immunometabolism: A future insight for targeted therapy in cancer. *Sleep Medicine Reviews, 80*, 102031. https://doi.org/10.1016/j.smrv.2024.102031.

Verheijen, F. W. M., Tran, T. N. M., Chang, J. C., Broere, F., Zaal, E. A., & Berkers, C. R. (2024). Deciphering metabolic crosstalk in context: lessons from inflammatory diseases. *Molecular Oncology, 18*(7), 1759–1776. https://doi.org/10.1002/1878-0261.13588, http://onlinelibrary.wiley.com/journal/10.1002/(ISSN)1878-0261.

Wang, R., Zhuang, J., Zhang, Q., Wu, W., Yu, X., Zhang, H., & Xie, Z. (2025). Decoding the metabolic dialogue in the tumor microenvironment: from immune suppression to precision cancer therapies. *Experimental Hematology & Oncology, 14*(1). https://doi.org/10.1186/s40164-025-00689-6.

Wang, X., Liao, Y., Liu, D., Zheng, J., & Shi, M. (2025). Presetting CAR-T cells during ex vivo biomanufacturing. *Molecular Therapy, 33*(4), 1380–1406. https://doi.org/10.1016/j.ymthe.2025.02.031.

Wang, Y., Chen, Y., & Wang, J. (2025). Role of tumor microenvironment in prostate cancer immunometabolism. *Biomolecules, 15*(6). https://doi.org/10.3390/biom15060826, http://www.mdpi.com/journal/biomolecules.

Wei, F., Wang, D., Wei, J., Tang, N., Tang, L., Xiong, F., Guo, C., Zhou, M., Li, X., Li, G., Xiong, W., Zhang, S., & Zeng, Z. (2021). Metabolic crosstalk in the tumor microenvironment regulates antitumor immunosuppression and immunotherapy resisitance. *Cellular and Molecular Life Sciences, 78*(1), 173–193. https://doi.org/10.1007/s00018-020-03581-0.

Wei, Y., Ding, J., Li, J., Cai, S., Liu, S., Hong, L., Yin, T., Zhang, Y., & Diao, L. (2021). Metabolic Reprogramming of Immune Cells at the Maternal-Fetal Interface and the Development of Techniques for Immunometabolism. *Frontiers in Immunology, 12*. https://doi.org/10.3389/fimmu.2021.717014.

Xia, Z, Tian, M, Cheng, Y, Yi, W, Du, Z, Li, T, Wen, Y, Li, L, Liu, Y, & Chen, C (2024). Preclinical evaluation of cyclophosphamide and fludarabine combined with CD19 CAR-T in the treatment of B-cell hematologic malignancies in vivo. *Oncology Research, 32*(6), 1109–1118. https://doi.org/10.32604/or.2024.049792.

Xiao, L., Xian, M., Zhang, C., Guo, Q., & Yi, Q. (2023). Lipid peroxidation of immune cells in cancer. *Frontiers in Immunology, 14*. https://doi.org/10.3389/fimmu.2023.1322746, https://www.frontiersin.org/journals/immunology#.

Yang, L., TeSlaa, T., Ng, S., Nofal, M., Wang, L., Lan, T., Zeng, X., Cowan, A., McBride, M., Lu, W., Davidson, S., Liang, G., Oh, T. G., Downes, M., Evans, R., Von Hoff, D., Guo, J. Y., Han, H., & Rabinowitz, J. D. (2022). Ketogenic diet and chemotherapy combine to disrupt pancreatic cancer metabolism and growth. *Med, 3*(2), 119. https://doi.org/10.1016/j.medj.2021.12.008.

Zeng, Y., Huang, Y., Tan, Q., Peng, L., Wang, J., Tong, F., & Dong, X. (2025). Influence of lactate in resistance to anti-PD-1/PD-L1 therapy: Mechanisms and clinical applications (Review). *Molecular Medicine Reports, 31*(2). https://doi.org/10.3892/mmr.2024.13413, https://www.spandidos-publications.com/10.3892/mmr.2024.13413.

Zhang, Y., Kang, Q., He, L., Chan, K. I., Gu, H., Xue, W., Zhong, Z., & Tan, W. (2024). Exploring the immunometabolic potential of Danggui Buxue Decoction for the treatment of IBD-related colorectal cancer. *Chinese Medicine, 19*(1). https://doi.org/10.1186/s13020-024-00978-y.

Zhao, Q., Zhong, X., Wang, X., Li, B., Xu, Y., Yu, J., & Wang, L. (2024). Clinical multi-dimensional prognostic nomogram for predicting the efficacy of immunotherapy in NSCLC. *Scientific Reports, 14*(1). https://doi.org/10.1038/s41598-024-72760-x.

Zhao, Y., Zhu, W., Dong, S., Zhang, H., & Zhou, W. (2025). Glucose Metabolism Reprogramming of Immune Cells in the Microenvironment of Pancreatic and Hepatobiliary Cancers. *Journal of Gastroenterology and Hepatology, 40*(2), 355–366. https://doi.org/10.1111/jgh.16873.

Zhou, N. J., Bao, W. Q., Zhang, C. F., Jiang, M. L., Liang, T. L., Ma, G. Y., Liu, L., Pan, H. D., & Li, R. Z. (2025). Immunometabolism and oxidative stress: roles and therapeutic strategies in cancer and aging. *npj Aging, 11*(1). https://doi.org/10.1038/s41514-025-00250-z, https://www.nature.com/npjamd/journal-information.

Zhou, Y., Wang, H., Luo, Y., Tuo, B., Liu, X., & Li, T. (2023). Effect of metabolism on the immune microenvironment of breast cancer. *Biochimica et Biophysica Acta (BBA) - Reviews on Cancer, 1878*(2), 188861. https://doi.org/10.1016/j.bbcan.2023.188861.

Zhu, C. X., Yan, K., Chen, L., Huang, R. R., Bian, Z. H., Wei, H. R., Gu, X. M., Zhao, Y. Y., Liu, M. C., Suo, C. X., Li, Z. K., Yang, Z. Y., Lu, M. Q., Hua, X. F., Li, L., Zhao, Z. B., Sun, L. C., Zhang, H. F., Gao, P., & Lian, Z. X. (2024). Targeting OXCT1-mediated ketone metabolism reprograms macrophages to promote antitumor immunity via CD8+ T cells in hepatocellular carcinoma. *Journal of Hepatology, 81*(4), 690–703. https://doi.org/10.1016/j.jhep.2024.05.007, https://www.sciencedirect.com/science/journal/01688278.

CHAPTER

10

Antineoplastic potential of nonsteroidal antiinflammatory drugs

Arkadiusz Surażyński, Magda Chalecka, and Jerzy Palka
Department of Medicinal Chemistry, Medical University of Białystok, Bialystok, Poland

10.1 Pivotal inflammatory pathways in cancer

Cancer development is promoted by inflammatory environment (Kapoor et al., 2025). The most important inflammatory pathways in cancer cells are mediated by nuclear factor-kappa B (NF-κB), Janus kinase/signal transducer and activator of transcription (JAK–STAT), mitogen-activated protein kinase, known also as extracellular signal-regulated kinases (MAPK/ERK1/2), phosphoinositide 3 kinase/protein kinase B/mammalian target of rapamycin (PI3K/AKT/mTOR), transforming growth factor-β/suppressor of mothers against decapentaplegic (TGF-β/Smad), and Wnt signalling. NF-κB pathway is pivotal in regulating the expression of proinflammatory genes (e.g., IL-1, TNFα, COX-2) (Rinkenbaugh & Baldwin, 2016). Upon activation, NF-κB translocates to the nucleus and binds to the specific DNA sequences, triggering the transcription of some genes involved in the regulation of cellular immunity, stress response, cell differentiation, proliferation, and apoptosis (Du & Geller, 2010). Proinflammatory signals activate STATs that regulate cell division, differentiation, apoptosis, and also angiogenesis and haematopoiesis (Brooks & Putoczki, 2020). The STAT family involves seven proteins (STAT1, STAT2, STAT3, STAT4, STAT5A, STAT5B, and STAT6). They are activated through phosphorylation mediated by JAK proteins (JAK1, JAK2, JAK3). JAK1/2 are expressed throughout the body, and JAK3, mainly in hematopoietic cells (Rodig et al., 1998). Phosphorylation of STATs by JAKs induces their dimerization and translocation into the nucleus, where they activate some genes (O'Shea et al., 2004; Villarino et al., 2014). Therefore STATs serve as the downstream targets of JAK and function as cytokine-activated transcription factors (Jung et al., 2015). In several solid tumors, STAT1, STAT3, and STAT5 were found to be overexpressed. JAK/STAT pathway, activated by inflammation, affects cell survival and proliferation.

MAPK/ERK1/2 signalling pathway is activated in response to different extracellular factors (e.g., growth factors, cytokines) and regulates cell proliferation, differentiation, migration, and

Inflammation in Tumorigenesis and Cancer Treatment
DOI: https://doi.org/10.1016/B978-0-443-36649-9.00003-7

apoptosis (Guo et al., 2020; Javan et al., 2019; Keshet & Seger, 2010). This pathway is known to induce expression of vascular endothelial growth factor (VEGF), a potent proangiogenic agent supporting metastasis (Kyriakis & Avruch, 2001). The ERK/MAPK signalling pathway also plays an important role in maintaining cytoskeletal architecture. Therefore persistent MAPK/ERK1/2 activation promotes tumorigenesis (Ma et al., 2020).

PI3K/AKT/mTOR signalling is involved in the regulation of cancer cell cycle, quiescence, metabolism, and proliferation (Almatroodi et al., 2021; Alzohairy et al., 2021; Rinkenbaugh & Baldwin, 2016). PI3Ks are a class of enzymes that phosphorylate phosphoinositides, producing phosphatidylinositol-3,4,5-trisphosphates (PIP3), which are involved in cell signalling. PIP3 at the membrane creates docking sites for signalling proteins like AKT. The mTOR complex 2 (mTORC2) facilitates the activation of AKT by phosphorylating it, which in turn stimulates the mTOR complex 1 (mTORC1), driving protein synthesis (Aziz et al., 2009). The PI3K pathway, activated by tyrosine kinase growth factor receptors, stimulates cellular growth, survival, and cancer cell metabolism (Vogt et al., 2010). PI3K/AKT pathway is often dysregulated in cancer cells and promotes cell survival and proliferation (Hodson et al., 2013).

Wnt signalling pathway is a highly conserved mechanism critical for embryonic development and tissue homeostasis, and coordinates function of other signalling pathways (Habas & Dawid, 2005; Yamaguchi, 2001). The term "Wnt" originates from a combination of wingless (a gene in *Drosophila*) and integrated (int-1), its vertebrate counterpart. The pathway consists of two cascades: the canonical (Wnt/β-catenin dependent) and the noncanonical (β-catenin-independent) pathway. Dysregulation of Wnt signalling is closely linked to invasion and resistance of cancer cells (Kohn & Moon, 2005).

TGF-β/SMAD pathway is initiated by binding of TGF-β to the serine/threonine kinase receptors and phosphorylation of the Smad proteins. The phosphorylated Smad proteins form complexes that translocate to the nucleus, inducing expression of several genes involved in the regulation of cell migration, differentiation, proliferation, and apoptosis (Hata & Chen, 2016). This pathway is also involved in the regulation of immune responses and modifications of tumor microenvironment (Proctor et al., 2010).

Cyclooxygenase-2 (COX-2) is an enzyme that mediates the release of inflammatory mediator, prostaglandin E2 (PGE2) from arachidonic acid. The COX-2/PGE2 pathway is implicated in the regulation of tumor growth, angiogenesis, immune evasion, and resistance to chemotherapy (Sun, 2017).

Targeting the inflammation-mediated cell signalling pathways has emerged as a promising strategy for cancer treatment; however, they did not bring the expected results (Kapoor et al., 2025). In this chapter, we present a novel experimental approach to cancer treatment by nonsteroidal antiinflammatory drugs (NSAIDs).

10.2 Experimental approach to understand antineoplastic potential of nonsteroidal antiinflammatory drugs

Promotion of cancer development by inflammatory environment is due to increased level of COX-2 and PGE_2 (Eibl et al., 2003; Hashemi Goradel et al., 2019; Kim et al., 2012;

Zappavigna et al., 2020) that stimulate proliferation, migration, and cell adhesion (Menter & Dubois, 2012; Pang et al., 2016). Pharmacoepidemiological data suggest that regular use of NSAIDs contributes to decrease in risk of some cancers, particularly gastric or colorectal cancer, but also lung, breast, and prostate cancers (Chan et al., 2005; Rothwell et al., 2010, 2012; Seetha et al., 2020; Shebl et al., 2014). Clinical data show that medication with aspirin and other inhibitors of COX-2 reduces the risk of colorectal cancer by about 20% (Arisan et al., 2018; Cheung et al., 2020; Rothwell et al., 2010). Similarly, regular use of nonselective COX-2 inhibitors (e.g., aspirin, ibuprofen) contributes to reduction in the risk of lung cancer by 69% (Harris et al., 2002). In fact, COX-2 is usually overexpressed in different cancers. For instance, treatment of HT-29 human colon cancer cells with sulindac, salicylate, or other NSAIDs induced apoptosis. Moreover, COX-2 inhibition impairs angiogenesis through attenuation of VEGF and metalloproteinases expression (Mazhar et al., 2005). However, some data suggest that the antineoplastic activity of NSAIDs may occur regardless of COX inhibition. Treatment of human prostate cancer cell lines, PC3 and LNCaP, lacking COX-2, with selective COX-2 inhibitor, celecoxib, inhibited the growth of both cell lines independently of PGE_2 level. The similar effect was observed in vivo. Prostaglandin-independent effects of NSAIDs were also found in both HT-29 cells expressing COX-1 and -2 as well as in HCT-15 cells lacking both isoforms of COX. However, NSAIDs concentration required for inhibition of COX expression and cancer cell proliferation are different. The concentration of NSAIDs required for inhibition of cell proliferation is relatively higher than for the inhibition of COX activity. NSAIDs induced COX-independent effects on cell proliferation, as shown in studies on chiral centers of ibuprofen and flurbiprofen. *S*-enantiomers of both drugs inhibit COX activity nonselectively, while *R*-enantiomers do not inhibit the enzyme's activity. However, both *S*- and *R*-enantiomers retain the same antiproliferative effect. The mechanism for antiproliferative effect of NSAIDs involves inhibition of cyclic guanosine monophosphate/phosphodiesterases (cGMP PDEs), Wnt/β-catenin, peroxisome proliferator-activated receptors (PPARs), receptor retinoid X, IKKβ/NF-κB, PDK-1/AKT, Akt/mTOR signaling, and upregulation of AMP-activated protein kinase (AMPK) (Akrami et al., 2018; Gurpinar et al., 2013, 2014).

Some data provide evidence that apoptosis induced by NSAIDs involves upregulation of 15-lipoxygenase-1 (15-LOX-1) activity, which, similar to COX, is involved in metabolism of polyunsaturated fatty acids (FAs). LOX metabolizes linoleic acid to eicosanoids (e.g., in colon). In adenocarcinomas, the expression of 15-LOX-1 gene and its product, 13-hydroxyoctadecadienoic acid (13-S-HODE), is significantly decreased, compared to normal mucosa. Treatment of COXs expressing colon cancer cells with some NSAIDs (e.g., sulindac) contributed to upregulation of 15-LOX-1 expression, increase in the formation of 13-S-HODE, and induction of apoptosis. This effect was confirmed in studies showing that LOX-dependent apoptosis in colon cancer cells could be counteracted by 15-LOX-1 inhibitor (e.g., caffeic acid). However, treatment of the cells with NSAID, 15-LOX-1 inhibitor, and 13-S-HODE augmented the apoptosis. The key factor in this process is 13-S-HODE because when substituted by linoleic acid, the apoptosis does not occur in these cells. Some data explain this effect as a consequence of reprogramming lipid metabolism by LOXs rather than COXs. Other authors suggest inhibitory function of LOX on PPARs. Increased level of 13-S-HODE, as a consequence of activation of 15-LOX-1 contributed to deregulation of PPARδ function. Such a mechanism was found in colon cancer cells (RKO and DLD-1). However, substrates for 15-LOX-1 (linoleic acid) do not evoke the same effect as 13-S-HODE and do not induce apoptosis in these cells (IL Lee et al., 2011). It has also been suggested that the interaction of 15-LOX-1 with tumor suppressor protein, p53. Products of 15-LOX-1 (13-S-HODE and other products of lipid oxidation) are also ligands of PPARγ, which, when activated, promote apoptosis in some cells (e.g., macrophages, HCT-116, KO1). These data led to the suggestion that NSAID-dependent proapoptotic activity could be mediated by PPARs. NSAIDs-dependent activation of PPARγ stimulates proapoptotic signaling mediated by AMPK or LOX-1 and suppresses prosurvival pathways mediated by Wnt/β-catenin and Akt/mTOR signaling (Fig. 10.1).

10.3 Molecular polymorphism and function of peroxisome proliferator-activated receptor

The PPARs belong to the family of nuclear hormone receptors. They represent nuclear transcription factors activated by natural or synthetic ligands. PPARs are involved in the regulation of lipid and glucose metabolism, adipogenesis (Okazaki et al., 2016), affecting inflammation, proliferation, differentiation, and carcinogenesis (Heudobler et al., 2018; Peters et al., 2012). Upon activation, PPAR in nucleus forms complex with retinoid X receptor (RXR), which binds to specific DNA motif (PPAR response element) in a target gene (Blitek & Szymanska, 2017). PPARs are represented by genetically different isoforms, PPARα (NR1C1), PPARβ/δ (NR1C2), and PPARγ (NR1C3) that are differentially expressed in different tissues (Zhao et al., 2016). They have similar structure, and four domains were determined: A/B, C, D, and E/F (Yousefi et al., 2016). The activity of A/B domain (ligand-independent transactivation function domain, AF-1) depends on phosphorylation or sumoylation. Domain C, containing two zinc finger motifs binding hormone response element, forms DNA-binding domain that recognizes promoter (peroxisome proliferator response element [PPRE]). Domain D represents docking site for cofactors, while E/F domain, containing ligand binding domain, activates interaction of PPAR with PPRE. This contributes to stimulation of target gene expression and activation function-2 (AF-2) (Zoete et al., 2007). In the absence of ligand, PPARs form complex with RXR, recruit corepressors (N-CoR, SMRT), bind to respective promoter of target gene, and inhibit the gene expression. In the presence of ligand, conformation of PPARs is changed, leading to dissociation of corepressor, interaction with coactivator, and initiation of gene expression (Viswakarma et al., 2010).

PPARα regulates the expression of genes involved in transport of cholesterol, metabolism of FAs, β-oxidation, and peroxisomal pathways (Tenenbaum et al., 2005). PPARα is particularly active in liver lipid metabolism. However, it is also expressed in skeletal muscle, brown adipose, kidney, heart, as well as in vascular and immune cells and hippocampal neurons (Corbett et al., 2015). Interestingly, statins (e.g., simvastatin) activate PPARα, leading to increase in expression of neurotrophins, nerve growth factors important in learning process.

PPARβ/δ is ubiquitously expressed in the intestine, liver, adipose tissue, and skeletal muscle. They play an important role in lipid and glucose metabolism (Liu et al., 2018).

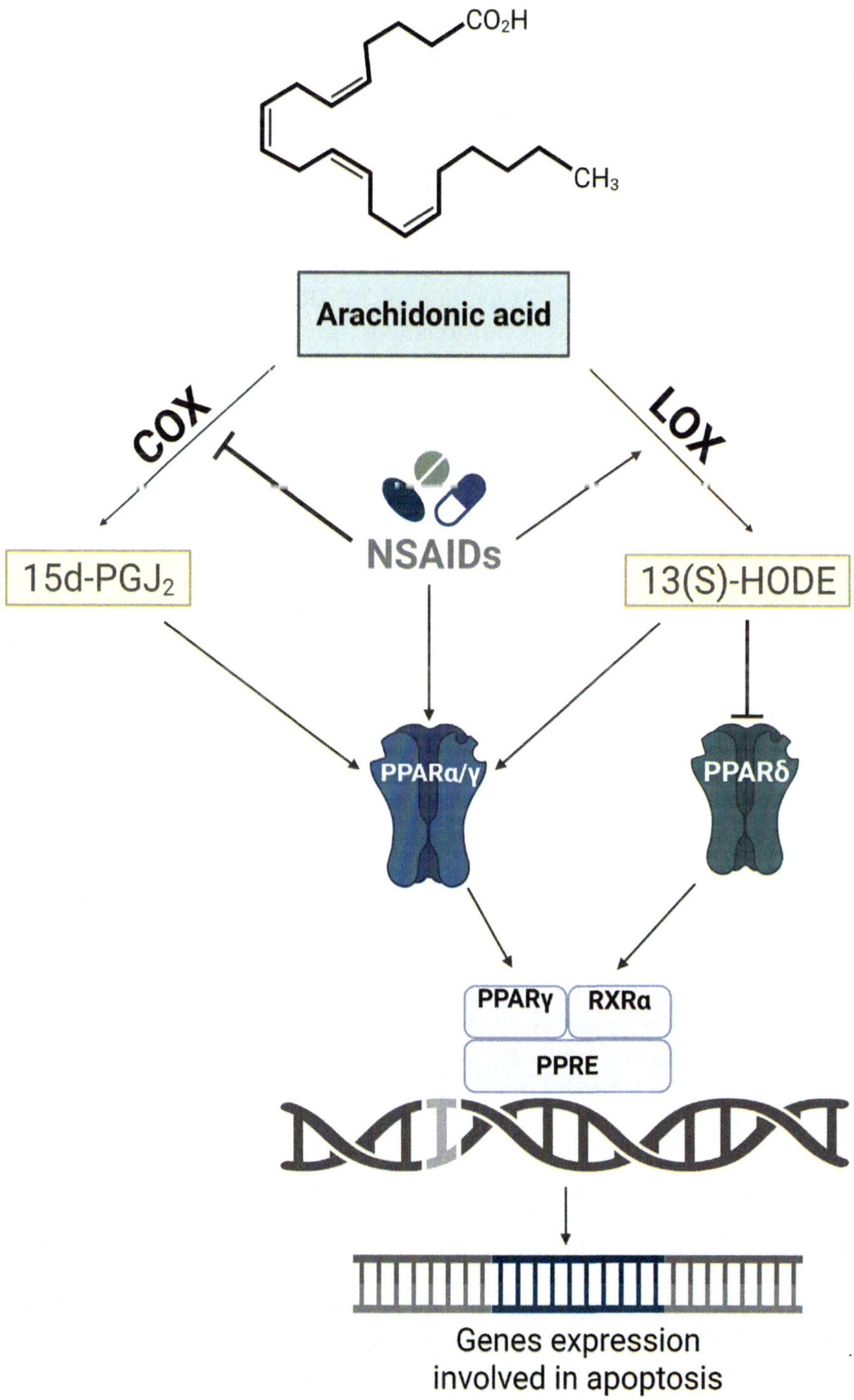

FIGURE 10.1 NSAIDs induce PPAR/γ-dependent apoptosis. *13(S)-HODE*, 13(S)-hydroxy-9Z,11E-octadecadienoic acid; *15d-PGJ2*, 15-deoxy-Δ12,14-prostaglandin J2; *COX*, cyclooxygenase; *LOX*, lipooxygenase; *NSAIDs*, nonsteroidal antiinflammatory drugs; *PPAR*, peroxisome proliferator-activated receptor; *PPRE*, peroxisome proliferator response element; *RXR*, retinoid X receptor alpha.

PPARβ/δ function differs from PPARα and PPARγ since, in its ligand-free form acts as a transcriptional repressor. PPARβ/δ can inhibit PPARα and PPARγ transcriptional activity by PPRE site competition mechanism. Activation of PPARβ/δ by FA-binding protein 5 (FABP5) augments prosurvival pathways in breast cancers. The interaction of FABP5 with PPARβ/δ activates cell proliferation mediated by epidermal growth factor receptor (EGFR). In fact, agonist of PPARβ/δ (GW501516) augmented tumor growth in vivo, while antagonist of this receptor inhibited expression of genes mediated by cell invasion in breast cancer MDA-MB-231 cells. Activation of PPARβ/δ in MCF-7 cells enhances cell migration and resistance to stress conditions (e.g., glucose shortage, hypoxia). The data suggest an important role of PPARβ/δ in adaptation to stress conditions in breast cancer cells (Müller, 2017). It was confirmed in other cancers showing PPARβ/δ-dependent stimulation of VEGF expression (angiogenesis), PI3K-Akt signaling, and tumor growth. In hematologic cancers, such as chronic lymphocytic leukemia, the overexpression of PPARδ contributes to stimulation of cell growth even in stress conditions (e.g., hypoxia, glucose shortage) (Li et al., 2017).

PPARγ is expressed abundantly in adipose tissue, spleen, and intestine. The receptor has three isoforms, γ1, γ2, γ3, transcribed on the same gene, but they are controlled by different promoters. Isoforms γ1 and γ3 are the same proteins; however, they are translated by different mRNAs. PPARγ1 is also expressed in liver, pancreas, kidney, and immune cells. Low expression of this isoform was found in cells of central nervous system (Marion-Letellier et al., 2016). PPARγ2 protein is larger than other isoforms due to an additional 30 amino acids on the N-terminal end of the protein. Among synthetic PPARγ agonists are thiazolidinedione group of drugs (e.g., pioglitazone, rosiglitazone) that are used for treatment of type 2 diabetes as well as colon, prostate, breast, liver, thyroid, and lung cancers. The effectiveness of these drugs is due to antiinflammatory potential of activated PPARs. Activated PPARγ was found to evoke antiinflammatory effects through inhibition of tumor necrosis factor α (TNF-α), interleukin 1β (IL-1β), interleukin 6 (IL-6), and PGE2 functions. In cancer cells, PPARγ is highly expressed in adenocarcinomas and liposarcomas. Upon activation, PPARγ inhibits proliferation and migration of endothelial cells, contributing to impairment of angiogenesis. Moreover, troglitazone-activated PPARγ promotes TRAIL-induced apoptosis in human lung cancer. Transfection of adenovirus gene with overexpression of PPARγ into SNU-668 gastric cancer cells resulted in apoptosis activation and upregulation of insulin-like growth factor-binding protein-3 (IGFBP-3). Tumor-suppressing activity of this protein was, however, not related to downregulation of insulin-like growth factor-I receptor (IGF-IR) signaling. Other studies show that activated PPARγ upregulates the expression of microRNA-125b (miR-125b), a tumor suppressor, inhibits expression of proto-oncogene B-cell lymphoma 3-encoded protein (BCL3), leading to inhibition of growth of ovarian cancers. In other cancers, such as bladder, breast, ovarian, and lung, miR-125b tumor suppressor expression is very low, affecting IGF-I, PI3K/Akt/mTOR, and MAPK signaling. These data suggest that activated PPARγ in cancer cells induces antineoplastic pathways; however, the molecular mechanism of these processes is not fully understood. One of the enzymes regulated by PPARγ and involved in cell death is proline dehydrogenase (PRODH)/proline oxidase (POX).

10.4 Proline dehydrogenase/proline oxidase–dependent apoptosis

Proline dehydrogenase (PRODH), also known as POX, is a mitochondrial flavin-dependent enzyme that catalyzes the conversion of L-proline (Pro) to Δ1-pyrroline-5-carboxylate (P5C). This process donates electrons through flavin adenine dinucleotide to the electron transport chain (ETC) for adenosine triphosphate (ATP) generation. From this point of view, the activity of PRODH/POX promotes cell survival. However, in certain microenvironmental conditions, the same electrons could be directly transferred to oxygen, forming reactive oxygen species (ROS), leading to apoptosis or prosurvival autophagy (Phang, 2019). Normal human tissues show different expression of PRODH/POX. High expression of this enzyme was found in kidney and liver, while low in brain and heart. In other tissues, PRODH/POX is very low or undetectable (Cappelletti et al., 2018). In most cancer cell lines, PRODH/POX expression and activity are low, while under low oxygen (hypoxia), the activity is increased, compared to normal conditions. In stress conditions (e.g., glucose shortage, hypoxia), PRODH/POX activity is increased due to AMPK-dependent prosurvival signaling. In conditions of glucose shortage, PRODH/POX contributes to the production of ATP, while in hypoxic conditions, PRODH/POXmediates, ROS generation resulting in protective autophagy. It suggests that the function of PRODH/POX depends on microenvironment of cancer tissue.

In general, catalytic activity of PRODH/POX, converting Pro into P5C, generates free electrons that support the ETC, producing ATP for cell survival (Phang, 2019). However, PRODH/POX can contribute to the apoptosis. The underlying mechanism of this function is PRODH/POX-dependent generation of ROS that is related to the deregulation of energetic metabolism in cancer cells. Due to Warburg's effect and high energy requirements of cancer cells, glucose metabolism is insufficient to cover energy requirements. Therefore degradation of extracellular matrix proteins (mainly collagen) serves as another source of energy, providing Pro as a substrate for PRODH/POX, resulting in ATP or ROS generation (Phang, 2019). However, the mechanism driving ROS generation is not fully understood.

The extent of PRODH/POX expression is considered a potential factor mediating ROS production. Such a function could play PPARγ. Activated PPARγ (e.g., by troglitazone) triggers PRODH/POX expression by specific binding to the PRODH/POX promoter. Increased expression and activity of PRODH/POX contributed to increase in ROS generation and cell death. It has been confirmed by using PPARγ inhibitor (GW9662) that recovered this effect (Pandhare et al., 2006). Another study shows that upregulation of PRODH/POX expression by doxycycline contributed to ROS-dependent apoptosis in colon cancer cells. This process was accompanied by significant reduction in COX-2 and PGE_2 levels in these cells. However, treatment of the cells with PGE_2 or neutralization of superoxide by stimulation of manganese superoxide dismutase (MnSOD) counteracted the induction of apoptosis. Interestingly, attenuation of COX-2 by doxycycline-dependent activation of PRODH/POX was reversed by EGFR signaling. inducing Wnt/β-catenin pathway.

It is well established that Pro plays an important role in the metabolism of cancer cells. In DLD-1 colon cancer cells expressing PRODH/POX, supplementation of culture media with 0.5 mM of Pro resulted in mitochondria-mediated apoptosis through activation of caspase-9, release of cytochrome *c*, and nuclear fragmentation, independently of p53. Therefore the studies on the role of Pro in apoptosis/survival were focused on enzymes metabolizing this amino acid and substrates for its synthesis. Substrates for Pro synthesis, ornithine and glutamate, are of special interest. These amino acids are converted into L-glutamate-γ-semialdehyde (GSAL) and reversibly into P5C. Ornithine is transferred to GSAL by ornithine δ-aminoacid transferase (OAT), while glutamate is converted into P5C with GSAL intermediate by P5C synthase (P5CS). The process of Pro biosynthesis with intermediate P5C takes place in mitochondria. However, P5C could be transferred to cytoplasm and reduced to Pro by cytosolic, nicotinamide adenine dinucleotide phosphate–dependent, P5C reductase (PYCRL). In mitochondria, two isoforms of PYCR originate, PYCR1 or PYCR2. Knockdown of PYCR1 contributed to decrease in cell proliferation in liver cancer cells. This phenomenon is linked to cellular energy production since Pro metabolite, glutamate, converting into α-ketoglutarate (αKG) by glutamate dehydrogenase, which enters the tricarboxylic acid (TCA) cycle. Metabolism of Pro is also linked to the pentose phosphate pathway, synthesizing precursors of nucleotides for DNA synthesis that contribute to biomass production and cell proliferation (Tanner et al., 2018). Although Pro could be synthesized from other amino acids, a large amount of Pro is derived from collagen degradation. Complex regulatory pathways of PRODH/POX–dependent ATP/ROS generation and PYCRL–dependent nucleotide synthesis are presented in Fig. 10.2.

Since about 25% of all amino acids in collagen subunits constitute hydroxyproline (Hyp) and Pro, the degradation of collagen may provide significant amount of substrates for PRODH/POX. The final process of collagen degradation, supporting intracellular Pro and Hyp concentrations, is catalyzed by prolidase.

10.5 The role of prolidase in proline dehydrogenase/proline oxidase–dependent apoptosis

Prolidase (PEPD, peptidase D or iminopeptidase) is imido-dipeptidase or imido-tripeptidase localized in the cytoplasm (Myara et al., 1984). The enzyme catalyzes hydrolysis of dipeptides and tripeptides containing C-terminal Pro or Hyp (Mock et al., 1990). The peptides are products of protein degradation, mainly derived from collagen degradation (Adibi & Mercer, 1973; Jackson et al., 1975). In native collagen, Pro forms 119 bonds with glycine (Gly) in α1 subunit of type I procollagen, and 106 such bonds in α2 subunit of this protein. However, most of the prolines in mature collagen are hydroxylated. Not-hydroxylated Pro in Gly–Pro sequence of type I collagen subunits occurs 25 times (Jackson et al., 1975). It suggests that degradation of collagen could significantly contribute to intracellular concentration of Pro and Hyp. The final stage of collagen degradation catalyzed by prolidase contributes to release of significant amount of Pro for recycling of this amino acid for collagen resynthesis or degradation by PRODH/POX. The key role of prolidase in collagen biosynthesis regulation was found in fibroblast treated with P5C, some antiinflammatory drugs (Miltyk et al., 1996), in fibroblasts subjected to experimental aging, in experimentally induced inflammation in chondrocytes, in fibroblasts with activated by type I collagen

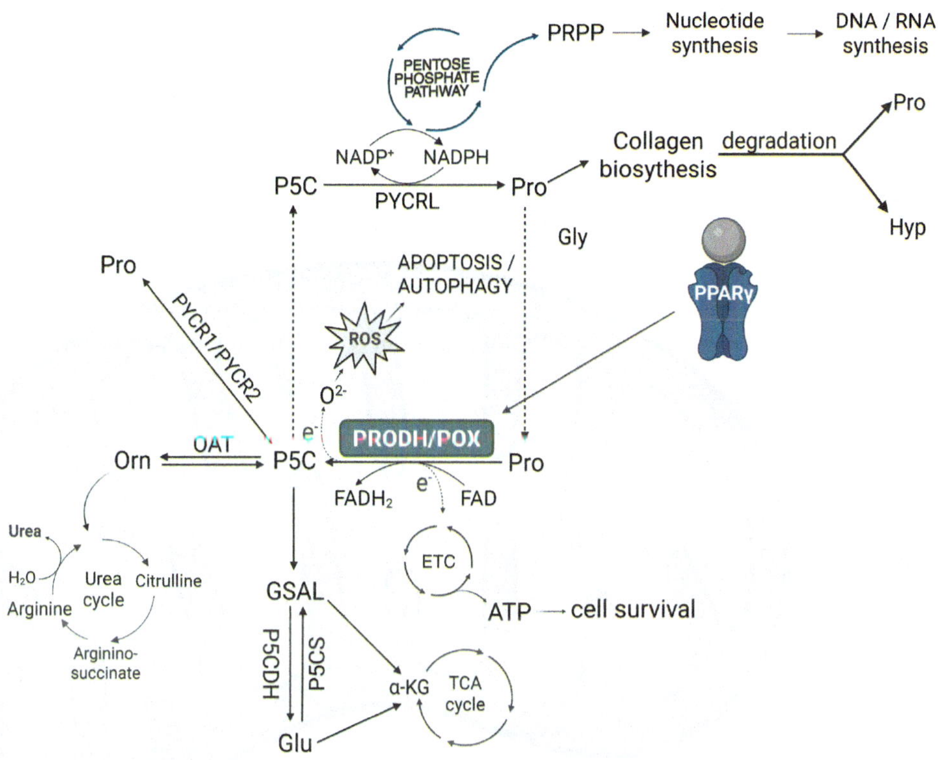

FIGURE 10.2 Regulatory pathways of PRODH/POX–dependent ATP/ROS generation and PYCRL-dependent nucleotide synthesis. *ATP*, Adenosine triphosphate; *ETC*, electron transport chain; *FAD*, oxidized form of flavin adenine dinucleotide; *FADH2*, reduced form of flavin adenine dinucleotide; *Glu*, glutamate; *Gly*, glycine; *GSAL*, L-glutamate-γ-semialdehyde; *Hyp*, hydroxyproline; *MMPs*, metalloproteinases; *NADP+*, oxidized form of nicotinamide adenine dinucleotide phosphate; *NADPH*, reduced form of nicotinamide adenine dinucleotide phosphate; *OAT*, ornithine aminotransferase; *ORN*, ornithine; *P5C*, Δ1-pyrroline-5-carboxylate; *P5CDH*, P5C dehydrogenase; *P5CS*, P5C synthase; *PPAR*, peroxisome proliferator-activated receptor gamma; *Pro*, proline; *PRODH/POX*, proline dehydrogenase/oxidase; *PRPP*, phosphoribosyl pyrophosphate; *PYCR1/2/L*, P5C reductase 1/2/L; *ROS*, reactive oxygen species; *TCA cycle*, tricarboxylic acid cycle; *α-KG*, α-ketoglutarate.

integrin receptor, in fibroblast-derived from patients with osteogenesis imperfecta and in several cancer tissues (Cechowska-Pasko et al., 2006; Karna et al., 2000, 2002). Prolidase is also involved in the regulation of transcription factors. Prolidase overexpression in colorectal cancer cells contributed to increase in expression of nuclear hypoxia inducible factor 1α (HIF-1α) as well as HIF-1α-regulated gene products (e.g., VEGF and glucose transporter-1 [Glut-1]) that contribute to cancer growth (Surazynski, Donald, et al., 2008). Increased HIF-1α transcriptional activity is due to downregulation of proteasomal degradation of HIF-1α and occurs when HIF-1α prolyl hydroxylase activity is inhibited. Interestingly, this enzyme is inhibited by Pro. Therefore increase in HIF-1α transcriptional activity could be result of increased Pro concentration in cytoplasm due to prolidase overexpression. Increase in HIF-1α transcriptional activity contributes to prosurvival phenotype of cancer cells mediated by inflammatory and proangiogenic factors, such as COX-2, IL-1, NF-κB, TNFα, and VEGF (Zareba et al., 2017). The data suggest that prolidase plays an important role in the regulation of transcriptional activity of HIF-1α.

Activation of PPARα/γ by NSAIDs induces expression of PRODH/POX, which catalytic activity conversion of Pro into P5C, generates ROS-inducing apoptosis. The rate-limiting factor in this process is Pro availability, which depends on prolidase activity (proline-releasing enzyme) and collagen biosynthesis (process of utilization of proline). Fig. 10.3 presents the role of prolidase in PRODH/POX and HIF-1α-dependent functions.

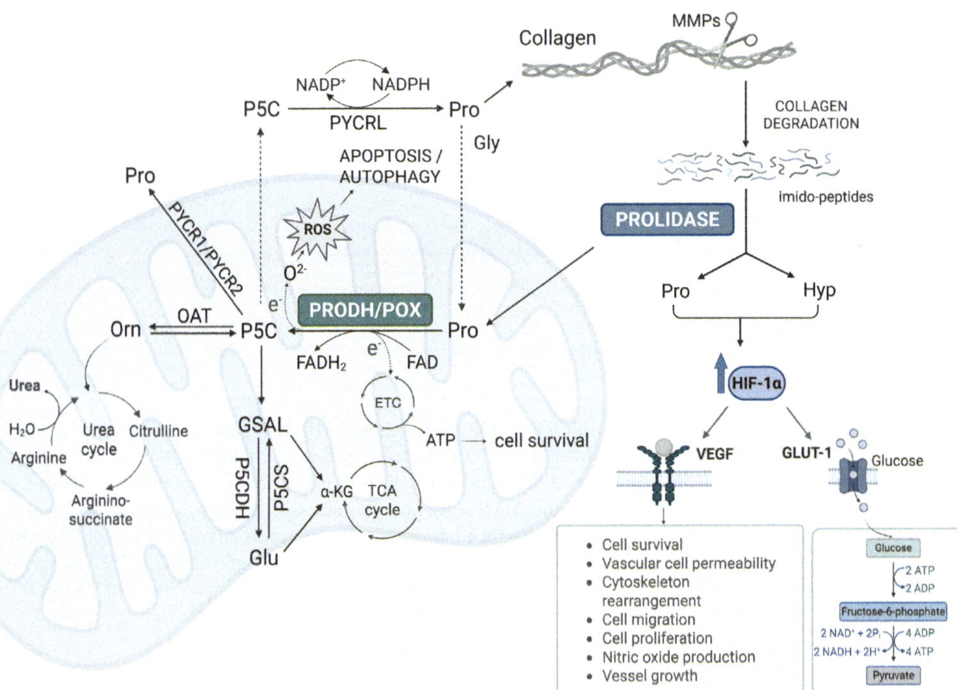

FIGURE 10.3 Prolidase induces PRODH/POX and HIF-1α - dependent functions. *ADP*, Adenosine diphosphate; *ATP*, adenosine triphosphate; *ETC*, electron transport chain; *FAD*, oxidized form of flavin adenine dinucleotide; *FADH2*, reduced form of flavin adenine dinucleotide; *Glu*, glutamate; *GLUT-1*, glucose transporter-1; *Gly*, glycine; *GSAL*, L-glutamate-γ-semialdehyde; *HIF-1α*, hypoxia-inducible factor 1α; *Hyp*, hydroxyproline; *MMPs*, metalloproteinases; *NAD+*, oxidized form of nicotinamide adenine dinucleotide; *NADH*, reduced form of nicotinamide adenine dinucleotide; *NADP+*, oxidized form of nicotinamide adenine dinucleotide phosphate; *NADPH*, reduced form of nicotinamide adenine dinucleotide phosphate; *OAT*, ornithine aminotransferase; *ORN*, ornithine; *P5C*, Δ1-pyrroline-5-carboxylate; *P5CDH*, P5C dehydrogenase; *P5CS*, P5C synthase; *PPAR*, peroxisome proliferator-activated receptor gamma; *Pro*, proline; *PRODH/POX*, proline dehydrogenase/oxidase; *PRPP*, phosphoribosyl pyrophosphate; *PYCR1/2/L*, P5C reductase 1/2/L; *ROS*, reactive oxygen species; *TCA cycle*, tricarboxylic acid cycle; *VEGF*, vascular endothelial growth factor; *α-KG*, α-ketoglutarate.

10.6 Nonsteroidal antiinflammatory drugs induce proline dehydrogenase/proline oxidase–dependent and proline dehydrogenase/proline oxidase–independent apoptosis in cancer cells

NSAID-induced PRODH/POX-dependent apoptosis was studied in breast cancer MCF-7 cells in which PRODH/POX was knocked out by CRISPR/Cas9 technology (MCF-7^{POX-KO} cells). Interestingly, studied NSAiDs (indomethacin, diclofenac) induced apoptosis in both MCF-7 and MCF-7^{POX-KO} cells. Unexpectedly, the NSAIDs-induced apoptosis was more pronounced in cells lacking PRODH/POX (Kazberuk, Chalecka, Palka, Bielawska, et al., 2022; Kazberuk, Chalecka, Palka, & Surazynski, 2022). The apoptosis in these cells was accompanied by low expression of mTOR (stimulator of growth) and high expression of p-AMPKα, a sensor of ATP level. It led to the suggestion that the mechanism for NSAIDs-dependent apoptosis in MCF7^{POX-KO} cells could be attributed to energetic shortage.

P5C, as a product of PRODH/POX activity, could be a sensor of energy production. Conversion of P5C into Glu (spontaneously in reversible reaction) and Glu into α-KG by glutamate dehydrogenase (GLUD 1/2) provides metabolite of TCA cycle (α-KG) supporting energy production. Another source of P5C could be derived from ornithine, a metabolite of the UC (Cappelletti et al., 2018). Since in MCF-7^{POX-KO} cells treated with NSAiDs, expression of GLUD1/2 is elevated, compared to control cells, therefore in these cells P5C could be derived from Glu or ornithine, supporting TCA cycle-generated energy (Phang, 2019). In NSAIDs-treated MCF-7 cells, increase in the expression of PRODH/POX (through PPARγ) was accompanied by increase in activity of PYCR1. In NSAIDs-treated MCF-7^{POX-KO}, the P5C production and PYCR1 expression were decreased, suggesting the mechanism for shortage of energy in these conditions and the role of P5C as a proenergetic precursor. Simultaneously, NSAIDs inhibit expression of PPARδ (energy-producing factor) and cancer cell growth (Blitek & Szymanska, 2017; Li et al., 2017; Liu et al., 2018; Müller, 2017; Schoonjans et al., 1996; Viswakarma et al., 2010; Zhao et al., 2016) facilitating proapoptotic pathways and attenuating cell proliferation, particularly in MCF-7^{POX-KO} cells (Kazberuk, Chalecka, Palka, Bielawska, et al., 2022; Kazberuk, Chalecka, Palka, & Surazynski, 2022).

Lack of PRODH/POX contributes to significant decrease in cell viability. Cytometric analysis of MCF-7^{POX-KO} cells showed 12% dead cells, compared to 1% dead cells in MCF-7 cells. Treatment of the cells with NSAIDs contributed to increase in early apoptotic and dead cells and decrease in DNA biosynthesis. In NSAIDs-treated cells, collagen biosynthesis is also inhibited (Cechowska-Pasko et al., 2006; Surazyński et al., 2004; Surazynski, Miltyk, et al., 2008). This process is more pronounced in NSAIDs-treated MCF-7^{POX-KO} cells. This activity of NSAIDs in cancer cells is desired because Pro, instead of being utilized for collagen biosynthesis is available for PRODH/POX-dependent ROS generation that induces apoptosis. Moreover, in NSAIDs-treated MCF-7^{POX-KO} cells, an increase in Pro level is harmful for the cells since the amino acid is a carrier of reducing potential (Cappelletti et al., 2018; Phang, 2019; Zareba et al., 2017). Interestingly, in MCF-7^{POK-KO} cells, prolidase expression and activity are elevated, contributing to the increase in intracellular Pro concentration. The functional significance of the processes is activation of apoptosis by PRODH/POX-dependent ROS generation. In MCF-7 cells, NSAIDs upregulate expression of active caspase 9 (marker of intrinsic apoptosis) and activated PARP (marker of DNA degradation) (Abeti & Duchen, 2012). DNA damage is mediated by different stressors, for example, oxidative stress, which is induced in cells treated with NSAIDs. Fluorescence analysis confirmed generation of ROS (using 2′,7′-dichlorofluorescin diacetate) in NSAIDs-treated cells. The study shows the functional significance of NSAIDs as a ligands of PPARγ that induce PRODH/POX-dependent ROS generation and mitochondrial apoptosis mediated by caspase-9. However, in MCF-7^{POX-KO} cells, the mechanism for NSAIDs-dependent apoptosis cannot be attributed to ROS formation since they were not detected. Expression of PARP was also very low in these cells, suggesting that in MCF-7^{POX-KO} cells, NSAIDs do not induce DNA degradation. However, these cells (MCF-7^{POX-KO}) evoke increased expression of caspase-8, suggesting induction of extrinsic pathway of apoptosis. Moreover, in NSAIDs-treated MCF-7^{POX-KO} cells, an increase in expression of BID was found, compared to NSAIDs-treated MCF-7 cells. An increase in the expression of BID induces mitochondrial caspase-9. However, some NSAIDs, particularly diclofenac, induce caspase 9 independently of BID expression. Similarly, treatment of both cell lines with NSAIDs did not induce expression of Beclin 1, Atg5, and Atg7 (autophagy markers), suggesting that autophagy-mediated cell death was not induced in the cells. Therefore it has been suggested that the mechanism of NSAID-induced apoptosis in MCF-7^{POX-KO} cells involves disturbances in energetic metabolism linked to the TCA, UC, and Pro cycles. As described above, knockout of PRODH/POX in breast cancer cells contributes to decrease in P5C concentration and deregulation of Pro, glutamine (Gln), α-KG, and ornithine interconversion, affecting the TCA and Urea cycles and energetic metabolism (Chalecka et al., 2025; Phang, 2019). In PRODH/POX knockout cells, intracellular concentration of Pro is increased due to inhibition of its degradation, increased prolidase activity, and inhibition of collagen biosynthesis. Moreover, Pro bearing reducing potential affects redox balance in the cells. It may explain the mechanism for PRODH/POX-independent apoptosis in breast cancer cells. The potential mechanism of NSAID-induced apoptosis in MCF-7^{POX-KO} cells is presented as Fig. 10.4.

It seems that the described mechanisms could be universal, particularly in cancer cells expressing PRODH/POX. However, some lines of evidence suggest that PRODH/POX-mediated apoptosis or survival in cancer cells is metabolic context dependent. An example is studies showing that metformin (potent PRODH/POX activator) induced apoptosis in both PRODH/POX expressing MCF-7 cells and the cells with PRODH/POX knockout cultured in glutamine (Gln) free medium. When the cells were cultured in the presence of Gln, they expressed a prosurvival phenotype. Metabolomic analysis shows metabolic context of this phenomenon, linking glycolysis, Gln, and Pro metabolism with cell energetic status and availability of Pro for PRODH/POX-dependent apoptosis or survival in these cells. It has been suggested that metformin contributes to starvation and proapoptotic phenotype in both cell lines cultured in the absence of Gln. Apoptosis in these cells was mediated by PARP and active caspase-7, which is executioner apoptotic enzyme activated by caspase-8 (extrinsic apoptosis) and caspase-9 (intrinsic apoptosis). It suggests different mechanisms for induction of apoptosis in either cells expressing PRODH/POX as well as cells with the absence or silencing of this enzyme. It seems that an important factor in the mechanism of

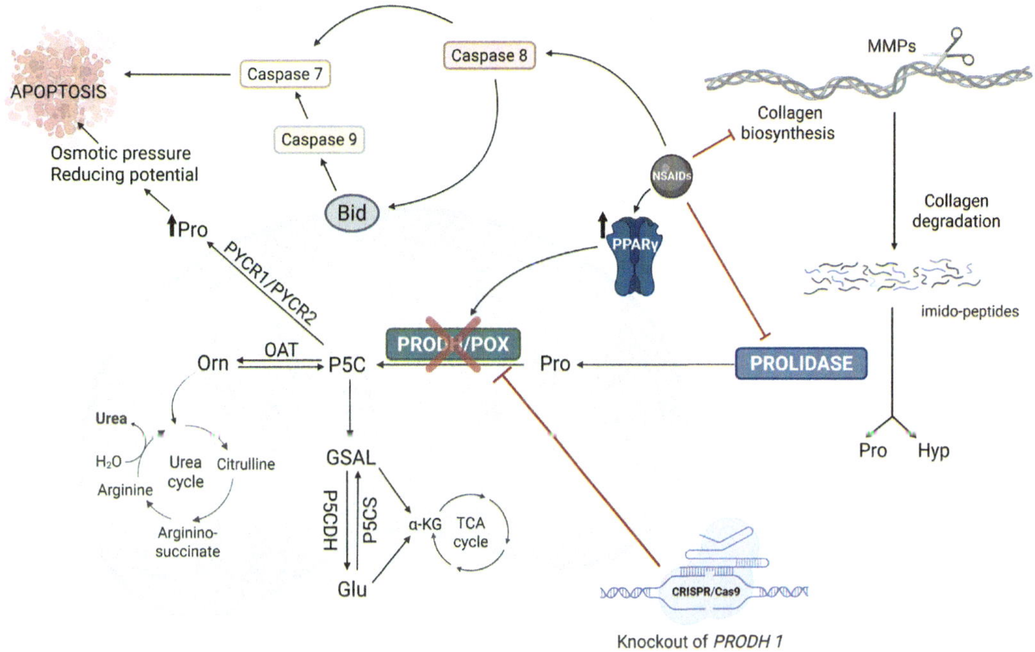

FIGURE 10.4 NSAIDs induced PRODH/POX-independent apoptosis. *GSAL*, L-Glutamate-γ-semialdehyde; *HIF-1α*, hypoxia-inducible factor 1α; *Hyp*, hydroxyproline; *MMPs*, metalloproteinases; *NSAIDs*, nonsteroidal antiinflammatory drugs; *OAT*, ornithine aminotransferase; *ORN*, ornithine; *P5C*, Δ1-pyrroline-5-carboxylate; *P5CDH*, P5C dehydrogenase; *P5CS*, P5C synthase; *PPAR*, peroxisome proliferator-activated receptor gamma; *Pro*, proline; *PRODH/POX*, proline dehydrogenase/oxidase; *PYCR1/2/L*, P5C reductase 1/2/L; *TCA cycle*, tricarboxylic acid cycle; *α-KG*, α-ketoglutarate.

apoptosis is the concentration in the cells. For instance, knockout of PRODH/POX in melanoma cells, which intensively synthesize collagen (the most potent process of Pro utilization), facilitates survival phenotype of the cells. It seems that in these cells, Pro concentration is too low to induce apoptosis by extrinsic pathway. In melanoma cells expressing PRODH/POX, metformin activates PRODH/POX-dependent ROS formation and apoptosis, while this effect was not shown in metformin-treated PRODH/POX knockout cells. Some studies suggested that estrogen receptors (ERα and ERβ) may play an important role in the mechanism of PRODH/POX-induced apoptosis. In studies on MCF-7 and MDA-MB-231 cells that differ in expression of ERα and ERβ, it has been found that troglitazone-activated PRODH/POX induced apoptosis only in ERβ-deficient MDA-MB-231 cells or in the absence of estradiol. It suggests that the PRODH/POX-dependent function (apoptosis or survival) in cancer cells is conditioned by the metabolic context. The data show complex regulatory mechanisms in cancer cells driving PRODH/POX-dependent and PRODH/POX-independent apoptosis (Fig. 10.5).

Summarizing, the data suggest that NSAIDs could induce apoptosis in cancer cells by intrinsic and extrinsic pathways, independent of COX activity. The mechanism for

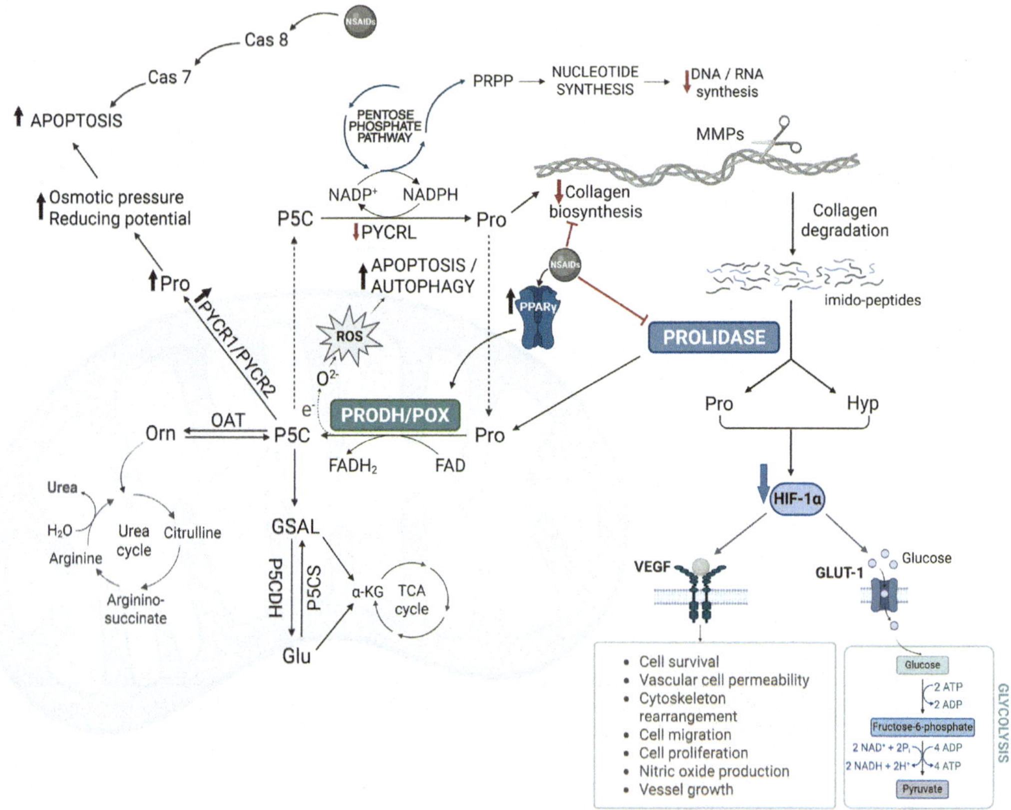

FIGURE 10.5 The molecular mechanisms creating PRODH/POX-dependent and PRODH/POX-independent apoptosis in cancer cells. *ADP*, Adenosine diphosphate; *ATP*, adenosine triphosphate; *Cas 7*, caspase 7; *Cas 8*, caspase 8; *FAD*, oxidized form of flavin adenine dinucleotide; *FADH2*, reduced form of flavin adenine dinucleotide; *Glu*, glutamate; *GLUT-1*, glucose transporter-1; *GSAL*, L-glutamate-γ-semialdehyde; *HIF-1α*, hypoxia-inducible factor 1α; *Hyp*, hydroxyproline; *MMPs*, metalloproteinases; *NAD+*, oxidized form of nicotinamide adenine dinucleotide; *NADH*, reduced form of nicotinamide adenine dinucleotide; *NADP+*, oxidized form of nicotinamide adenine dinucleotide phosphate; *NADPH*, reduced form of nicotinamide adenine dinucleotide phosphate; *NSAIDs*, nonsteroidal anti-inflammatory drugs; *OAT*, ornithine aminotransferase; *ORN*, ornithine; *P5C*, Δ1-pyrroline-5-carboxylate; *P5CDH*, P5C dehydrogenase; *P5CS*, P5C synthase; *PPAR*, peroxisome proliferator-activated receptor gamma; *Pro*, proline; *PRODH/POX*, proline dehydrogenase/oxidase; *PRPP*, phosphoribosyl pyrophosphate; *PYCR1/2/L*, P5C reductase 1/2/L; *ROS*, reactive oxygen species; *TCA cycle*, tricarboxylic acid cycle; *VEGF*, vascular endothelial growth factor; *α-KG*, α-ketoglutarate.

antineoplastic activity of NSAIDs is metabolic context dependent and involves PPARγ, PRODH/POX, proline metabolism, energetic metabolism, estrogenic status, and oncogenic factors (Heudobler et al., 2018; Okazaki et al., 2016; Peters et al., 2012; Varga et al., 2011; Yousefi et al., 2016). NSAIDs, as ligands of PPARγ, induce PRODH/POX-dependent apoptosis (ROS-induced intrinsic pathway) and PRODH/POX-independent apoptosis (death receptor-induced extrinsic pathway). The experimental data presented in this review constitute basis for undertaking *in vivo* studies on anticancer activity of NSAIDs.

References

Abeti, R., & Duchen, M. R. (2012). Activation of PARP by Oxidative Stress Induced by β-Amyloid: Implications for Alzheimer's Disease. *Neurochemical Research, 37*, 2589–2596. https://doi.org/10.1007/s11064-012-0895-x.

Adibi, S. A., & Mercer, D. W. (1973). Protein Digestion in Human Intestine as Reflected in Luminal, Mucosal, and Plasma Amino Acid Concentrations after Meals. *Journal of Clinical Investigation, 52*, 1586–1594. https://doi.org/10.1172/JCI107335.

Akrami, H., Moradi, B., Borzabadi Farahani, D., & Mehdizadeh, K. (2018). Ibuprofen reduces cell proliferation through inhibiting Wnt/β catenin signaling pathway in gastric cancer stem cells. *Cell Biology International, 42*, 949–958. https://doi.org/10.1002/cbin.10959.

Almatroodi, S. A., Alnuqaydan, A. M., Alsahli, M. A., Khan, A. A., & Rahmani, A. H. (2021). Thymoquinone, the most prominent constituent of nigella sativa, attenuates liver damage in streptozotocin-induced diabetic rats via regulation of oxidative stress, inflammation and cyclooxygenase-2 protein expression. *Applied Sciences (Switzerland), 11*(7). https://doi.org/10.3390/app11073223, https://www.mdpi.com/2076-3417/11/7/3223/pdf.

Alzohairy, M. A., Khan, A. A., Ansari, M. A., Babiker, A. Y., Alsahli, M. A., Almatroodi, S. A., & Rahmani, A. H. (2021). Protective effect of quercetin, a flavonol against benzo(A)pyrene-induced lung injury via inflammation, oxidative stress, angiogenesis and cyclooxygenase-2 signalling molecule. *Applied Sciences (Switzerland), 11*(18). https://doi.org/10.3390/app11188675, https://www.mdpi.com/2076-3417/11/18/8675/pdf.

Arisan, E. D., Ergül, Z., Bozdağ, G., Rencüzoğulları, Ö., Çoker-Gürkan, A., Obakan-Yerlikaya, P., Coşkun, D., & Palavan-Ünsal, N. (2018). Diclofenac induced apoptosis via altering PI3K/Akt/MAPK signaling axis in HCT 116 more efficiently compared to SW480 colon cancer cells. *Molecular Biology Reports, 45*(6), 2175–2184. https://doi.org/10.1007/s11033-018-4378-2.

Aziz, S. A., Davies, M., Pick, E., Zito, C., Jilaveanu, L., Camp, R. L., Rimm, D. L., Kluger, Y., & Kluger, H. M. (2009). Phosphatidylinositol-3-kinase as a therapeutic target in melanoma. *Clinical Cancer Research, 15*(9), 3029–3036. https://doi.org/10.1158/1078-0432.CCR-08-2768, http://clincancerres.aacrjournals.org/cgi/reprint/15/9/3029.

Blitek, A., & Szymanska, M. (2017). Peroxisome proliferator-activated receptor (PPAR) isoforms are differentially expressed in peri-implantation porcine conceptuses. *Theriogenology, 101*, 53–61. https://doi.org/10.1016/j.theriogenology.2017.06.013.

Brooks, A. J., & Putoczki, T. (2020). Jak-stat signalling pathway in cancer. *Cancers, 12*(7), 1–3. https://doi.org/10.3390/cancers12071971, https://www.mdpi.com/2072 6694/12/7/1971/pdf.

Cappelletti, P., Tallarita, E., Rabattoni, V., Campomenosi, P., Sacchi, S., & Pollegioni, L. (2018). Proline oxidase controls proline, glutamate, and glutamine cellular concentrations in a U87 glioblastoma cell line. *PLoS One, 13*, e0196283. https://doi.org/10.1371/journal.pone.0196283.

Cechowska-Pasko, M., Pałka, J., & Wojtukiewicz, M. Z. (2006). Enhanced prolidase activity and decreased collagen content in breast cancer tissue. *International Journal of Experimental Pathology, 87*, 289–296. https://doi.org/10.1111/j.1365-2613.2006.00486.x.

Chalecka, M., Hermanowicz, J. M., Palka, J., & Surazynski, A. (2025). The new insight into the role of hydroxyproline in metabolism of cancer cells. *Front Cell Dev Biol, 13*. https://doi.org/10.3389/fcell.2025.1556770.

Chan, A. T., Giovannucci, E. L., Meyerhardt, J. A., Schernhammer, E. S., & Curhan, G. C. (2005). C.S. Fuchs, Long-term use of aspirin and nonsteroidal anti-inflammatory drugs and risk of colorectal cancer. *JAMA: the Journal of the American Medical Association, 294*(8), 914–923. https://doi.org/10.1001/jama.294.8.914, http://jama.ama-assn.org/cgi/reprint/294/8/914.

Cheung, K. S., Chen, L., Chan, E. W., Seto, W. K., Wong, I. C. K., & Leung, W. K. (2020). Nonsteroidal anti-inflammatory drugs but not aspirin are associated with a lower risk of post-colonoscopy colorectal cancer. *Alimentary Pharmacology and Therapeutics, 51*(9), 899–908. https://doi.org/10.1111/apt.15693, http://onlinelibrary.wiley.com/journal/10.1111/(ISSN)1365-2036.

Corbett, G. T., Gonzalez, F. J., & Pahan, K. (2015). Activation of peroxisome proliferator-activated receptor α stimulates ADAM10-mediated proteolysis of APP. *Proceedings of the National Academy of Sciences, 112*, 8445–8450. https://doi.org/10.1073/pnas.1504890112.

Du, Q., & Geller, D. A. (2010). Cross-regulation between wnt and NF-κB signaling pathways. *Forum on Immunopathological Diseases and Therapeutics, 1*(3), 155–181. https://doi.org/10.1615/ForumImmunDisTher.v1.i3.10, http://www.dl.begellhouse.com/download/article/327512e1296113a3/FIDT0103%20(155-181).pdf.

Eibl, G., Bruemmer, D., Okada, Y., Duffy, J. P., Law, R. E., Reber, H. A., & Hines, O. J. (2003). PGE2 is generated by specific COX-2 activity and increases VEGF production in COX-2-expressing human pancreatic cancer cells. *Biochemical and Biophysical Research Communications, 306*(4), 887–897. https://doi.org/10.1016/S0006-291X(03)01079-9, http://www.sciencedirect.com/science/journal/0006291X.

Guo, Y.-J., Pan, W.-W., Liu, S.-B., Shen, Z.-F., Xu, Y., & Hu, L.-L. (2020). ERK/MAPK signalling pathway and tumorigenesis (Review). *Experimental and Therapeutic Medicine, 19*(3). https://doi.org/10.3892/etm.2020.8454.

Gurpinar, E., Grizzle, W. E., & Piazza, G. A. (2013). COX-Independent Mechanisms of Cancer Chemoprevention by Anti-Inflammatory Drugs. *Front Oncol, 3*. https://doi.org/10.3389/fonc.2013.00181.

Gurpinar, E., Grizzle, W. E., & Piazza, G. A. (2014). NSAIDs Inhibit Tumorigenesis, but How? *Clinical Cancer Research, 20*, 1104–1113. https://doi.org/10.1158/1078-0432.CCR-13-1573.

Habas, R., & Dawid, I. B. (2005). Dishevelled and Wnt signaling: Is the nucleus the final frontier? *Journal of Biology, 4*(1). https://doi.org/10.1186/jbiol22.

Harris, R. E., Beebe-Donk, J., & Schuller, H. M. (2002). Chemoprevention of lung cancer by non-steroidal anti-inflammatory drugs among cigarette smokers. *Oncol Rep 9, 693–5.*

Hashemi Goradel, N., Najafi, M., Salehi, E., Farhood, B., & Mortezaee, K. (2019). Cyclooxygenase-2 in cancer: A review. *Journal of Cellular Physiology, 234*(5), 5683–5699. https://doi.org/10.1002/jcp.27411, http://onlinelibrary.wiley.com/journal/10.1002/(ISSN)1097-4652.

Hata, A., & Chen, Y. G. (2016). TGF-β signaling from receptors to smads. *Cold Spring Harbor Perspectives in Biology, 8*(9). https://doi.org/10.1101/cshperspect.a022061, http://cshperspectives.cshlp.org/content/8/9/a022061.full.pdf.

Heudobler, D., Rechenmacher, M., Lüke, F., Vogelhuber, M., Pukrop, T., Herr, W., et al. (2018). Peroxisome Proliferator-Activated Receptors (PPAR)γ Agonists as Master Modulators of Tumor Tissue. *Int J Mol Sci, 19*, 3540. https://doi.org/10.3390/ijms19113540.

Hodson, L. J., Chua, A. C. L., Evdokiou, A., Robertson, S. A., & Ingman, W. V. (2013). Macrophage phenotype in the mammary gland fluctuates over the course of the estrous cycle and is regulated by ovarian steroid hormones. *Biology of Reproduction, 89*(3). https://doi.org/10.1095/biolreprod.113.109561.

Jackson, S. H., Dennis, A. W., & Greenberg, M. (1975). Iminodipeptiduria: a genetic defect in recycling collagen; a method for determining prolidase in erythrocytes. *Canadian Medical Association Journal, 113*, 759, 762–3.

Javan, M. R., Khosrojerdi, A., & Moazzeni, S. M. (2019). New Insights Into Implementation of Mesenchymal Stem Cells in Cancer Therapy: Prospects for Anti-angiogenesis Treatment. *Front Oncol, 9*. https://doi.org/10.3389/fonc.2019.00840.

Jung, I. H., Choi, J. H. K., Chung, Y. Y., Lim, G. L., Park, Y. N., & Park, S. W. (2015). Predominant Activation of JAK/STAT3 Pathway by Interleukin-6 Is Implicated in Hepatocarcinogenesis. *Neoplasia (United States), 17*(7), 586–597. https://doi.org/10.1016/j.neo.2015.07.005, http://www.journals.elsevier.com/neoplasia/.

Kapoor, G., Prakash, S., Jaiswal, V., & Singh, A. K. (2025). Chronic Inflammation and Cancer: Key Pathways and Targeted Therapies. *Cancer Investigation, 43*, 1–23. https://doi.org/10.1080/07357907.2024.2437614.

Karna, E., Surazynski, A., Orłowski, K., łaszkiewicz, J., Puchalski, Z., Nawrat, P., et al. (2002). Serum and tissue level of insulin-like growth factor-I (IGF-I) and IGF-I binding proteins as an index of pancreatitis and pancreatic cancer. *International Journal of Experimental Pathology, 83*, 239–246. https://doi.org/10.1046/j.1365-2613.2002.00237.x.

Karna, E., Surazynski, A., & Palka, J. A. (2000). Collagen metabolism disturbances are accompanied by an increase in prolidase activity in lung carcinoma planoepitheliale. *International Journal of Experimental Pathology, 81*, 341–347. https://doi.org/10.1111/j.1365-2613.2000.00168.x.

Kazberuk, A., Chalecka, M., Palka, J., Bielawska, K., & Surazynski, A. (2022). NSAIDs Induce Proline Dehydrogenase/Proline Oxidase-Dependent and Independent Apoptosis in MCF7 Breast Cancer Cells. *Int J Mol Sci, 23*, 3813. https://doi.org/10.3390/ijms23073813.

Kazberuk, A., Chalecka, M., Palka, J., & Surazynski, A. (2022). Nonsteroidal Anti-Inflammatory Drugs as PPARγ Agonists Can Induce PRODH/POX-Dependent Apoptosis in Breast Cancer Cells: New Alternative Pathway in NSAID-Induced Apoptosis. *Int J Mol Sci, 23*, 1510. https://doi.org/10.3390/ijms23031510.

Keshet, Y., & Seger, R. (2010). The MAP kinase signaling cascades: a system of hundreds of components regulates a diverse array of physiological functions. *Methods in molecular biology (Clifton, N.J.), 661*, 3–38. https://doi.org/10.1007/978-1-60761-795-2_1.

Kim, H. S., Moon, H. G., Han, W., Yom, C. K., Kim, W. H., Kim, J. H., & Noh, D. Y. (2012). COX2 overexpression is a prognostic marker for Stage III breast cancer. *Breast Cancer Research and Treatment, 132*(1), 51–59. https://doi.org/10.1007/s10549-011-1521-3.

Kohn, A. D., & Moon, R. T. (2005). Wnt and calcium signaling: β-Catenin-independent pathways. *Cell Calcium, 38*(3-4), 439–446. https://doi.org/10.1016/j.ceca.2005.06.022, http://www.elsevier-international.com/journals/ceca/.

Kyriakis, J. M., & Avruch, J. (2001). Mammalian mitogen-activated protein kinase signal transduction pathways activated by stress and inflammation. *Physiological Reviews, 81*(2), 807–869. https://doi.org/10.1152/physrev.2001.81.2.807, physrev.physiology.org.

IL Lee, S., Zuo, X., & Shureiqi, I. (2011). 15-Lipoxygenase-1 as a tumor suppressor gene in colon cancer: is the verdict in? *Cancer and Metastasis Reviews, 30*, 481–491. https://doi.org/10.1007/s10555-011-9321-0.

Li, Y.-J., Sun, L., Shi, Y., Wang, G., Wang, X., Dunn, S. E., et al. (2017). PPAR-delta promotes survival of chronic lymphocytic leukemia cells in energetically unfavorable conditions. *Leukemia: Official Journal of the Leukemia Society of America, Leukemia Research Fund, U.K, 31*, 1905–1914. https://doi.org/10.1038/leu.2016.395.

Liu, Y., Colby, J. K., Zuo, X., Jaoude, J., Wei, D., & Shureiqi, I. (2018). The Role of PPAR-δ in Metabolism, Inflammation, and Cancer: Many Characters of a Critical Transcription Factor. *Int J Mol Sci, 19*, 3339. https://doi.org/10.3390/ijms19113339.

Ma, Q., Wu, H., Xiao, Y., Liang, Z., & Liu, T. (2020). Upregulation of exosomal microRNA-21 in pancreatic stellate cells promotes pancreatic cancer cell migration and enhances Ras/ERK pathway activity. *International Journal of Oncology, 56*(4), 1025–1033. https://doi.org/10.3892/ijo.2020.4986, https://www.spandidos-publications.com/10.3892/ijo.2020.4986.

Marion-Letellier, R., Savoye, G., & Ghosh, S. (2016). Fatty acids, eicosanoids and PPAR gamma. *European Journal of Pharmacology, 785*, 44–49. https://doi.org/10.1016/j.ejphar.2015.11.004.

Mazhar, D., Gillmore, R., & Waxman, J. (2005). COX and cancer. *QJM: An International Journal of Medicine, 98*, 711–718. https://doi.org/10.1093/qjmed/hci119.

Menter, D. G., & Dubois, R. N. (2012). Prostaglandins in cancer cell adhesion, migration, and invasion. *International Journal of Cell Biology*. https://doi.org/10.1155/2012/723419.

Miltyk, W., Karna, E., & Pałka, J. (1996). Inhibition of prolidase activity by non-steroid antiinflammatory drugs in cultured human skin fibroblasts. *Polish Journal of Pharmacology, 48*, 609–613.

Mock, W. L., Green, P. C., & Boyer, K. D. (1990). Specificity and pH dependence for acylproline cleavage by prolidase. *The Journal of Biological Chemistry, 265*, 19600–19605.

Myara, I., Charpentier, C., & Lemonnier, A. (1984). Prolidase and prolidase deficiency. *Life Sciences, 34*, 1985–1998. https://doi.org/10.1016/0024-3205(84)90363-1.

Müller, R. (2017). PPARβ/δ in human cancer. *Biochimie, 136*, 90–99. https://doi.org/10.1016/j.biochi.2016.10.019.

O'Shea, J. J., Pesu, M., Borie, D. C., & Changelian, P. S. (2004). A new modality for immunosuppression: Targeting the JAK/STAT pathway. *Nature Reviews. Drug Discovery, 3*(7), 555–564. https://doi.org/10.1038/nrd1441, http://www.nature.com/nrd/index.html.

Okazaki, S., Shioi, R., Noguchi-Yachide, T., Ishikawa, M., Makishima, M., Hashimoto, Y., et al. (2016). Structure–activity relationship studies of non-carboxylic acid peroxisome proliferator-activated receptor α/δ (PPARα/δ) dual agonists. *Bioorganic & Medicinal Chemistry, 24*, 5455–5461. https://doi.org/10.1016/j.bmc.2016.08.067.

Pandhare, J., Cooper, S. K., & Phang, J. M. (2006). Proline Oxidase, a Proapoptotic Gene, Is Induced by Troglitazone. *Journal of Biological Chemistry, 281*, 2044–2052. https://doi.org/10.1074/jbc.M507867200.

Pang, L. Y., Hurst, E. A., & Argyle, D. J. (2016). Cyclooxygenase-2: A Role in Cancer Stem Cell Survival and Repopulation of Cancer Cells during Therapy. *Stem Cells Int, 2016*. https://doi.org/10.1155/2016/2048731.

Peters, J. M., Shah, Y. M., & Gonzalez, F. J. (2012). The role of peroxisome proliferator-activated receptors in carcinogenesis and chemoprevention. *Nature Reviews. Cancer, 12*, 181–195. https://doi.org/10.1038/nrc3214.

Phang, J. M. (2019). Proline Metabolism in Cell Regulation and Cancer Biology: Recent Advances and Hypotheses. *Antioxidants & Redox Signaling, 30*, 635–649. https://doi.org/10.1089/ars.2017.7350.

Proctor, M. J., Talwar, D., Balmar, S. M., O'Reilly, D. S. J., Foulis, A. K., Horgan, P. G., Morrison, D. S., & McMillan, D. C. (2010). The relationship between the presence and site of cancer, an inflammation-based prognostic score and biochemical parameters. Initial results of the Glasgow Inflammation Outcome Study. *British Journal of Cancer, 103*(6), 870–876. https://doi.org/10.1038/sj.bjc.6605855.

Rinkenbaugh, A., & Baldwin, A. (2016). The NF-κB Pathway and Cancer Stem Cells. *Cells, 5*, 16. https://doi.org/10.3390/cells5020016.

Rodig, S. J., Meraz, M. A., White, J. M., Lampe, P. A., Riley, J. K., Arthur, C. D., King, K. L., Sheehan, K. C. F., Yin, L., Pennica, D., Johnson, E. M., & Schreiber, R. D. (1998). Disruption of the Jak1 gene demonstrates obligatory and nonredundant roles of the Jaks in cytokine-induced biologic responses. *Cell, 93*(3), 373–383. https://doi.org/10.1016/S0092-8674(00)81166-6, https://www.sciencedirect.com/journal/cell.

Rothwell, P. M., Price, J. F., Fowkes, F. G. R., Zanchetti, A., Roncaglioni, M. C., Tognoni, G., Lee, R., Belch, J. F. F., Wilson, M., Mehta, Z., & Meade, T. W. (2012). Short-term effects of daily aspirin on cancer incidence, mortality, and non-vascular death: Analysis of the time course of risks and benefits in 51 randomised controlled trials. *The Lancet, 379*(9826), 1602–1612. https://doi.org/10.1016/S0140-6736(11)61720-0, http://www.journals.elsevier.com/the-lancet/.

Rothwell, P. M., Wilson, M., Elwin, C. E., Norrving, B., Algra, A., Warlow, C. P., & Meade, T. W. (2010). Long-term effect of aspirin on colorectal cancer incidence and mortality: 20-year follow-up of five randomised trials. *The Lancet, 376*(9754), 1741–1750. https://doi.org/10.1016/S0140-6736(10)61543-7, http://www.journals.elsevier.com/the-lancet/.

Schoonjans, K., Staels, B., & Auwerx, J. (1996). The peroxisome proliferator activated receptors (PPARs) and their effects on lipid metabolism and adipocyte differentiation. *Biochimica et Biophysica Acta (BBA) - Lipids and Lipid Metabolism, 1302*, 93–109. https://doi.org/10.1016/0005-2760(96)00066-5.

Seetha, A., Devaraj, H., & Sudhandiran, G. (2020). Indomethacin and juglone inhibit inflammatory molecules to induce apoptosis in colon cancer cells. *Journal of Biochemical and Molecular Toxicology, 34*. https://doi.org/10.1002/jbt.22433.

Shebl, F. M., Hsing, A. W., Park, Y., Hollenbeck, A. R., Chu, L. W., Meyer, T. E., & Koshiol, J. (2014). Non-steroidal anti-inflammatory drugs use is associated with reduced risk of inflammation-associated cancers: NIH-AARP study. *PLoS One, 9*(12). https://doi.org/10.1371/journal.pone.0114633, http://www.plosone.org/article/fetchObject.action?uri=info:doi/10.1371/journal.pone.0114633&representation=PDF.

Sun, S. C. (2017). The non-canonical NF-κB pathway in immunity and inflammation. *Nature Reviews. Immunology, 17*(9), 545–558. https://doi.org/10.1038/nri.2017.52, http://www.nature.com/nri/index.html.

Surazynski, A., Donald, S. P., Cooper, S. K., Whiteside, M. A., Salnikow, K., Liu, Y., et al. (2008). Extracellular matrix and HIF-1 signaling: The role of prolidase. *International Journal of Cancer. Journal International du Cancer, 122*, 1435–1440. https://doi.org/10.1002/ijc.23263.

Surazynski, A., Miltyk, W., Palka, J., & Phang, J. M. (2008). Prolidase-dependent regulation of collagen biosynthesis. *Amino Acids, 35*, 731–738. https://doi.org/10.1007/s00726-008-0051-8.

Surazyński, A., Pałka, J., & Wołczyński, S. (2004). Acetylsalicylic acid-dependent inhibition of collagen biosynthesis and beta1-integrin signaling in cultured fibroblasts. *Medical Science Monitor: International Medical Journal of Experimental and Clinical Research, 10*, BR175–BR179.

Tanner, J. J., Fendt, S.-M., & Becker, D. F. (2018). The Proline Cycle As a Potential Cancer Therapy Target. *Biochemistry, 57*, 3433–3444. https://doi.org/10.1021/acs.biochem.8b00215.

Tenenbaum, A., Motro, M., & Fisman, E. Z. (2005). Dual and pan-peroxisome proliferator-activated receptors (PPAR) co-agonism: the bezafibrate lessons. *Cardiovascular Diabetology, 4*, 14. https://doi.org/10.1186/1475-2840-4-14.

Varga, T., Czimmerer, Z., & Nagy, L. (2011). PPARs are a unique set of fatty acid regulated transcription factors controlling both lipid metabolism and inflammation. *Biochimica et Biophysica Acta (BBA) - Molecular Basis of Disease, 1812*, 1007–1022. https://doi.org/10.1016/j.bbadis.2011.02.014.

Villarino, A. V., Kanno, Y., Ferdinand, J. R., & O'Shea, J. J. (2014). Mechanisms of Jak/STAT Signaling in Immunity and Disease. *The Journal of Immunology, 194*, 21–27. https://doi.org/10.4049/jimmunol.1401867.

Viswakarma, N., Jia, Y., Bai, L., Vluggens, A., Borensztajn, J., Xu, J., et al. (2010). Coactivators in PPAR-Regulated Gene Expression. *PPAR Research, 2010*, 1–21. https://doi.org/10.1155/2010/250126.

Vogt, P. K., Hart, J. R., Gymnopoulos, M., Jiang, H., Kang, S., Bader, A. G., Zhao, L., & Denley, A. (2010). Phosphatidylinositol 3-kinase: The oncoprotein. *Current Topics in Microbiology and Immunology, 347*(1), 79–104. https://doi.org/10.1007/82-2010-80.

Yamaguchi, T. P. (2001). Heads or tails: Wnts and anterior-posterior patterning. *Current Biology, 11*(17), R713. https://doi.org/10.1016/S0960-9822(01)00417-1, http://www.elsevier.com/journals/current-biology/0960-9822.

Yousefi, B., Samadi, N., Baradaran, B., Shafiei-Irannejad, V., & Zarghami, N. (2016). Peroxisome Proliferator-Activated Receptor Ligands and Their Role in Chronic Myeloid Leukemia: Therapeutic Strategies. *Chemical Biology & Drug Design, 88*, 17–25. https://doi.org/10.1111/cbdd.12737.

Zappavigna, S., Cossu, A. M., Grimaldi, A., Bocchetti, M., Ferraro, G. A., Nicoletti, G. F., Filosa, R., & Caraglia, M. (2020). Anti-inflammatory drugs as anticancer agents. *International Journal of Molecular Sciences, 21*(7). https://doi.org/10.3390/ijms21072605, https://www.mdpi.com/1422-0067/21/7/2605/pdf.

Zareba, I., Surazynski, A., Chrusciel, M., Miltyk, W., Doroszko, M., Rahman, N., et al. (2017). Functional Consequences of Intracellular Proline Levels Manipulation Affecting PRODH/POX-Dependent Pro-Apoptotic Pathways in a Novel in Vitro Cell Culture Model. *Cellular Physiology and Biochemistry, 43*, 670–684. https://doi.org/10.1159/000480653.

Zhao, S., Kanno, Y., Li, W., Wakatabi, H., Sasaki, T., Koike, K., et al. (2016). Picrasidine N Is a Subtype-Selective PPARβ/δ Agonist. *Journal of Natural Products, 79*, 879–885. https://doi.org/10.1021/acs.jnatprod.5b00909.

Zoete, V., Grosdidier, A., & Michelin, O. (2007). Peroxisome proliferator-activated receptor structures: Ligand specificity, molecular switch and interactions with regulators. *Biochimica et Biophysica Acta (BBA) - Molecular and Cell Biology of Lipids, 1771*, 915–925. https://doi.org/10.1016/j.bbalip.2007.01.007.

CHAPTER

11

Immunotherapy and inflammation management

Yuyu Xie[1], *Mowei Kong*[2], *and Junfeng Yu*[1]

[1]Department of Dermatology, Chengdu Fifth People's Hospital, Chengdu, Sichuan, P.R. China

[2]Department of Cardiology, The Affiliated Hospital of Southwest Medical University, Luzhou, Sichuan, P.R. China

11.1 The tumor microenvironment

Malignant tumors are diseases driven by the accumulation of numerous gene mutations. Tumor cells exhibit abnormal growth and invasive capabilities. Gene mutations and abnormally activated signaling pathways in tumor cells are recognized as crucial factors contributing to tumor treatment resistance and poor prognosis in cancer patients (Xiao & Yu, 2021; Xie et al., 2021).

Tumors are considered to be an evolving ecosystem. The continuous and dynamic interactions between tumor cells and the tumor microenvironment (TME) play a significant role in tumorigenesis and tumor progression (Goenka et al., 2023). The TME is a complex system consisting of nontumor host cells, noncellular components, the vascular system, and soluble products surrounding tumor cells. Among these, nontumor host cells include immune cells and stromal cells. Noncellular components mainly refer to the extracellular matrix (ECM). Soluble products are primarily composed of chemokines, cytokines, growth factors, and extracellular vesicles. The vascular system is mainly made up of endothelial cells, which form new tumor blood vessels under the induction of angiogenic factors.

Research has revealed that the TME plays a crucial role in the pathogenesis of tumors. It influences tumorigenesis and development through multiple mechanisms, including the release of continuous proliferative signals, resistance to cell death, induction of angiogenesis, activation of tumor cell invasion and metastasis, promotion of inflammatory responses, and facilitation of immune escape (Xiao & Yu, 2021). In the TME of breast cancer, components such as immune cells, fibroblasts, and vascular tissues possess diagnostic and prognostic value and are closely associated with the prognosis of breast cancer patients. Moreover, tumor-associated macrophages (TAMs) can attenuate the treatment efficacy in

Inflammation in Tumorigenesis and Cancer Treatment
DOI: https://doi.org/10.1016/B978-0-443-36649-9.00006-2

breast cancer patients. They do this by releasing chemotherapy resistance factors or indirectly modulating the drug resistance of tumor stem cells.

In human lung cancer samples, CD10+GPR77+ cancer-associated fibroblasts provide a survival niche for lung tumor stem cells by secreting interleukin (IL)-6 and IL-8. This ultimately leads to the formation of lung tumors and the emergence of chemotherapy resistance (Su et al., 2018). In various murine tumor models, inhibiting the remodeling and crosslinking of the ECM or reducing matrix stiffening can decelerate tumor development. Numerous studies have indicated that, compared with the genomic instability of tumor cells, the stability and vulnerability of the TME endow TME-targeted therapies with an edge over direct tumor cell-targeted therapies (de Visser & Joyce, 2023; Xiao & Yu, 2021). Existing research has demonstrated that tumor therapies targeting the TME are effective. TAMs can impede the cytotoxic CD8+ T cells from killing tumor cells, further rendering the antiprogrammed death-ligand 1 (PD-L1) immunotherapy ineffective. TAM-targeted drugs such as PLX3397 and nivolumab can significantly suppress TAMs in animal tumor models or in tumor patients, thereby enhancing the treatment outcome (Cassetta & Pollard, 2018; David & Brian, 2019). Another study has shown that vascular endothelial growth factor A, angiopoietin-2, and CD40 agonist antibodies can target chemotherapy-resistant colorectal tumor cells, disrupt tumor fibrosis, and induce T cell-mediated cytotoxicity. In many instances, targeting only the TME components may not be adequate to achieve comprehensive and durable treatment effects (Xiao & Yu, 2021). This implies that TME-targeted therapies may need to be integrated with other treatment modalities to optimize the therapeutic efficacy and benefit a greater number of patients.

In the TME, nutrients such as glucose and glutamine are consumed by tumor cells in large quantities, and a large number of metabolic by-products such as lactic acid, tryptophan, and ammonia are produced. To create a tumor metabolic microenvironment characterized by "nutrient deprivation" and "metabolic waste accumulation." Antitumor T cells are in a state of nutritional deficiency for a long time, which leads to their low antitumor immune effect. Moreover, the tumor immunosuppressive microenvironment created by metabolic reprogramming of tumor cells is an important factor leading to the low efficacy of antitumor T cells. Therefore it is urgent to explore the metabolic rules and molecular mechanisms of antitumor T cells in the TME and to develop immunotherapy strategies targeting the metabolism of T cells in the TME. In this review, we summarize the recent research progress on the immunometabolism mechanism of tumor immunosuppression and the regulation of immunometabolism in tumor immunotherapy and prospect the possible research directions of immunometabolism in tumor immunotherapy in the future.

11.2 Glycolysis

Even in the cases with enough oxygen, cancer cells will also use aerobic glycolysis, using a lot of glucose and lactic acid. Oxidative phosphorylation (OXPHOS) rate is relatively low, namely, the Warburg effect. The upregulation of aerobic glycolysis in tumor cells is to prepare for the adaptation to the hypoxic environment and make corresponding changes to adapt to the low glucose concentration and acidic environment brought by glycolysis, such as glucose transporters (GLUT), especially the upregulation of GLUT1 and H^+ transporters (Corbet & Feron, 2017). Aerobic glycolysis and acidic TME affect antitumor immunity. CASCONE found that increased tumor glycolytic activity was associated with decreased T cell effects. The glycolytic activity of regulatory T cells (Treg cells) in TME is enhanced, and glucose uptake and consumption are increased (Cascone et al., 2018; Liu et al., 2020). Low glucose and high acid environment will not affect the proliferation of Treg cells and inhibit immune function (Angelin et al., 2017). However, low glucose induces senescence of CD4+ T cells and CD8+ T cells and also leads to T thinning.

The activity of mammalian target of rapamycin and the production of interferon-gamma are reduced. Lactic acid, the glycolytic metabolite, inhibits T cell and monocyte differentiation and immune response, inhibits natural killer (NK) cell function, and promotes T cell apoptosis, and TAM M2 polarization. Inhibition of type I IFN production (Husain et al., 2013). Lactate can also activate G-protein-coupled receptor 81 (GPR81) through autocrine and paracrine pathways to promote angiogenesis and immune escape. The key enzymes and transporters of tumor glycolysis pathway are important targets for the development of tumor immunotherapy drugs.

Deoxy-D-glucose (2-DG), a hexokinase (HK) II inhibitor, effectively suppresses glycolysis by inhibiting HK-mediated phosphorylation, thereby limiting tumor cell proliferation (Sun et al., 2017). Treatment strategies involving 2-DG and its derivatives, in combination with other antitumor immunotherapeutic approaches, warrant further investigation. In addition, pyruvate kinase M2 (PKM2), which catalyzes the production of pyruvate during glycolysis, is frequently overexpressed in tumor cells and has been shown to promote tumor proliferation, metastasis, and macrophage differentiation. Based on these findings, the roles of PKM2 inhibitors and agonizts in tumor immunotherapy have become a subject of increasing interest. PKM2 inhibitors, such as Benserazide and compound 3k (C3k), can inhibit the proliferation of melanoma, cervical cancer, and breast cancer cells (Zhou et al., 2020). PKM2 agonizts, including ML-265, Tepp-46, and parthenolide (PTL5), activate the tetrameric form of PKM2, thereby promoting OXPHOS and suppressing tumor progression. LI et al. (Xiao & Yu, 2021) demonstrated that combining PKM2 agonizts with programmed death-1/ligand (PD-1/PD-L1) immune checkpoint inhibitors may enhance antitumor responses by promoting tumor cell elimination and reducing aerobic glycolysis and PD-L1 expression in immune cells, thereby alleviating metabolic stress and immunosuppression within the TME. Further research is needed to explore the combination of PKM2-targeted agents with immune checkpoint inhibitors in cancer therapy.

The use of lactate dehydrogenase A (LDHA) inhibitors can reduce the level of lactate produced by tumor cells. Studies have shown that pretreatment of melanoma cells with LDHA inhibitors can enhance the antitumor immune response mediated by T cells, and it has also been found that melanoma patients with low serum LDHA levels may have a better therapeutic response to the anti-PD-1 antibody pembrolizumab. The above research results suggest that perhaps reducing the production of lactate can enhance the efficacy of tumor immunotherapy, but the selectivity of small-molecule LDHA inhibitors is limited. High levels of monocarboxylate transporters (MCT) in tumor cells are rapid transport carriers of lactate, and their blockade will lead to intracellular lactate accumulation, inhibit glycolysis, and inhibit tumor cell growth and proliferation. AZD3965 can effectively inhibit MCT1 and has MCT2 activity. It shows an inhibitory effect on tumor growth in hematological tumors and can further increase the antitumor effect when combined with rituximab, providing a new treatment strategy for hematological tumors (Curtis et al., 2017; Hsu and Hung, 2018).

11.3 Amino acid

Amino acids are one of the main nutritional substrates for the human body. They are essential structural components for cell growth, differentiation, and function and also play a significant role in the tumor ecosystem. They can serve as both carbon and nitrogen sources, providing raw materials for the synthesis of biological macromolecules necessary for the rapid proliferation of tumor cells. At the same time, they can also be taken up by immune cells in the TME, promoting their proliferation and activation, thereby exerting antitumor effects. Rapidly proliferating tumor cells compete with other cells in the TME, such as fibroblasts and immune cells, for the uptake of amino acids and other nutrients, leading to nutritional deprivation in the TME and promoting tumor progression and immune escape. Therefore targeting amino acids in the TME is an effective approach to limit tumor growth. Recent studies have shown that changes in amino acid metabolism and its products in the TME can affect the biological functions of various cell populations and participate in the occurrence and development of tumors (Chen et al., 2024).

Arginine metabolism plays an important role in T cell activation and the regulation of immune responses. During the resolution of inflammation, immunomodulatory cells promote arginine hydrolysis by expressing arginase 1 (ARGase1), thereby limiting the utilization of arginine by T cells and inhibiting tumor immunity (Grohmann et al., 2017). Therefore arginine supplementation and prevention of arginine hydrolysis are effective ways to reactivate T- and NK cell-mediated immune responses. In vitro experiments, increasing arginine is beneficial to T cells and NK cells to produce cytotoxic effects and stimulate the production of effector cytokines (He et al., 2017). Arginine supplementation during the in vitro expansion of T cells can promote their differentiation into memory T cells with antitumor activity (Geiger et al., 2016). Notably, studies have found that ARGase1 inhibitors have synergistic effects with anti-PD-1 therapy because ARGase1-targeted immunotherapy induces Th1-related inflammation, which is beneficial for PD-L1 expression in TME (Aaboe Jørgensen et al., 2021). PEGylated arginine deiminase (ADI-PEG20), a new anticancer drug, can inhibit the growth of arginine-auxotrophic cancers by depleting arginine in the TME (Werner et al., 2017). The specific tumor types for which ARGase1 inhibitors and ADI-PEG20 are applicable remain to be further studied. TME with low arginine can also affect the proliferation of chimeric antigen receptors (CAR) T cells, thereby reducing the clearance of blood and solid malignant tumors by CAR-T cells (Mussai et al., 2019). Therefore metabolic modification of CAR-T cell therapy according to the characteristics of arginine in TME is a new idea for tumor treatment. Tryptophan metabolism also plays an important role in the development of tumors. It has the properties of inhibiting antitumor immune response and increasing the malignancy of cancer cells, mainly because of the tryptophan-degrading enzyme indoleamine 2,3-bis in tumor cells. High levels of indoleamine 2,3-dioxygenase 1 (IDO1), IDO2, and tryptophan 2,3-dioxygenase (TDO) reduce the availability of tryptophan in TME. Thus it inhibits T cell function and promotes tumor development (Platten et al., 2019).

TAMs can exert antitumor effects by recognizing and eliminating tumor cells, or promote tumor progression by enhancing tumor growth, invasion, and metastasis. During the progression of the purine metabolic pathway, tryptophan is ultimately metabolized into nicotinamide adenine dinucleotide (NAD+), pyridine nucleotides, adenosine triphosphate (ATP), and carbon dioxide (CO_2), all of which play distinct roles in the antiinflammatory functions of macrophages. For instance, NAD+ has been shown to suppress inflammation and enhance endocytosis (Minhas et al., 2019). Activation of the aryl hydrocarbon receptor (AhR) in TAMs not only relies on tryptophan metabolism within macrophages but also requires the conversion of tryptophan by Lactobacillus into indole, which subsequently drives TAMs toward an immunosuppressive phenotype. Elevated AhR activity in gliomas correlates with reduced overall survival, and inhibition of tryptophan metabolism has been shown to improve survival outcomes (Panitz et al., 2021). Branched-chain amino acids have both proinflammatory and antiinflammatory effects in macrophages. The cytosolic branched chain amino acid transaminase 1 (BCAT1) can regulate the inflammatory response, and its inhibitory effect has been proven to be able to suppress the proinflammatory activity of macrophages. In breast cancer, sepicetrin (a precursor of tetrahydrobiopterin) as a cofactor of nitric oxide synthase can redirect the metabolism of arginine in macrophages, shifting it from polyamine synthesis to the production of nitric oxide. This transformation promotes the transformation of M2-type macrophages to M1-type macrophages, inhibits tumor growth, and inhibits the expression of PD-L1 dependent on signal transducer and activator of transcription 3 (STAT3). The downregulation of α-ketoglutaric acid is regulated by isocitrate dehydrogenase, which is a downstream target of the nuclear receptor Nur77 (Nr4a1). Glutamine has been proven to enhance the antiinflammatory function of macrophages through Nur77-mediated transcriptional enhancement.

11.4 Lipid metabolism

Lipid is one of the three major nutrients and metabolic substances in the human body. In addition to serving as a primary structural component of cells, lipids also function as crucial second messengers and play essential roles in energy supply and storage (Long et al., 2018; Koundouros & Poulogiannis, 2020). Unlike normal cells, tumor cells can not only meet their demands for unlimited proliferation by reprogramming their metabolism to generate ATP and macromolecules, but they can also release microenvironmental mediators under stress conditions to activate immune cells. This enables tumor cells to alter their own metabolic patterns, thereby jointly influencing tumor initiation and progression within the microenvironment (Long et al., 2018). Reprogramming of lipid metabolism in tumors constitutes a key aspect of overall tumor metabolic reprogramming, which primarily involves abnormal fatty acid (FA) transport, enhanced de novo FA synthesis (FAS), accumulation of lipid droplets, and altered FA β-oxidation. These metabolic alterations are regulated by oncogenic signaling pathways and are part of a complex regulatory network shaped by multiple factors, including the upregulation of FA transporters and related genes, epigenetic modifications, changes in lipid metabolism-related enzyme networks, and transcription factors (Koundouros & Poulogiannis, 2020). Among these, the de novo FAS pathway is a critical metabolic process required for the survival of tumor cells. The substantial amounts of FAs and other metabolites generated through this pathway can act as signaling molecules that influence the differentiation and functional activities of immune cells (Röhrig & Schulze, 2016).

Tumor cells activate the de novo synthesis of large amounts of FAs in response to their high metabolic requirements, and the presence of adipocytes and adipocyte-associated fibroblasts also increases the lipid content in TME (Bochet et al., 2013). There were also differences in the way of TAM lipid metabolism in different subgroups. FAS is dominant in M1 macrophages, while M2 macrophages depend on FA oxidation (FAO) for their bioenergy requirements. The high FA content in TME is also conducive to the M2 polarization of TAM (Geeraerts et al., 2017). Interfering with the lipid metabolism of TAM by inhibiting lipid uptake mediated by FA transporters, such as CD36 and FAO, may achieve the effect of enhancing antitumor immunity. Lipid species in the TME may alter the infiltration pattern of CD4+ T cells and determine the efficacy of targeting lipid metabolic pathways in cancer therapy. The increased FA content in TME activated CD8+ tumor infiltrating lymphocyte (TIL) peroxisome proliferator-activated receptor alpha signaling, thereby upregulating FAO and promoting effector T cell differentiation (Chowdhury et al., 2018). LIN et al. proposed that CD8+ tissue-resident memory T (Trm) cells in gastric adenocarcinoma are TILs that depend on FAO for survival (Lin et al., 2020). Blocking PD-L1 can reduce the expression of FA binding protein in tumor cells, thereby increasing the uptake of FAs by Trm and enhancing the antitumor immune activity of Trm.

Since the 1970s the health benefits of ω-3 polyunsaturated FAs (PUFAs) have increasingly drawn extensive attention in the academic community. A substantial body of research, encompassing in vitro experiments at the cellular level, animal tumor models, epidemiological surveys, and clinical trials, has firmly established that ω-3 PUFAs exert a positive influence in the prevention of various malignancies, including colorectal cancer (CRC), breast cancer, and prostate cancer (Berquin et al., 2008). Put simply, ω-3 PUFAs possess certain antitumor properties. Conversely, evidence suggests that excessive dietary intake of ω-6 PUFAs is closely associated with an elevated risk of tumor development (Montecillo-Aguado et al., 2022).

Dydjow-Bendek and Zagożdżon (2020) conducted a case–control study that found that when the ratio of ω-6 to ω-3 PUFAs in the diet was greater than 5, the risk of breast cancer would be twice that of the general population. Another case–control study in Toulouse, France, showed that the ratio of ω-6 to ω-3 PUFAs in breast fat tissue was significantly negatively correlated with the risk of breast cancer (Maillard et al., 2002). A metaanalysis that included six prospective nested case–control studies and five cohort studies found that a lower ratio of ω-6 to ω-3 PUFAs could effectively reduce the risk of breast cancer in women (Yang et al., 2014). A large amount of epidemiological evidence indicates that the intake of ω-3 PUFAs is closely related to CRC(Zhu et al., 2017; Schnekenburger et al., 2017). Some studies have pointed out that a higher intake of fish can effectively reduce the risk of CRC. A random double-blind study in Japan showed that additional supplementation of a certain amount of eicosapentaenoic acid (EPA), compared with the control group, had significantly fewer abnormal crypt lesions in the colon. Gastric cancer is also significantly related to the intake of ω-3 PUFAs. Animal experiments have shown that (Otto et al., 2008), for mice with gastric cancer transplants, additional supplementation of ω-3 PUFAs can inhibit tumor growth. There are also corresponding clinical trials showing that additional supplementation of ω-3 PUFAs can improve postoperative recovery rates and significantly reduce the incidence of complications (Ruiz-Tovar et al., 2019; Zhao & Wang, 2018).

Currently, the relationship between ω-3 PUFAs and lung cancer is a new research hotspot. Yin et al. (2017) found that docosahexaenoic acid (DHA) can inhibit the invasion and metastasis of nonsmall cell lung cancer cells and downregulate the levels of their metastasis-related proteins. Deniz et al. (2019) discovered in a prospective study that a higher ratio of ω-6 to ω-3 PUFAs would lead to a high inflammatory state in lung cancer patients after lung lobe resection, increasing the possibility of persistent pulmonary leakage after surgery. The results of two prospective trials by Van Der Meij et al. (2010, 2012) showed that the addition of an immune nutritional preparation containing ω-3 PUFAs was beneficial for maintaining the patient's weight, physical strength, fat accumulation, reducing the resting energy consumption of the patient, and reducing the production of inflammatory factors. It may have a positive impact on the quality of life, work status, and physical activity of patients with stage III nonsmall cell lung cancer. The incidence of prostate cancer ranks at the top among all male tumors worldwide, causing great pain to patients. Therefore it is necessary to take intervention measures against prostate cancer. Current research shows that the level of ALA is also highly correlated with the risk of prostate cancer (Yan et al., 2024). A case–control study by Williams et al. (2011) clearly pointed out that the risk of prostate cancer is related to the ratio of ω-6 to ω-3 PUFAs, but not to the levels of ω-3 PUFAs or ω-6 PUFAs alone.

Current research suggests that controlling the ratio of omega-6 and omega-3 PUFAs plays a crucial role in the development of chronic diseases such as cardiovascular diseases, tumors, and inflammation and is more important than merely supplementing omega-3 PUFAs (D'Angelo, Motti and Meccariello, 2020). Simopoulos (2002) believes that when the ratio of omega-6 to omega-3 PUFAs in the human body is 4:1, the mortality rate can be reduced by 70% after a 2-year follow-up. The prognosis of breast cancer patients is inversely proportional to the ratio of omega-6 and omega-3 PUFAs in the body. Strictly controlling the ratio of omega-6 and omega-3 PUFAs in the body can significantly reduce the prevalence of chronic diseases. Based on a large amount of clinical research data, the National Institutes of Health in the United States proposed that the ratio of omega-6 and omega-3 PUFAs in a healthy person's diet should be around 4:1. The World Health Organization recommends that the ratio of omega-6 and omega-3 PUFAs in the human body should be less than 4:1. The International Fatty Acids and Lipid Society recommends the optimal ratio as 1:1.

11.5 Gut microbiota and immunotherapy

Since the intestinal microbiota is a crucial component of the digestive process, food residues, as well as compounds produced by the host and the microbiota, are all fermented by the intestinal microbiota, thereby generating a large amount of metabolites. The intestinal microbiota and its metabolites also interact with host cells through the single layer of intestinal epithelial cells and participate in the host's immune activities and the development of cancer. Moreover, the composition of the microbiota has also been linked to the efficacy of immune checkpoint blockade therapy in patients with melanoma or epithelial tumors (Gopalakrishnan et al., 2018; Routy et al., 2018). Alternatively, the existing data indicate that nearly half of the plasma metabolites have a close connection with bacteria, suggesting that the microbiome plays a crucial role in the human metabolic process (Martin et al., 2007). Furthermore, bacterial metabolites, including short-chain FAs, AhR ligands, secondary bile acids, polyamines, and polysaccharides, may be involved in the development of cancer and the efficacy of anticancer treatments by influencing the host's immune system.

Abnormal intestinal microbiota has been recognized as one of the key hallmarks of tumorigenesis (Hanahan, 2022). Accumulating evidence indicates that the intestinal microbiota plays a crucial role in the initiation and progression of various types of tumors (Manor et al., 2020). Among them, CRC represents the most extensively studied intestinal malignancy. Notably, an increasing number of studies have also revealed significant associations between extraintestinal cancers, such as hepatocellular carcinoma and breast cancer, and alterations in the intestinal microbiota (Qin et al., 2024; Wong & Yu, 2023; Ponziani et al., 2019; Zhang et al., 2021; Ma et al., 2022; Yang et al., 2021; Yu et al., 2024). Although the underlying molecular mechanisms remain incompletely understood, current findings suggest that oncogenic microorganisms may contribute to tumor development through multiple pathways. Microbial-derived bioactive molecules, including the microbiota-associated metabolites discussed in detail below, can directly interact with tumor cells, inducing genomic DNA damage, epigenetic modifications, impairing DNA damage response, and activating protumorigenic signaling pathways. Furthermore, these molecules may also modulate tumor progression indirectly by influencing immune cell function and shaping the tumor-immune microenvironment (Zhao et al., 2023).

New knowledge about the modulation of the responsiveness of the gut microbiota to immunotherapy offers new possibilities to improve its efficacy by targeting the microbiota (Vétizou et al., 2015; Sivan et al., 2015). In the ileum and colon, CTLA-4 antagonists alter the composition of the gut microbiota and induce T cell-mediated mucosal injury. "In tumor-bearing mouse models, treatment with CTLA-4 antagonists reduces *Bacteroides* and *Burkholderia* (e.g., *Bacteroides* pleomorphic and monomorphic and *Burkholderia cepacia*), while increasing *Clostridium*." By promoting the maturation of intratumoral dendritic cells (DCS) and inducing a Th1 response in tumor-draining lymph nodes, oral administration of *Bacteroides plebeius* or *Bacteroides fragilis* to mice deficient in the microbiota restored the anti-CTLA-4 therapeutic response, suggesting that anti-CTLA-4 treatment may alter the composition of the gut microbiota, which would favor its antitumor activity in some patients. Similarly, PD-1/PD-L1 inhibitors also alter the composition of the gut microbiota, thereby influencing the antitumor immune response. Moreover, the fecal microbiota samples of patients receiving checkpoint blockade immunotherapy showed significantly higher alpha diversity and relative abundance of rumen bacillus species. The results of the immune spectrum analysis indicated that patients with a favorable gut microbiota and those who received fecal transplants from responsive patients in germ-free mice had enhanced systemic and antitumor immunity. Additionally, the metagenomic analysis of patient fecal samples obtained at the time of diagnosis revealed that the abundance of the Acinetobacter mucoid type was closely related to the clinical response to immune checkpoint inhibitors. By increasing the recruitment of CCR9+ CXCR3+ CD4+ T lymphocytes to tumor beds in mice, oral administration of Akkermanella mucophila restored the efficacy of PD-1 blockade after transplantation with fecal microbiota from the feces of nonresponsive patients. Roberti also found that Bacteroides fragilis and Erysiotrichosis near the ileal crypt induce DC to activate the immune response of follicular helper T cells, which is helpful for immune monitoring of colon cancer and thereby enhances the antitumor effects of chemotherapy and immunotherapy. Similarly, the use of Shigella sonnei containing phages can also activate the T cell response after chemotherapy or immunotherapy. The mechanism by which changes in the gut microbiota alter the systemic immune mechanism is currently under investigation, but Tanaka demonstrated in several mouse models that inoculating mice with a combination of 11 bacterial strains from healthy human donors promoted the immune response mediated by CD8+ T cells. Some believe that this combination of 11 strains is related to the increase in metabolites such as mevalonate and dimethylglycine in the colon and throughout the body, which may potentially enhance immune function.

Based on the interaction between the microbiota and the host, the effect of using antibiotics to regulate the microbiota during the cancer immunotherapy process is complex. Oral vancomycin can improve the efficacy of cancer immunotherapy targeting CTLA-4 by eliminating Gram-positive coccobacilli. Similarly, the thistreptoplain produced by Streptomyces percyanus and laurentiae can synergize with chemotherapy drugs to enhance the immunogenicity of antitumor immunity (Wang et al., 2020). However, antibiotics inhibit the effect of ICIs in advanced cancers, suggesting that antibiotic-mediated effects may be environmental. Thus natural antibiotics with a narrow range of activity may be suitable for the removal of specific harmful microbial species. There is evidence that the use of antianaerobic drugs, including carbapenem, cefmetazole, flumoxifloxacin, cefpirome, cefepime, clindamycin, and pajufloxacin, is associated with poor prognosis. Therefore targeted use of specific antibiotics and/or probiotics, rather than short-term or repeated use of broad-spectrum antibiotics to adjust the composition of the microbiome, may be more favorable for oncological therapeutic effects.

11.6 Current status and challenges of research

In recent years, the field of cancer immunometabolism has attracted much attention (Leone & Powell, 2020). Studies on the metabolic aspects of the TME have shown that cancer cells have an extremely strong adaptability, being able to obtain the nutrients necessary for growth and survival even under the most adverse conditions. In contrast, nonmalignant cells are more sensitive to the lack of nutrients and the accumulation of metabolic waste. Both tumor cells and antitumor immune cells consume large amounts of glucose and glutamine, but tumor cells are more tolerant and even utilize lactic acid and hypoxic environments, which are detrimental to antitumor immune cells but beneficial to immune regulatory cells. These differences provide an opportunity to target metabolism. Tumor immunotherapy promotes the immune system to exert antitumor immune response, but most patients still cannot benefit from immunotherapy, which may be due to the immunosuppressive TME that limits the transformation of protumor immune response to antitumor immune response. Metabolic alterations are one of the important characteristics of tumor tissue. Tumor cells reprogram the metabolism of sugars, amino acids, and lipids to form a microenvironment that is conducive to tumor proliferation and metastasis. By interacting with immune cells and competing for nutrients, tumor cells induce metabolic changes in immune cells, promote the transformation of immune cells to an immune tolerance phenotype, and impair their antitumor immune response. In addition, while enhancing T cell activation signals, immune checkpoints also regulate the metabolic fitness of T cells. Therefore the utilization of drugs that target immune metabolism may synergistically enhance the effect of immunotherapy through metabolic reprogramming of the TME. However, we must be vigilant about potential therapeutic toxicity, as tumor cells and immune cells often utilize the same metabolic pathways for proliferation. Therefore multiple strategies can be employed to overcome this limitation: (1) Strategy one involves developing novel drug delivery methods to selectively alter the metabolic processes of specific immune cell subsets or phenotypes. It is important to consider that there may be differences in the expression of amino acid and nutrient transport proteins between tumor cells and lymphocytes, especially when there are excessive metabolic carriers involved. Identifying the metabolic targets selectively utilized by tumor cells will significantly enhance antitumor immunity and avoid harmful effects on immune cells, and identify these differences may help to selectively inhibit the metabolic pathways in tumor cells. (2) The second strategy is to combine metabolic intervention with CAR T cell therapy, which can precisely clarify changes in metabolic pathways through genetic means. Additionally, tumors that respond or do not respond to immune checkpoint inhibitors have different metabolic characteristics. Therefore the relative utilization of glucose, amino acids, oxygen, or other nutrients may also vary, and studies aimed at determining the metabolic characteristics of immune checkpoint-resistant tumors may help identify metabolic pathways in tumor cells, thereby providing targets to influence the efficacy of immune checkpoint inhibitors.

References

Aaboe Jørgensen, M., Ugel, S., Linder Hübbe, M., Carretta, M., Perez-Penco, M., Weis-Banke, S. E., Martinenaite, E., Kopp, K., Chapellier, M., Adamo, A., De Sanctis, F., Frusteri, C., Iezzi, M., Zocca, M.-B., Hargbøll Madsen, D., Wakatsuki Pedersen, A., Bronte, V., & Andersen, M. H. (2021). Arginase 1–based immune modulatory vaccines induce anticancer immunity and synergize with anti–PD-1 checkpoint blockade. *Cancer Immunology Research, 9*(11), 1316–1326. https://doi.org/10.1158/2326-6066.cir-21-0280.

Angelin, A., Gil-de-Gómez, L., Dahiya, S., Jiao, J., Guo, L., Levine, M. H., Wang, Z., Quinn, W. J., Kopinski, P. K., Wang, L., Akimova, T., Liu, Y., Bhatti, T. R., Han, R., Laskin, B. L., Baur, J. A., Blair, I. A., Wallace, D. C., Hancock, W. W., & Beier, U. H. (2017). Foxp3 reprograms T cell metabolism to function in low-glucose, high-lactate environments. *Cell Metabolism, 25*(6), 1282. https://doi.org/10.1016/j.cmet.2016.12.018.

Berquin, I. M., Edwards, I. J., & Chen, Y. Q. (2008). Multi-targeted therapy of cancer by omega-3 fatty acids. *Cancer Letters, 269*(2), 363–377. https://doi.org/10.1016/j.canlet.2008.03.044, www.elsevier.com/locate/canlet.

Bochet, L., Lehuédé, C., Dauvillier, S., Wang, Y. Y., Dirat, B., Laurent, V., Dray, C., Guiet, R., Maridonneau-Parini, I., Le Gonidec, S., Couderc, B., Escourrou, G., Valet, P., & Muller, C. (2013). Adipocyte-derived fibroblasts promote tumor progression and contribute to the desmoplastic reaction in breast cancer. *Cancer Research, 73*(18), 5657–5668. https://doi.org/10.1158/0008-5472.can-13-0530.

Cascone, T., McKenzie, J. A., Mbofung, R. M., Punt, S., Wang, Z., Xu, C., Williams, L. J., Wang, Z., Bristow, C. A., Carugo, A., Peoples, M. D., Li, L., Karpinets, T., Huang, L., Malu, S., Creasy, C., Leahey, S. E., Chen, J., Chen, Y., ... Peng, W. (2018). Increased tumor glycolysis characterizes immune resistance to adoptive T cell therapy. *Cell Metabolism, 27*(5), 977. https://doi.org/10.1016/j.cmet.2018.02.024, http://www.cellmetabolism.org/.

Cassetta, L., & Pollard, J. W. (2018). Targeting macrophages: Therapeutic approaches in cancer. *Nature Reviews Drug Discovery, 17*(12), 887–904. https://doi.org/10.1038/nrd.2018.169.

Chen, J., Cui, L., Lu, S., & Xu, S. (2024). Amino acid metabolism in tumor biology and therapy. *Cell Death and Disease, 15*(1). https://doi.org/10.1038/s41419-024-06435-w, https://www.nature.com/cddis/.

Chowdhury, P. S., Chamoto, K., Kumar, A., & Honjo, T. (2018). PPAR-induced fatty acid oxidation in T cells increases the number of tumor-reactive CD^{8+} T cells and facilitates anti–PD-1 therapy. *Cancer Immunology Research, 6*(11), 1375–1387. https://doi.org/10.1158/2326-6066.CIR-18-0095, http://cancerimmunolres.aacrjournals.org/content/6/11/1375.full-text.pdf.

Corbet, C., & Feron, O. (2017). Tumour acidosis: From the passenger to the driver's seat. *Nature reviews. Cancer, 17*(10), 577–593. https://doi.org/10.1038/nrc.2017.77.

Curtis, N. J., Mooney, L., Hopcroft, L., Michopoulos, F., Whalley, N., Zhong, H., Murray, C., Logie, A., Revill, M., Byth, K. F., Benjamin, A. D., Firth, M. A., Green, S., Smith, P. D., & Critchlow, S. E. (2017). Pre-clinical pharmacology of AZD3965, a selective inhibitor of MCT1: DLBCL, NHL and Burkitt's lymphoma anti-tumor activity. *Oncotarget, 8*(41), 69219–69236. https://doi.org/10.18632/oncotarget.18215, http://www.impactjournals.com/oncotarget/index.php?journal=oncotarget&page=article&op=download&path%5B%5D=18215&path%5B%5D=58390.

David, G. D., & Brian, R. (2019). Macrophages as regulators of tumour immuniy and immunotherapy[J]. *Nature Reviews Immunology, 19*(6), 369–382.

Deniz, C., Ramos, R., Macía, I., et al. (2019). Effects of the omega-6/ omega-3 ratio on postoperative complications after lung resection: Preliminary results. *Journal of Thoracic Oncology, 14*(10), S887.

Dydjow-Bendek, D., & Zagożdżon, P. (2020). Total dietary fats, fatty acids, and omega-3/omega-6 ratio as risk factors of breast cancer in the Polish population - A case-control study. *International Institute of Anticancer Research, Poland In Vivo, 34*(1), 423–431. https://doi.org/10.21873/invivo.11791, http://iv.iiarjournals.org/content/34/1/423.full.pdf.

D'Angelo, S., Motti, M. L., & Meccariello, R. (2020). ω-3 and ω-6 Polyunsaturated fatty acids, obesity and cancer. *Nutrients, 12*(9), 2751. https://doi.org/10.3390/nu12092751.

Geeraerts, X., Bolli, E., Fendt, S. M., & Van Ginderachter, J. A. (2017). Macrophage metabolism as therapeutic target for cancer, atherosclerosis, and obesity. *Frontiers Research Foundation, Belgium Frontiers in Immunology, 8*. https://doi.org/10.3389/fimmu.2017.00289, www.frontiersin.org/Immunology.

Geiger, R., Rieckmann, J. C., Wolf, T., Basso, C., Feng, Y., Fuhrer, T., Kogadeeva, M., Picotti, P., Meissner, F., Mann, M., Zamboni, N., Sallusto, F., & Lanzavecchia, A. (2016). L-Arginine modulates T cell metabolism and enhances survival and anti-tumor activity. *Cell, 167*(3), 829. https://doi.org/10.1016/j.cell.2016.09.031, https://www.sciencedirect.com/journal/cell.

Goenka, A., Khan, F., Verma, B., Sinha, P., Dmello, C. C., Jogalekar, M. P., Gangadaran, P., & Ahn, B.-C. (2023). Tumor microenvironment signaling and therapeutics in cancer progression. *Cancer Communications, 43*(5), 525–561. https://doi.org/10.1002/cac2.12416.

Gopalakrishnan, V., Spencer, C. N., Nezi, L., Reuben, A., Andrews, M. C., Karpinets, T. V., Prieto, P. A., Vicente, D., Hoffman, K., Wei, S. C., Cogdill, A. P., Zhao, L., Hudgens, C. W., Hutchinson, D. S., Manzo, T., Petaccia De Macedo, M., Cotechini, T., Kumar, T., Chen, W. S., ... Wargo, J. A. (2018). Gut microbiome modulates response to anti-PD-1 immunotherapy in melanoma patients. *Science, 359*(6371), 97–103. https://doi.org/10.1126/science.aan4236, http://science.sciencemag.org/content/359/6371/97/tab-pdf.

Grohmann, U., Mondanelli, G., Belladonna, M. L., Orabona, C., Pallotta, M. T., Iacono, A., Puccetti, P., & Volpi, C. (2017). Amino-acid sensing and degrading pathways in immune regulation. *Cytokine and Growth Factor Reviews, 35*, 37–45. https://doi.org/10.1016/j.cytogfr.2017.05.004, www.elsevier.com/inca/publications/store/8/6/8/index.htt.

Hanahan, D. (2022). Hallmarks of cancer: New dimensions. *Cancer Discovery, 12*(1), 31–46. https://doi.org/10.1158/2159-8290.cd-21-1059.

He, X., Lin, H., Yuan, L., & Li, B. (2017). Combination therapy with L-arginine and α-PD-L1 antibody boosts immune response against osteosarcoma in immunocompetent mice. *Cancer Biology and Therapy, 18*(2), 94–100. https://doi.org/10.1080/15384047.2016.1276136, http://www.tandfonline.com/loi/kcbt20.

Hsu, M. C., & Hung, W. C. (2018). Pyruvate kinase M2 fuels multiple aspects of cancer cells: from cellular metabolism, transcriptional regulation to extracellular signaling. *Molecular Cancer, 17*(1), 35.

Husain, Z., Huang, Y., Seth, P., & Sukhatme, V. P. (2013). Tumor-derived lactate modifies antitumor immune response: Effect on myeloid-derived suppressor cells and NK cells. *The Journal of Immunology, 191*(3), 1486–1495. https://doi.org/10.4049/jimmunol.1202702.

Koundouros, N., & Poulogiannis, G. (2020). Reprogramming of fatty acid metabolism in cancer. *British Journal of Cancer, 122*(1), 4–22. https://doi.org/10.1038/s41416-019-0650-z.

Leone, R. D., & Powell, J. D. (2020). Metabolism of immune cells in cancer. *Nature Reviews Cancer, 20*(9), 516–531. https://doi.org/10.1038/s41568-020-0273-y.

Lin, R., Zhang, H., Yuan, Y., He, Q., Zhou, J., Li, S., Sun, Y., Li, D. Y., Qiu, H.-B., Wang, W., Zhuang, Z., Chen, B., Huang, Y., Liu, C., Wang, Y., Cai, S., Ke, Z., & He, W. (2020). Fatty acid oxidation controls CD8+ tissue-resident memory T-cell survival in gastric adenocarcinoma. *Cancer Immunology Research, 8*(4), 479–492. https://doi.org/10.1158/2326-6066.cir-19-0702.

Liu, X., Hoft, D. F., & Peng, G. (2020). Senescent T cells within suppressive tumor microenvironments: Emerging target for tumor immunotherapy. *Journal of Clinical Investigation, 130*(3), 1073–1083. https://doi.org/10.1172/JCI133679, https://www.jci.org/articles/view/133679/pdf.

Long, Zhang, Zhu, et al. (2018). Lipid metabolism and car cinogenesis，cancer development［ *American Journal of Cancer Research, 8*, 778–791.

Ma, Z., Qu, M., & Wang, X. (2022). Analysis of gut microbiota in patients with breast cancer and benign breast lesions. *Polish Journal of Microbiology, 71*(2), 217–226. https://doi.org/10.33073/PJM-2022-019, https://www.sciendo.com/article/10.33073/pjm-2022-019.

Maillard, V., Bougnoux, P., Ferrari, P., Jourdan, M.-L., Pinault, M., Lavillonnière, F., Body, G., Le Floch, O., & Chajès, V. (2002). N-3 and N-6 fatty acids in breast adipose tissue and relative risk of breast cancer in a case-control study in Tours, France. *International Journal of Cancer, 98*(1), 78–83. https://doi.org/10.1002/ijc.10130.

Manor, O., Dai, C. L., Kornilov, S. A., Smith, B., Price, N. D., Lovejoy, J. C., Gibbons, S. M., & Magis, A. T. (2020). Health and disease markers correlate with gut microbiome composition across thousands of people. *Nature Communications, 11*(1). https://doi.org/10.1038/s41467-020-18871-1, http://www.nature.com/ncomms/index.html.

Martin, F. P. J., Dumas, M. E., Wang, Y., Legido-Quigley, C., Yap, I. K. S., Tang, H., Zirah, S., Murphy, G. M., Cloarec, O., Lindon, J. C., Sprenger, N., Fay, L. B., Kochhar, S., Van Bladeren, P., Holmes, E., & Nicholson, J. K. (2007). A top-down systems biology view of microbiome-mammalian metabolic interactions in a mouse model. *Molecular Systems Biology, 3*. https://doi.org/10.1038/msb4100153.

van der Meij, B. S., Langius, J. A. E., Spreeuwenberg, M. D., Slootmaker, S. M., Paul, M. A., Smit, E. F., & van Leeuwen, P. A. M. (2012). Oral nutritional supplements containing n-3 polyunsaturated fatty acids affect quality of life and functional status in lung cancer patients during multimodality treatment: An RCT. *European Journal of Clinical Nutrition, 66*(3), 399–404. https://doi.org/10.1038/ejcn.2011.214.

Minhas, P. S., Liu, L., Moon, P. K., Joshi, A. U., Dove, C., Mhatre, S., Contrepois, K., Wang, Q., Lee, B. A., Coronado, M., Bernstein, D., Snyder, M. P., Migaud, M., Majeti, R., Mochly-Rosen, D., Rabinowitz, J. D., & Andreasson, K. I. (2019). Macrophage de novo NAD+ synthesis specifies immune function in aging and inflammation. *Nature Immunology, 20*(1), 50–63. https://doi.org/10.1038/s41590-018-0255-3.

Montecillo-Aguado, M., Tirado-Rodriguez, B., Antonio-Andres, G., Morales-Martinez, M., Tong, Z., Yang, J., Hammock, B. D., Hernandez-Pando, R., & Huerta-Yepez, S. (2022). Omega-6 polyunsaturated fatty acids enhance tumor aggressiveness in experimental lung cancer model: Important role of oxylipins. *International Journal of Molecular Sciences, 23*(11), 6179. https://doi.org/10.3390/ijms23116179.

Mussai, F., Wheat, R., Sarrou, E., Booth, S., Stavrou, V., Fultang, L., Perry, T., Kearns, P., Cheng, P., Keeshan, K., Craddock, C., & De Santo, C. (2019). Targeting the arginine metabolic brake enhances immunotherapy for leukaemia. *International Journal of Cancer, 145*(8), 2201–2208. https://doi.org/10.1002/ijc.32028.

Otto, C., Kaemmerer, U., Illert, B., Muehling, B., Pfetzer, N., Wittig, R., Voelker, H. U., Thiede, A., & Coy, J. F. (2008). Growth of human gastric cancer cells in nude mice is delayed by a ketogenic diet supplemented with omega-3 fatty acids and medium-chain triglycerides. *BMC cancer, 8*(1). https://doi.org/10.1186/1471-2407-8-122.

Panitz, V., Končarević, S., Sadik, A., Friedel, D., Bausbacher, T., Trump, S., Farztdinov, V., Schulz, S., Sievers, P., Schmidt, S., Jürgenson, I., Jung, S., Kuhn, K., Pflüger, I., Sharma, S., Wick, A., Pfänder, P., Selzer, S., Vollmuth, P., ... Opitz, C. A. (2021). Tryptophan metabolism is inversely regulated in the tumor and blood of patients with glioblastoma. *Theranostics, 11*(19), 9217–9233. https://doi.org/10.7150/thno.60679.

Platten, M., Nollen, E. A. A., Röhrig, U. F., Fallarino, F., & Opitz, C. A. (2019). Tryptophan metabolism as a common therapeutic target in cancer, neurodegeneration and beyond. *Nature reviews. Drug discovery, 18*(5), 379–401. https://doi.org/10.1038/s41573-019-0016-5, http://www.nature.com/nrd/index.html.

Ponziani, F. R., Bhoori, S., Castelli, C., Putignani, L., Rivoltini, L., Del Chierico, F., Sanguinetti, M., Morelli, D., Paroni Sterbini, F., Petito, V., Reddel, S., Calvani, R., Camisaschi, C., Picca, A., Tuccitto, A., Gasbarrini, A., Pompili, M., & Mazzaferro, V. (2019). Hepatocellular carcinoma is associated with gut microbiota profile and inflammation in nonalcoholic fatty liver disease. *Hepatology, 69*(1), 107–120. https://doi.org/10.1002/hep.30036, http://aasldpubs.onlinelibrary.wiley.com/hub/journal/10.1002/(ISSN)1527-3350/.

Qin, Y., Tong, X., Mei, W. J., Cheng, Y., Zou, Y., Han, K., Yu, J., Jie, Z., Zhang, T., Zhu, S., Jin, X., Wang, J., Yang, H., Xu, X., Zhong, H., Xiao, L., & Ding, P. R. (2024). Consistent signatures in the human gut microbiome of old- and young-onset colorectal cancer. *Nature Communications, 15*(1). https://doi.org/10.1038/s41467-024-47523-x, https://www.nature.com/ncomms/.

Routy, B., Le Chatelier, E., Derosa, L., Duong, C. P. M., Alou, M. T., Daillère, R., Fluckiger, A., Messaoudene, M., Rauber, C., Roberti, M. P., Fidelle, M., Flament, C., Poirier-Colame, V., Opolon, P., Klein, C., Iribarren, K., Mondragón, L., Jacquelot, N., Qu, B., ... Zitvogel, L. (2018). Gut microbiome influences efficacy of PD-1-based immunotherapy against epithelial tumors. *Science, 359*(6371), 91–97. https://doi.org/10.1126/science.aan3706, http://science.sciencemag.org/content/359/6371/91/tab-pdf.

Ruiz-Tovar, J., Blanca, M., Garcia, A., Gonzalez, J., Gutierrez, S., Paniagua, A., Prieto, M. J., Ramallo, L., Llanos, L., & Duran, M. (2019). Preoperative administration of Omega-3 fatty acids on postoperative pain and acute phase reactants in patients undergoing Roux-en-Y gastric bypass: A randomized clinical trial. *Clinical Nutrition, 38*(4), 1588–1593. https://doi.org/10.1016/j.clnu.2018.07.026, http://www.elsevier-international.com/journals/clnu/.

Röhrig, F., & Schulze, A. (2016). The multifaceted roles of fatty acid synthesis in cancer. *Nature reviews. Cancer, 16*(11), 732–749. https://doi.org/10.1038/nrc.2016.89.

Schnekenburger, M., Goffin, E., Lee, J. Y., Jang, J. Y., Mazumder, A., Ji, S., Rogister, B., Bouider, N., Lefranc, F., Miklos, W., Mathieu, V., De Tullio, P., Kim, K. W., Dicato, M., Berger, W., Han, B. W., Kiss, R., Pirotte, B., & Diederich, M. (2017). Discovery and characterization of R/S-N-3-cyanophenyl-N′-(6-tert-butoxycarbonylamino-3,4-dihydro-2,2-dimethyl-2H-1-benzopyran-4-yl)urea, a new histone deacetylase class III inhibitor exerting antiproliferative activity against cancer cell lines. *Journal of Medicinal Chemistry, 60*(11), 4714–4733. https://doi.org/10.1021/acs.jmedchem.7b00533, http://pubs.acs.org/jmc.

Simopoulos, A. P. (2002). The importance of the ratio of omega-6/omega-3 essential fatty acids. *Biomedicine & Pharmacotherapy, 56*(8), 365–379. https://doi.org/10.1016/s0753-3322(02)00253-6.

Sivan, A., Corrales, L., Hubert, N., Williams, J. B., Aquino-Michaels, K., Earley, Z. M., Benyamin, F. W., Lei, Y. M., Jabri, B., Alegre, M. L., Chang, E. B., & Gajewski, T. F. (2015). Commensal Bifidobacterium promotes antitumor immunity and facilitates anti-PD-L1 efficacy. *Science, 350*(6264), 1084–1089. https://doi.org/10.1126/science.aac4255, http://www.sciencemag.org/content/350/6264/1084.full.pdf.

Su, S., Chen, J., Yao, H., Liu, J., Yu, S., Lao, L., Wang, M., Luo, M., Xing, Y., Chen, F., Huang, D., Zhao, J., Yang, L., Liao, D., Su, F., Li, M., Liu, Q., & Song, E. (2018). CD10+GPR77+ cancer-associated fibroblasts promote cancer formation and chemoresistance by sustaining cancer stemness. *Cell, 172*(4), 841. https://doi.org/10.1016/j.cell.2018.01.009, https://www.sciencedirect.com/journal/cell.

Sun, S., Li, H., Chen, J., & Qian, Q. (2017). Lactic acid: No longer an inert and end-product of glycolysis. *Physiology, 32*(6), 453–463. https://doi.org/10.1152/physiol.00016.2017.

Van Der Meij, B. S., Langius, J. A. E., Smit, E. F., Spreeuwenberg, M. D., Von Blomberg, B. M. E., Heijboer, A. C., Paul, M. A., & Van Leeuwen, P. A. M. (2010). Oral nutritional supplements containing (n-3) polyunsaturated fatty acids affect the nutritional status of patients with stage III non-small cell lung cancer during multimodality treatment. *Journal of Nutrition, 140*(10), 1774–1780. https://doi.org/10.3945/jn.110.121202Netherlands, http://jn.nutrition.org/cgi/reprint/140/10/1774.

de Visser, K. E., & Joyce, J. A. (2023). The evolving tumor microenvironment: From cancer initiation to metastatic outgrowth. *Cancer cell, 41*(3), 374–403. https://doi.org/10.1016/j.ccell.2023.02.016.

Vétizou, M., Pitt, J. M., Daillère, R., Lepage, P., Waldschmitt, N., Flament, C., Rusakiewicz, S., Routy, B., Roberti, M. P., Duong, C. P. M., Poirier-Colame, V., Roux, A., Becharef, S., Formenti, S., Golden, E., Cording, S., Eberl, G., Schlitzer, A., Ginhoux, F., ... Zitvogel, L. (2015). Anticancer immunotherapy by CTLA-4 blockade relies on the gut microbiota. *Science, 350*(6264), 1079–1084. https://doi.org/10.1126/science.aad1329, http://www.sciencemag.org/content/350/6264/1079.full.pdf.

Wang, Y., Xie, W., Humeau, J., Chen, G., Liu, P., Pol, J., Zhang, Z., Kepp, O., & Kroemer, G. (2020). Autophagy induction by thiostrepton improves the efficacy of immunogenic chemotherapy. *Journal for Immunotherapy of Cancer, 8*(1), e000462. https://doi.org/10.1136/jitc-2019-000462.

Werner, A., Koschke, M., Leuchtner, N., Luckner-Minden, C., Habermeier, A., Rupp, J., Heinrich, C., Conradi, R., Closs, E. I., & Munder, M. (2017). Reconstitution of T cell proliferation under arginine limitation: Activated human T cells take up citrulline via L-type amino acid transporter 1 and use it to regenerate arginine after induction of argininosuccinate synthase expression. *Frontiers in immunology, 8*. https://doi.org/10.3389/fimmu.2017.00864.

Williams, C. D., Whitley, B. M., Hoyo, C., Grant, D. J., Iraggi, J. D., Newman, K. A., Gerber, L., Taylor, L. A., McKeever, M. G., & Freedland, S. J. (2011). A high ratio of dietary n-6/n-3 polyunsaturated fatty acids is associated with increased risk of prostate cancer. *Nutrition Research, 31*(1), 1–8. https://doi.org/10.1016/j.nutres.2011.01.002.

Wong, C. C., & Yu, J. (2023). Gut microbiota in colorectal cancer development and therapy. *Nature Reviews Clinical Oncology, 20*(7), 429–452. https://doi.org/10.1038/s41571-023-00766-x, https://www.nature.com/nrclinonc/archive/.

Xiao, Y., & Yu, D. (2021). Tumor microenvironment as a therapeutic target in cancer. *Pharmacology & Therapeutics, 221*, 107753. https://doi.org/10.1016/j.pharmthera.2020.107753.

Xie, Q., Ding, J., & Chen, Y. (2021). Role of CD8+ T lymphocyte cells: Interplay with stromal cells in tumor microenvironment. *Acta Pharmaceutica Sinica B, 11*(6), 1365–1378. https://doi.org/10.1016/j.apsb.2021.03.027.

Yan, H., Zhang, S., Yang, L., Jiang, M., Xin, Y., Liao, X., Li, Y., & Lu, J. (2024). The antitumor effects of α-linolenic acid. *Journal of Personalized Medicine, 14*(3), 260. https://doi.org/10.3390/jpm14030260.

Yang, B., Ren, X. L., Fu, Y. Q., Gao, J. L., & Li, D. (2014). Ratio of n-3/n-6 PUFAs and risk of breast cancer: A meta-analysis of 274135 adult females from 11 independent prospective studies. *BMC cancer, 14*(1). https://doi.org/10.1186/1471-2407-14-105, http://www.biomedcentral.com/1471-2407/14/105.

Yang, P., Wang, Z., Peng, Q., Lian, W., & Chen, D. (2021). Comparison of the gut microbiota in patients with benign and malignant breast tumors: A pilot study. *Evolutionary Bioinformatics, 17*. https://doi.org/10.1177/11769343211057573.

Yin, Y., Sui, C., Meng, F., et al. (2017). The omega-3 polyunsaturated fat ty acid docosahexaenoic acid inhibits proliferation and progression of non-small cell lung cancer cells through the reactive oxygen spe cies-mediated inactivation of the PI3K /Akt pathway. *Lipids in Health and Disease, 16*(1), 87–95.

Yu, X., Ou, J., Wang, L., Li, Z., Ren, Y., Xie, L., Chen, Z., Liang, J., Shen, G., Zou, Z., Zhao, C., Li, G., & Hu, Y. (2024). Gut microbiota modulate CD^{8+} T cell immunity in gastric cancer through Butyrate/GPR109A/HOPX. *Gut Microbes, 16*(1). https://doi.org/10.1080/19490976.2024.2307542.

Zhang, N., Gou, Y., Liang, S., Chen, N., Liu, Y., He, Q., Zhang, J., & Wang, L. (2021). Dysbiosis of gut microbiota promotes hepatocellular carcinoma progression by regulating the immune response. *Journal of Immunology Research, 2021*, 1–13. https://doi.org/10.1155/2021/4973589.

Zhao, L. Y., Mei, J. X., Yu, G., Lei, L., Zhang, W. H., Liu, K., Chen, X. L., Kołat, D., Yang, K., & Hu, J. K. (2023). Role of the gut microbiota in anticancer therapy: From molecular mechanisms to clinical applications. *Signal Transduction and Targeted Therapy, 8*(1). https://doi.org/10.1038/s41392-023-01406-7, https://www.nature.com/sigtrans.

Zhao, Y., & Wang, C. (2018). Effect of ω-3 polyunsaturated fatty acid-supplemented parenteral nutrition on inflammatory and immune function in postoperative patients with gastrointestinal malignancy. *Medicine, 97*(16), e0472. https://doi.org/10.1097/md.0000000000010472.

Zhou, Y., Huang, Z., Su, J., Li, J., Zhao, S., Wu, L., Zhang, J. L., He, Y., Zhang, G., Tao, J., Zhou, J., Chen, X., & Peng, C. (2020). Benserazide is a novel inhibitor targeting PKM2 for melanoma treatment. *International Journal of Cancer, 147*(1), 139–151. https://doi.org/10.1002/ijc.32756.

Zhu, M. L., Wang, C. Y., Xu, C. M., Bi, W. P., & Zhou, X. Y. (2017). Evaluation of 6-chloro-N-[3,4-disubstituted-1,3-thiazol-2(3H)-ylidene]-1,3-benzothiazol-2-amine using drug design concept for their targeted activity against colon cancer cell lines HCT-116, HCT15, and HT29. *Medical Science Monitor, 23*, 1146–1155. https://doi.org/10.12659/MSM.899646, http://www.medscimonit.com/download/index/idArt/899646.

Index

Note: Page numbers followed by *f* indicate figures, *t* indicate tables.

U

V

W

Printed and bound by CPI Group (UK) Ltd, Croydon, CR0 4YY
14/09/2026
02216409-0009